Pediatric Health Conditions in Schools

Pediatric Health Conditions in Schools

A Clinician's Guide for Working with Children, Families, and Educators

EDITED BY ALLISON G. DEMPSEY

Oxford University Press is a department of the University of Oxford. It furthers
the University's objective of excellence in research, scholarship, and education
by publishing worldwide. Oxford is a registered trade mark of Oxford University
Press in the UK and certain other countries.

Published in the United States of America by Oxford University Press
198 Madison Avenue, New York, NY 10016, United States of America.

Library of Congress Control Number: 2019950590
ISBN 978-0-19-068728-1

9 8 7 6 5 4 3 2 1

Printed by Marquis, Canada

For Isla

CONTENTS

CONTRIBUTORS

Ana Arenivas, PhD
TIRR Memorial Hermann

Amy K. Barton, MEd
Department of Psychological
Health & Learning Sciences
University of Houston

Elizabeth Bennett, PhD
Department of Pediatrics
University of Colorado School of
Medicine
Children's Hospital Colorado

Rashmi P. Bhandari, PhD
Department of Anesthesiology
Perioperative and Pain Medicine
Stanford University Medical Center

Grai Bluez
Department of Disability and
Psychoeducational Studies
University of Arizona

Kathy L. Bradley-Klug, PhD
Department of Educational and
Psychological Studies
University of South Florida

Angela I. Canto, PhD
Southeastern Behavioral Health

Stephanie Chapman, PhD
Department of Pediatrics
Baylor College of Medicine
Texas Children's Hospital

David J. Chesire, PhD
Department of Surgery
Division of Trauma-Critical Care
University of Florida Health
Science Center

Abigail C. Demianczyk, PhD
Department of Child and Adolescent
Psychiatry and Behavioral Sciences
The Children's Hospital of
Philadelphia

Allison G. Dempsey, PhD
Department of Psychiatry
University of Colorado School of
Medicine
Children's Hospital Colorado

Jack Dempsey, PhD
Department of Pediatrics
University of Colorado School of
Medicine
Children's Hospital Colorado

Christina L. Duncan, PhD
Department of Psychology
West Virginia University

Kristine Durkin, MS
Department of Psychology
West Virginia University

Michael M. Etzl, Jr., MD
Center for Cancer and Blood
Disorders
Phoenix Children's Hospital

Rachel Fein, PhD
Department of Pediatrics
Baylor College of Medicine
Texas Children's Hospital

Sara S. Frye, PhD
Department of Disability and
Psychoeducational Studies
University of Arizona

Katherine A. S. Gallagher, PhD
Department of Pediatrics
Baylor College of Medicine
Texas Children's Hospital

M. Cullen Gibbs, PhD
TIRR Memorial Hermann

Amy Goetz, PhD
Center for Child Behavior and
    Nutrition Research
Cincinnati Children's Hospital
    Medical Center

Jane Gray, PhD
Department of Educational
    Psychology
University of Texas

Carolyn Ha, PhD
Katy Psychological Services PLLC

Lyla E. Hampton, PhD
Department of Child and Adolescent
    Psychiatry and Behavioral Sciences
The Children's Hospital of
    Philadelphia

Jennifer L. Harman, PhD
Department of Psychology
St. Jude Children's Research Hospital

Sayward E. Harrison, PhD
South Carolina SmartState Center for
    Healthcare Quality
Department of Health Promotion,
    Education, and Behavior, Arnold
    School of Public Health
University of South Carolina

Lisa Hayutin, PhD
Department of Pediatrics
University of Colorado School of
    Medicine
Children's Hospital Colorado

Ryan M. Hill, PhD
Department of Pediatrics
Baylor College of Medicine
Texas Children's Hospital

Marisa E. Hilliard, PhD
Department of Pediatrics
Baylor College of Medicine
Texas Children's Hospital

Casey Hoffman, PhD
Department of Child and Adolescent
    Psychiatry and Behavioral Sciences
The Children's Hospital of Philadelphia

Samantha E. Huestis, PhD
Department of Anesthesiology
Perioperative and Pain Medicine
Stanford University Medical Center

Lisa Hynes, PhD
Department of Psychology
West Virginia University

Sasha D. Jaquez, PhD
University of Texas at Austin
Dell Medical School

Randa G. Jarrar, MD
Barrow Neurological Institute at
    Phoenix Children's Hospital

Niki Jurbergs, PhD
Department of Psychology
St. Jude Children's Research Hospital

Grace S. Kao, PhD
Department of Anesthesiology
Perioperative and Pain Medicine
Baylor College of Medicine
Texas Children's Hospital

Julie B. Kaplow, PhD
Department of Pediatrics
Baylor College of Medicine
Texas Children's Hospital

Milena A. Keller-Margulis, PhD
Department of Psychological
Health & Learning Sciences
University of Houston

Alison J. Lee, LCSW
Department of Educational
    Psychology
University of Texas at Austin

Ashlie Llorens, PhD
Department of Pediatrics
McGovern Medical School
University of Texas Health Science
    Center at Houston

Courtney Lynn, PhD
Emory University School of Medicine
Children's Healthcare of Atlanta

Shannon McKee, EdS
Department of Psychological
Health & Learning Sciences
University of Houston

Ariel McKinney
Department of Disability and
    Psychoeducational Studies
University of Arizona

Sarah S. Mire, PhD
Department of Psychological
Health & Learning Sciences
University of Houston

Evelyn C. Monico, MD
Department of Anesthesiology
Perioperative and Pain Medicine
Baylor College of Medicine
Texas Children's Hospital

Kerri P. Nowell, PhD
Health Professions Division
Thompson Center for Autism &
    Neurodevelopmental Disorders
University of Missouri

Sarah Ochs, PhD
Department of Psychology
Western Kentucky University

Puja G. Patel, PhD
University of Texas at Austin
Dell Medical School

Michelle M. Perfect, PhD
Department of Disability and
    Psychoeducational Studies
University of Arizona

Stephen Pont, MD, MPH
Office of Science and
    Population Health
Texas Department of State Health
    Services

Thea L. Quinton, PhD
Dayton Children's Hospital

Madeline Racine, MEd
Department of Psychological
Health & Learning Sciences
University of Houston

Ashley N. Ramclam, EdS
Department of Psychological
Health & Learning Sciences
University of Houston

Kimberly Rennie, PhD
Department of Pediatrics
McGovern Medical School
University of Texas Health Science
    Center at Houston

Van Michelle Ruda, MD
Department of Pediatrics
McGovern Medical School
University of Texas Health Science
    Center at Houston

Robin J. Sakakini, PsyD
Oaks Christian School

Nicole M. Schneider, PhD
Department of Pediatrics
Baylor College of Medicine
Texas Children's Hospital

Kimberly D. Schoger, PhD
Department of Psychological
Health & Learning Sciences
University of Houston

Michael C. Selbst, PhD, BCBA-D
Behavior Therapy Associates

**Glenn M. Sloman, PhD,
BCBA-D, NCSP**
Florida Psychological Center PLLC

Michael L. Sulkowski, PhD
Departments of Disability and
    Psychoeducational Studies and
    Psychiatry
University of Arizona

Elizabeth Vincent, PhD
TIRR Memorial Hermann

Rebecca Wagner, PhD
Private Practice

Christy M. Walcott, PhD
Department of Psychology
East Carolina University

Caitlin E. Walsh, PhD
Department of Pediatrics
University of Colorado School of
    Medicine
Children's Hospital Colorado

Katherine L. Wesley, PhD
Department of Psychology
Nationwide Children's Hospital

Megan L. Wilkins, PhD
Departments of Psychology &
    Infectious Diseases
St. Jude Children's Research Hospital

Desireé N. Williford, MS
Department of Psychology
West Virginia University

David L. Wodrich, PhD
Department of Disability and
    Psychoeducational Studies
University of Arizona

Jaclyn Wolf
Department of Disability and
    Psychoeducational Studies
University of Arizona

Rachel Wolfe, PhD
Department of Pediatrics
Baylor College of Medicine
Texas Children's Hospital

C. Baker Wright, PhD, BCBA-D
Behavior Management
    Consultants, Inc.

Cortney T. Zimmerman, PhD
Department of Pediatrics
Baylor College of Medicine
Texas Children's Hospital

General Issues

S ection I provides a broad overview of school-related issues for children with chronic health conditions. This includes a review of common medical conditions and terminology and cross-cutting issues related to social and emotional and academic functioning, as well as the role of the school-based professional in collaborating across systems of care. The section also reviews legal and policy issues and alternative educational settings for students with chronic health needs.

Childhood Chronic Illnesses in the Schools

KIMBERLY RENNIE, MADELINE RACINE, AND VAN MICHELLE RUDA ■

The definition of chronic illness is not consistent among agencies or organizations that address issues surrounding chronic illness, nor is the definition consistent across the literature. The American Academy of Pediatrics (AAP) defines chronic illness based upon the length of time that symptoms have been present (AAP, 2018). A review of the literature shows that the length of time can vary from as little as 1 month or more to more than 12 months (Bernell & Howard, 2016). The World Health Organization (WHO) defines chronic illness as a condition that is "not passed from person to person. It is of long duration and generally slow progression" (WHO, 2017). However, this definition differs from other organizations' definitions in that it excludes infectious diseases, such as human immunodeficiency virus (HIV) infection, which can be transmitted from person to person. It is important to note that in none of the definitions is chronic illness defined as solely pertaining to physical health. Instead, there seems to be a general consensus among providers and researchers alike that a chronic pediatric health condition is defined as "any physical, emotional, or mental condition that [prevents a child] from attending school regularly, doing regular schoolwork, or doing usual childhood activities or that requires frequent attention or treatment from a doctor or other health professional, regular use of any medication, or use of special equipment" (Van Cleave, Gortmaker, & Perrin, 2010, p. 624). For purposes of this book, chronic illness is defined as "any physical, emotional, or mental condition" that is of "long duration and generally slow progression." Emotional and mental illnesses are covered extensively in other texts (McCabe & Shaw, 2010); thus, the focus of this book is on physical health conditions.

PREVALENCE OF CHRONIC PEDIATRIC HEALTH CONDITIONS IN THE SCHOOLS

Over the course of the 20th century, the United States saw an increasing number of children living with chronic health conditions (Perrin, Anderson, & Van Cleave, 2014; Van Cleave et al., 2010). The increases in the prevalence of chronic health conditions appear to be secondary to declining rates of mortality and morbidity, in part due to advances in medical knowledge leading to earlier detection and improved treatments of various health conditions. For instance, HIV/acquired immunodeficiency syndrome (AIDS) used to be considered a "death sentence," but it is now considered a chronic illness (Bernell & Howard, 2016). Specialized treatments and technology-enhanced care have also led to declining mortality rates for conditions like childhood cancers, congenital heart disease, neural tube defects (e.g., spina bifida), cystic fibrosis, and sickle cell disease. Improvements in neonatal care and the development of specialized neonatal intensive care programs have led to drastically increased rates of extremely preterm infants (i.e., infants born at 28 weeks or less) and consequently an increase in long-term complications and neurodevelopmental disabilities associated with prematurity.

As rates of morbidity and mortality have declined, the number of children living with chronic illness has increased. Data from the 2007 National Survey of Children's Health (Bethell et al., 2011) estimated that approximately 43% of children in the United States have at least one chronic health condition, whereas the 2003 version of the survey estimated that 20% of school-aged children had a "special health care need." (Bethell, Read, Blumberg, & Newacheck, 2008, p.1) Whereas a review of the literature shows that estimates of the number of children living with chronic health conditions can vary based upon the definition of a chronic health condition, the data are clear that the numbers are increasing.

Along with the rising rates of children with chronic health conditions, the United States has also seen changes in education law requiring public school systems to provide a free and appropriate public education to all children. Consequently, school systems across the country have also seen a rise in the number of children with chronic health conditions enrolling in schools, and many of these children have specialized needs.

OVERVIEW OF SPECIALTIES AND COMMON CONDITIONS WITHIN SPECIALTIES

In children 17 years old and younger, the most common health conditions are asthma, allergies, chronic respiratory diseases, emotional/behavioral disorders, visual impairments, migraines, chronic diseases of the esophagus, dental and jaw difficulties, and diabetes (Gerteis et al., 2014). According to Van Cleave et al. (2010), one in ten children has asthma and one in 20 has epilepsy. Recent estimates indicate that 17% of children ranging in age from 2 to 19 years old are obese (Ogden, Carroll, Fryar, & Flegal, 2015), and, although diabetes is rare in children, rates of type 2 diabetes are increasing with the rise in childhood obesity (Ogden, Carroll, Curtin, Lamb, & Flegal, 2010). Moreover, cancer is the leading disease-related cause of death in children, with approximately 15,000 children diagnosed with cancer in 2017 and almost 1,800 of them dying from cancer. In the United States, the most prevalent types of cancer are leukemias, tumors of the central nervous system, lymphomas, soft tissue sarcomas, and kidney tumors (Siegel, Miller, & Jemal, 2017). Table 1.1 lists the most common medical specialties and the common pediatric conditions that may be managed by each specialty. Table 1.2 lists common medical terms and procedures.

Table 1.1. DESCRIPTION OF SPECIALTIES AND COMMON CONDITIONS

Specialty	Description	Common Conditions
Allergy-Immunology	Disorders involving the immune system	• Asthma • Seasonal allergic rhinitis (hay fever) • Anaphylaxis to foods, drugs, and insect bites • Eczema
Cardiovascular	Diseases involving the heart and blood vessels	• Congenital heart disease • Arrhythmias
Endocrinology	Disorders of hormones and their actions	• Diabetes mellitus • Thyroid disorders • Growth failure
Gastroenterology	Diseases of the digestive organs	• Abdominal pain • Ulcers • Diarrhea • Inflammatory bowel disease
Hematology/Oncology	Blood disorders and cancerous diseases	• Anemia • Sickle cell disease • Leukemia
Infectious Disease	Infectious disease of all types in all organ systems	• HIV/AIDS • Tuberculosis
Nephrology	Diseases of the kidneys and urinary tract	• Hypertension • Urinary incontinence
Neurology	Diseases of the nerves and nervous system	• Seizures/epilepsy • Cerebral palsy • Migraines
Pulmonology	Diseases of the lungs and airways	• Asthma • Cystic fibrosis • Sleep disorders
Rheumatology	Diseases of joints, muscles, bones, and tendons	• Arthritis • Collagen disease

Table 1.2. COMMON MEDICAL TERMS, PROCEDURES, AND TREATMENTS

ALLERGY-IMMUNOLOGY	
Adenoidectomy	Surgical removal of adenoids to help prevent blockage of the pharynx (back of throat) or eustachian tubes. The procedure may help prevent ear infections.
Anaphylaxis	Severe, life-threatening allergic response that may include symptoms of swelling, hives, wheezing, difficulty breathing, vomiting, diarrhea, and lowered blood pressure.
Epinephrine	Medicine used to treat severe allergic reactions. Also known as adrenaline.
Immunotherapy	Allergy desensitization or allergy shots used to increase tolerance of, or reduce sensitivity to, a substance.
Myringotomy with tubes	Surgical procedure in which metal or plastic tubes are inserted through the eardrum to equalize pressure between the middle and outer ear.
RAST (radioallergosorbent test)	Blood test used to identify substances that may be causing allergy symptoms.
CARDIOVASCULAR	
Cardiac catheterization	Procedure that provides information on the structure and function of the heart; the catheter is usually inserted through the femoral artery.
Echocardiogram	Noninvasive test that uses ultrasound waves to look at the structures of the heart.
Electrocardiogram (EKG)	Test that records the electrical activity of the heart. Leads with sticky pads are placed on the chest.
Stress test	Test to measure blood pressure, breathing, heart rate, and functioning during exercise (usually on a treadmill) to see how the heart muscle reacts.
ENDOCRINOLOGY	
Acanthosis nigricans	Gray or black discoloration of the skin, usually seen on the neck, underarms, and groin. It is a sign of insulin resistance.
Growth hormone deficiency	Condition due to the pituitary gland's not making enough growth hormone for the body. A child with this deficiency will look younger and be smaller than children of the same age.
Growth hormone replacement therapy	Daily shot that is given for growth hormone deficiency or growth failure.
Gynecomastia	Enlargement of one or both breasts in boys. It can be caused by a hormone imbalance or sometimes by too much fatty tissue in overweight boys.

Table 1.2. CONTINUED

ENDOCRINOLOGY	
Insulin	Hormone made in the pancreas that has many functions. One important function is helping the body control blood sugar levels.
Insulin resistance	Condition in which the body needs more insulin than normal to control blood sugar. It increases a person's risk of diabetes and heart disease and it is usually associated with obesity.
Metformin	Oral medication that has been shown to improve the body's response to insulin. It is most commonly used in patients with type 2 diabetes mellitus, polycystic ovarian syndrome, and obesity.
Type 1 diabetes mellitus	Chronic condition that develops when the body no longer produces enough insulin.
Type 2 diabetes mellitus	Condition that develops when the insulin the body makes does not work effectively.
GASTROENTEROLOGY	
Air-contrast barium enema	X-ray examination of the entire large intestine (colon) and rectum in which barium and air are introduced gradually into the colon by a rectal tube.
Appendectomy	Surgical removal of the appendix to treat appendicitis.
Cholecystectomy	Surgical removal of the gallbladder.
Colonoscopy	Outpatient procedure in which a physician inserts a scope (a long, flexible instrument about ½ inch in diameter) in the rectum and advances it to the large intestine (colon) to view the rectum and entire colon.
Colectomy	Surgical removal of part or all of the colon, performed to treat cancer of the colon, necrosis (dead bowel), or severe, chronic ulcerative colitis.
Endoscopy	Method of physical examination using a lighted, flexible instrument that allows a physician to see the inside of the digestive tract. The endoscope can be passed through the mouth or through the anus, depending on which part of the digestive tract is being examined.
Enema	Injection of fluid into the rectum and colon to induce a bowel movement, used for severe/chroic constipation.
Fecal occult blood test	Stool testing for blood.
Inflammatory bowel disease	Diseases that cause inflammation of the bowel, including Crohn's disease and ulcerative colitis.

(*continued*)

Table 1.2. CONTINUED

GASTROENTEROLOGY	
Inguinal hernia	Abnormal bulge or protrusion that can be seen and felt in the groin area (area between the abdomen and thigh). An inguinal hernia develops when a portion of an internal organ, such as the intestine, bulges through a weakened area in the muscular wall of the abdomen. Male athletes can develop an inguinal hernia during playing sports; therefore, they should be screened at their yearly sports physical.
Irritable bowel syndrome	Condition in which the colon muscle contracts more readily and causes abdominal pain and cramps, excess gas, bloating, and a change in bowel habits that alternates between diarrhea and constipation. It can be related to anxiety.
Laparoscopy	Method of surgery that is much less invasive than traditional surgery. Tiny incisions are made to create a passageway for a special instrument called a laparoscope, then a miniature video camera and light source are used to transmit images to a video monitor. The surgeon watches the video screen while performing the procedure with small instruments that pass through small tubes placed in the incisions.
Ultrasound	Technique used to diagnose a wide range of diseases and conditions in which high-frequency sound waves are transmitted through body tissues. The echoes vary according to tissue density and are recorded and translated into video or photographic images that are displayed on a monitor.
Urea breath test	Test to detect urease, an enzyme produced by *Helicobacter pylori* (*H. pylori*), a type of bacteria that usually infects the stomach or duodenum (first part of the small intestine) and that can cause ulcers.
HEMATOLOGY/ONCOLOGY	
Anticoagulant	Drug that prevents blood clots from forming.
Biopsy	Removal of a sample of tissue from the body for further examination. A biopsy helps doctors make a diagnosis and choose the right treatment.
Blood transfusion	Procedure in which blood collected from a donor is transferred to another person.
Bone marrow transplant	Procedure that involves replacing unhealthy bone marrow with healthy bone marrow cells from a donor.
CAT scan (also called computed tomography or CT scan)	Type of X-ray examination in which a machine rotates around the patient and creates a picture of the inside of the body from different angles.

Table 1.2. CONTINUED

HEMATOLOGY/ONCOLOGY	
Chemotherapy	Special medicines used to treat cancer. Often, several chemotherapy drugs are combined to attack the cancer cells in different ways.
Complementary therapy	Use of alternative treatments together with conventional therapies.
Hospice	Special type of care for people who are in the last phase of an illness. Hospice care can be either inpatient or outpatient.
Magnetic resonance imaging (MRI)	Test that uses a magnetic field and radio waves to produce detailed pictures of the body's organs and structures.
Port	Medical device inserted under the skin and attached to a vein that allows medications, blood products, and nutrients to be given intravenously. A port eliminates the need for repeated needle sticks to start an IV line or to draw blood.
Radiation therapy	One of the most common forms of cancer treatment in which high-energy radiation from X-rays, gamma rays, or other sources is used to kill cancer cells and shrink tumors. Radiation therapy prevents cells from growing or reproducing by destroying them.
Stem cell transplant	Procedure that involves introducing stem cells (cells found primarily in the bone marrow and from which all types of blood cells develop) into the body in the hope that the new cells will rebuild the immune system.
INFECTIOUS DISEASE	
Culture	Laboratory test that involves growing bacteria or other microorganisms to aid in diagnosis.
Nephrology	
Dialysis	Process of cleansing and achieving chemical balance in the blood of kidney failure patients.
Voiding cystourethrogram	Test to evaluate whether bladder function is normal.
NEUROLOGY	
Electroencephalography (EEG)	Test that is used to study brain wave activity. It is most useful to evaluate the seizure disorders
Electromyography/ nerve conduction study (EMG/NCV)	Test that is used to study the nerves and muscles to help diagnose disorders that can affect them. A small needle is placed in the muscle in the EMG, while electrical conduction is studied in the NCV. The results are seen on a screen and are compared to normal values.

(*continued*)

Table 1.2. CONTINUED

NEUROLOGY	
Lumbar puncture (also known as a spinal tap)	Procedure that involves removing some of the cerebrospinal fluid from the base of the spine; the fluid is obtained from the spinal area using a small needle and a syringe.
PULMONOLOGY	
Albuterol	Common rescue medication that is delivered with an inhaler or nebulizer.
Bronchoscopy	Procedure that allows the doctor to examine the airways; a flexible endoscope is inserted through the nose or mouth and through the windpipe down into each lung.
Dry powder inhaler (DPI)	Device for inhaling medicines in powder form.
Peak flow meter	Handheld device that measures how fast air comes out of your lungs.
Metered dose inhaler (MDI)	Aerosol canister that releases a mist of medicine; many asthma medicines are taken using an MDI.
Nebulizer	Machine that changes liquid medicine into droplets that can be inhaled through a mask or mouthpiece.
Spacer	Chamber with a 1-way valve that is used with a metered dose inhaler; it makes the inhaler easier to use and helps more medicine get into the airways.
Spirometry	Basic lung function test that measures how fast and how much air can be breathed out of the lungs.
Wheezing	High-pitched whistling sound of air moving through narrow airways.

COMMON ISSUES RELATED TO SYMPTOM MANAGEMENT

Children with chronic illnesses may feel different from other children. They are more likely to require frequent doctor and hospital visits, which can lead to chronic absenteeism. Poor school attendance, along with having other needs, can cause them to struggle with academic achievement. Children with chronic illnesses may also undergo procedures that are painful and stress-inducing. They may have to take medications and/or receive treatments during the school day, which draws more attention to their absence from class. Their activities may be limited or restricted, and they can also be put on special diets, factors causing them to feel isolated from their peers. Included below are examples of some common chronic illnesses that occur in school-age children and the potential issues that frequently arise throughout their management. Each of the conditions is described in much more detail in individual chapters in this book, but the case examples serve to illustrate the common themes and variations in the challenges and needs of children with chronic health conditions in schools.

Asthma

Timothy is an 8-year-old boy in the third grade with asthma and seasonal allergies. He has been hospitalized three times for asthma attacks and is followed by a pulmonologist every 3 to 6 months. Timothy's asthma is usually triggered by respiratory infections (such as the common cold) and exercise. He has a rescue inhaler in the nurse's office in case his symptoms flare up and has to take two puffs from his inhaler before exercising, playing sports, and physical education class. At home, Timothy takes an allergy pill, an allergy nasal spray, and another inhaler in the morning and night to control his asthma and allergy symptoms. He has an asthma action plan (AAP) that was prepared by his pulmonologist and that is to be used at home and at school. The AAP shows Timothy's daily treatment, such as what kind of medicines to take and when to take them. The plan describes long-term control of asthma and how to handle worsening asthma or acute attacks. The plan also explains when to call the doctor or go to the emergency department (ED).

Asthma is one of the leading causes of absence due to illness. It is estimated that approximately 3 students in a classroom of 30 currently have asthma (National Heart, Lung, and Blood Institute, 2018). School staff should have basic knowledge of asthma, including common triggers, symptoms, and how to respond to emergencies. The school-based clinician should have an up-to-date AAP for every child with asthma. The plan can change throughout the school year depending on how well the child's symptoms are controlled. Children with asthma may have activity restrictions, and physical education instructors and coaches should know how to prevent exercise-induced asthma.

Congenital Heart Disease

Allison is a 16-year-old girl in the eleventh grade who was born with an abnormal heart that required multiple surgeries and a long hospital stay after birth. She has had many hospitalizations and doctor visits due to complications of her heart defect. She had a feeding tube when she was younger due to her poor growth, and she developed learning difficulties, probably as a result of her multiple heart surgeries. Allison has been fairly healthy over the past few years but is still on daily heart medications and has poor stamina during physical activity. While she has not been held back and is in regular classes, she has been diagnosed with ADHD and requires accommodations for her schoolwork. Allison is very small for her age and often gets bullied by her peers.

Most children with simple heart defects do not require special care in school. Children with more complex heart disease may require special attention to certain signs (such as cyanosis, fatigue, and small stature). School staff should have a basic understanding of the child's heart condition. For example, the child may require heart surgery that could disrupt schoolwork and have physical, cognitive, and behavioral effects. The child may have restrictions on physical exercise and sports participation that should be clarified with his or her physician. The child may also need additional time to travel to classes. Medication is usually taken at home, although some children may require medication during school hours. School coordination with parents and the child's physician can help children with heart conditions succeed.

Diabetes Mellitus (Type 1 Diabetes)

Zachary is a 12-year-old boy in the seventh grade who was diagnosed with diabetes 1 year earlier. He has been hospitalized only once, when he was initially diagnosed. Zachary checks his blood sugar four times a day (breakfast, lunch, dinner, and bedtime) by pricking his finger and using a metered device. He has to give himself a certain amount of insulin via a needle injection after each blood sugar check depending on how high his level is. Zachary also has to give himself another long-acting insulin injection at bedtime regardless of his blood sugar level. He and his family have been taught how to count his carbohydrates and he is only allowed a certain amount at each meal and snack time. Zachary can feel bad if his blood sugar level is too low or too high. If his blood sugar gets very low, he could experience serious complications, such as having a seizure or passing out. If his blood sugar gets too high, he could go into diabetic ketoacidosis, which can be very dangerous and lead to hospitalization. Zachary is followed very closely by an endocrinologist and he has a diabetes medical management plan. Zachary checks his blood sugar and administers his insulin in the nurse's office at school and is supervised by his parents at home. Zachary has recently become frustrated with his illness and has stated that he just wants to be normal.

Type 1 diabetes is one of the most common childhood chronic illnesses. It is a lifelong illness that requires intensive daily management. Some children have more difficulty adjusting to living with diabetes than others. The needs and management of a child with diabetes change over time, so close monitoring of the child's physical and psychosocial needs is imperative.

Diabetes control should be well managed at home and at school. School clinicians and/or designated staff should have a basic understanding of the disease, blood glucose goals, management tasks, and symptoms of low and high blood glucose that may require intervention during school-related activities. School coordination with parents, managing physician, and diabetic educator is essential in promoting success and safety at school.

Seizures/Epilepsy

Samantha is a 15-year-old girl in the ninth grade who has a seizure disorder. Her seizures are well controlled on a daily antiepileptic medication. Samantha had a seizure in class when she was in the seventh grade and she had to be given a rectal gel medication emergently by the school nurse. The school called 9-1-1 and Samantha was taken to the local children's hospital. Her last seizure was 1 year ago at home. Samantha sees her neurologist one or two times a year. She has a seizure action plan for school. Samantha is nervous about getting her driver's license because she has to be seizure-free for a specified period of time and she has to be deemed safe to drive by her doctor.

Although epilepsy is well controlled with medication in many children and the children can participate in activities and perform academically, studies show that children with epilepsy miss more school, have more difficulties in classes, and participate less in extracurricular activities than children with other medical conditions. Academic difficulties faced by children with epilepsy can be related to the seizures themselves and the impact of seizures on neurocognitive development or they can be secondary to medications. School staff should have a basic understanding of epilepsy, its treatment, how to prevent triggers (e.g., flashing lights), and administering first aid and rescue medications. Staff should also monitor for mental-health concerns, such as depression, and social risk factors like bullying.

Sickle Cell Disease

Lane is a 13-year-old male in the eighth grade with sickle cell disease that was diagnosed on his newborn screen. He has had multiple hospitalizations and ED visits for pain crises that required opioid medications to help relieve the pain. Lane is at risk for infections because of disease-related damage to his spleen. Until he was 5 years old, he had to take a daily antibiotic to help prevent serious infections. Lane is also at high risk for strokes and needs to remember to drink water throughout the day in order to stay hydrated. He does not have a learning disorder but he tires easily in school and has to rest in the nurse's office.

Teachers, nurses, and administrators play an important role in supporting children living with sickle cell disease. Children with sickle cell disease may experience variable levels of daily pain, which may cause them to reduce social, school, and sport activities when pain intensity is high. School staff should ensure the child has adequate access to water/hydration throughout the day in order to prevent pain episodes and other health problems. Additionally, staff should allow accommodations during physical education and recess activities, including less strenuous activities and frequent breaks, to help monitor for fatigue. School staff should also be aware of increased risk for stroke in children with sickle cell disease. Learning difficulties (e.g., decline in academic achievement, difficulty maintaining attention, delays in vocabulary development) may be caused by stroke-related brain injuries. Teachers should notify parents if they notice changes in school performance so that the child can be evaluated by a doctor. Further, children with sickle cell disease may benefit from educational testing to determine if they have learning difficulties caused by stroke.

Summary of Challenges and Considerations Across Conditions

The examples above highlight some of the issues that children with chronic health conditions face in the school setting. Most of these children experience commonalities that affect their academic functioning, including attending medical appointments, managing treatment in the school setting, and managing emotional or behavioral reactions to their condition, which may make them feel isolated from their peers. Depending on the condition, many children experience cognitive, behavioral, and emotional symptoms that can arise directly from their conditions and treatments (e.g., fatigue, potential cognitive effects from strokes, emotional distress from living with a chronic illness), may require emergency plans or protocols in the school setting, and may have activity or dietary restrictions. Thus, it is important for school personnel to understand the cognitive, behavioral, and emotional effects of chronic illness and its treatments on a child's well-being and academic functioning.

Many children living with the health conditions discussed in this book will "look okay" physically (e.g., they may be able to walk, or they may have age-appropriate stature). However, many of them will have cognitive complications resulting from their chronic illness that will affect their ability to succeed academically. For instance, while undergoing treatment, children with cancer may "look sick," especially if they experience hair loss. Following treatment, they may recover their hair and no longer appear ill. However, the side effects of chemotherapy agents and other treatments associated with cancer adversely affect neurocognitive functioning, resulting in academic difficulties. As a result of their chronic health conditions, these children may require 504 accommodations or special education services from their school. It is critical for schools to meet the needs of these children, because the literature has shown that children with chronic health conditions are at higher risk of disengaging from education (Crump et al., 2013) than children without chronic health conditions.

CULTURAL CONSIDERATIONS

Research consistently indicates racial and ethnic disparities in chronic health conditions among U.S. children. For example, black and Hispanic children have a greater chance of having a chronic health condition (e.g., obesity, asthma, other physical condition, or behavior/learning problems) than non-Hispanic white children (Van Cleave et al., 2010). Similarly, a study using data from the National Survey of Children's Health found a higher prevalence of chronic health conditions, such as asthma, hearing impairment, vision impairment, joint/bone/muscle problems, brain injury, and other illness, among black children than among white children

(Kitsantas, Kornides, Cantiello, & Wu, 2013). Other cultural factors, such as gender and socioeconomic status, also contribute to disparities in chronic health conditions. Male children have a 50% higher rate of chronic health conditions and have a higher prevalence of asthma, autism spectrum disorder, physical disability, and behavior or learning problems than female children (Van Cleave et al., 2010). Children living in a single-parent household, regardless of race or ethnicity, are more likely to have any health condition, such as asthma, than children living in a two-parent household (Kitsantas et al., 2013). Additionally, research consistently shows there is a greater risk of a chronic health condition among children who live at or below the federal poverty level than among children who are not living in poverty (Kitsantas et al., 2013; Larson, Russ, Crall, & Halfon, 2008). Given these disparities, it is important that practitioners continually recognize the relationship between culture and the risk of chronic illness.

Culture is also an essential determinant of how an individual and family respond to a severe medical condition. Many ethnic and minority populations do not define or address a chronic illness in the same way that mainstream American culture does (Groce & Zola, 1993). An individual's culture often influences beliefs about the cause of the chronic illness, which plays a significant role in how the family and community perceive the illness and seek out treatment. Furthermore, culture affects family and community expectations for a child with the chronic illness, which may significantly affect his or her education, social functioning, and independence (Groce & Zola, 1993).

Given the cultural disparities among children with chronic health conditions and the increasing diversity of U.S. schools, it is imperative that practitioners engage in culturally competent practices to better serve children with chronic illness. Cultural competence is defined as the ability to work effectively with people from a variety of cultural, ethnic, economic, and religious backgrounds (Miranda, 2014). Practitioners who are knowledgeable and sensitive to an individual's cultural background, values, beliefs, religions, languages, and notions of healthcare are better equipped to offer culturally competent interventions. Within a school setting, consultative services and assessment procedures can have significant implications for the placement and the services a child receives. Therefore, culturally competent practices within the school setting are essential to providing successful services and support in the context of a child's culture.

FUTURE IMPLICATIONS

With continued advances in medicine, the numbers of children with chronic health conditions attending traditional schools will continue to increase. As mortality rates decline among the sickest of children with physical illness, without similar rates in declining morbidity, the specialized needs of these children are likely to increase. Thus, it is important that schools address the needs of current children living with chronic health conditions while also preparing to meet the needs of the increasing numbers of chronically ill children entering schools in the years to come. This book aims to be useful to professionals working within school systems and to allow both educators and administrators to prepare for and better address the increasing numbers of, and needs of, children with chronic health conditions.

REFERENCES

American Academy of Pediatrics. (2018). *Chronic conditions.* Retrieved from https://www.healthychildren.org/English/health-issues/conditions/chronic/Pages/default.aspx

Bernell, S., & Howard, S. W. (2016). Use your words carefully: What is a chronic disease? *Frontiers in Public Health, 4,* 1–3.

Bethell, C. D., Kogan, M. D., Strickland, B. B., Schor, E. L., Robertson, J., & Newacheck, P. W. (2011). A national and state profile of leading health problems and health care quality for US children: Key insurance disparities and across-state variations. *Academic Pediatrics, 11*(3S) S22–S33.

Bethell, C. D., Read, D., Blumberg, S. J., & Newacheck, P. W. (2008). What is the prevalence of children with special health care needs? Toward an understanding of variations in findings and methods across three national surveys. *Maternal and Child Health Journal, 12,* 1–14.

Crump, C., Rivera, D., London, R., Landau, M., Erlendson, B., & Rodriguez, E. (2013). Chronic health conditions and school performance among children and youth. *Annals of Epidemiology, 23,* 179–184.

Gerteis, J., Izrael, D., Deitz, D., LeRoy, L., Ricciardi, R., Miller, T., & Basu, J. (2014). *Multiple chronic conditions chartbook: 2010 MEPS data* (pp. 1–45). Rockville, MD: Agency for Healthcare Research and Quality.

Groce, N. E., & Zola, I. K. (1993). Multiculturalism, chronic illness, and disability. *Pediatrics, 91,* 1048–1055.

Kitsantas, P., Kornides, M. L., Cantiello, J., & Wu, H. (2013). Chronic physical health conditions among children of different racial/ethnic backgrounds. *Public Health, 127*(6), 546–553.

Larson, K., Russ, S. A., Crall, J. J., & Halfron, N. (2008). Influence of multiple social risks on children's health. *Pediatrics, 121*(2), 337–344.

McCabe, P. C., & Shaw, S. R. (2010). *Pediatric disorders: Current topics and interventions for educators.* Thousand Oaks, CA: Corwin Press.

Miranda, A. H. (2014). Best practices in increasing cross-cultural competency. In P. L. Harrison & A. Thomas (Eds.), *Best practices in school psychology* (pp. 9–19). Bethesda, MD: National Association of School Psychologists.

National Heart, Lung, and Blood Institute. (2014). *Managing asthma.* Retrieved from https://www.nhlbi.nih.gov

Ogden, C. L., Carroll, M. D., Curtin, L. R., Lamb, M. M., & Flegal, K. M. (2010). Prevalence of high body mass index in US children and adolescents, 2007–2008. *JAMA, 303*(3), 242–249.

Ogden, C. L., Carroll, M. D., Fryar, C. D., & Flegal, K. M. (2015). *Prevalence of obesity among adults and youth: United States, 2011–2014* (pp. 1–8). Washington, DC: U.S.

Department of Health and Human Services, Centers for Disease Control and Prevention, National Center for Health Statistics.

Perrin, J. M., Anderson, E., & Van Cleave, J. (2014). The rise in chronic conditions among infants, children, and youth can be met with continuous health system innovations. *Health Affairs, 33*(12), 2099–2105.

Siegel, R. L., Miller, K. D., & Jemal, A. (2017). Cancer statistics, 2017. *CA: A Cancer Journal for Clinicians, 67*(1), 7–30.

Van Cleave, J., Gortmaker, S. L., & Perrin, J. M. (2010). Dynamics of obesity and chronic health conditions among children and youth. *JAMA, 303*(7), 623–630.

World Health Organization. (2017). *Noncommunicable diseases.* Retrieved from https:// afro.who.int/health-topics/noncommunicable-diseases

Social and Emotional Issues Related to Chronic Health Conditions

ASHLIE LLORENS, SHANNON MCKEE,
AND ALLISON G. DEMPSEY ■

Antonio is a 14-year-old male in his freshman year of high school. When he was 10 years old, he was diagnosed with type 1 diabetes. Antonio lives with his father, who is his primary caregiver and works long hours at two jobs. Since Antonio's diagnosis, Antonio and his father have had difficulties managing his diabetes and Antonio frequently experiences hyperglycemia. From ages 11 to 14 years, Antonio experienced seven hospitalizations for diabetic ketoacidosis. During his middle school years, Antonio had poor attendance and missed an average of 35 days of school per year. Antonio had a 504 plan with accommodations to visit the nurse daily to check his blood glucose levels, but he tended to visit the nurse only if he was feeling ill, which typically signaled elevated blood glucose levels. At home, Antonio was not checking his blood glucose, administering insulin, or monitoring carbohydrate intake as recommended by his endocrinologist. Antonio often reported to his father that he did not like visiting the nurse during the school day to receive insulin, because he did not want classmates to ask questions about why he was leaving class, to feel sorry for him, or to feel like they have to take care of him. So, Antonio often either skipped lunch or ate lunch without checking his blood glucose and administering necessary insulin. Antonio's attendance continued to decline following each hospitalization, as did his grades.

Antonio was most recently hospitalized 1 month into his freshman year with complications from diabetes. During his 4-day hospital stay, Antonio reported to the social worker that he was not looking forward returning to school because he would have to answer questions from his classmates and teacher about his absences and

missing assignments, and that made him feel "weird." Antonio noted that school was
very stressful because he often felt tired during class, had a hard time concentrating,
and did not like talking to the kids in his class because they "probably think I'm
weird." He shared that he sometimes gets stomach aches the night before school, and
on these days it is easy for him to stay in bed at home because his dad has already
left for work. The hospital social worker decides to reach out to Antonio's school to
discuss his return to school.

The processes of obtaining an initial diagnosis and managing the ongoing treatment of a chronic health condition can be unexpected and often can involve
a degree functional impairment for the children and their families. Whereas
each medical condition presents its own unique challenges, facing ongoing
stressors associated with having a condition is a shared experience among youth
and families with chronic health conditions. This stress, in combination with
the typical challenges of child and adolescent development, can lead to social
and emotional difficulties for some children that manifest in various areas of
the child's life. For example, stressors related to a chronic health condition can
(1) affect social interactions with peers, siblings, and parents; (2) create or exacerbate academic difficulties; and (3) cause emotional difficulties in responding
to general stress—all domains of functioning that affect functioning within the
school environment.

Not only can having a condition place a child at increased risk for social and
emotional difficulties (Bilfield, Wildman, & Karazsia, 2005; Pinquart & Shen,
2011), but also a bidirectional relationship exists in which the social and emotional
difficulties in turn negatively affect the child's health. The presence of a chronic
health condition acts as a stressor for youth and families, and stress is known
to negatively affect general physical health, in addition to emotional functioning
(Juster, McEwen, & Lupien, 2010). Additionally, treatment nonadherence is a
common experience among children and adolescents, with one of the significant
outcomes being an increase in symptoms, medical visits, and school absences
(Lemanek, Kamps, & Chung, 2001). This may further exacerbate the severity of
the health condition and lead to more social, emotional, and medical difficulties.

ROLE OF THE SCHOOL-BASED PROFESSIONAL

For youth with chronic health conditions, many variables are involved in the identification and treatment of psychosocial difficulties (Wildman, Stancin, Golden, &
Yerkey, 2004). In the United States, there has been a push to address unmet mental
health needs among youth by integrating mental health providers into primary
and specialty care medical clinics (Wissow, van Ginneken, Chandna, & Rahman,
2016). While many medical clinics have behavioral health specialists who assist in detecting and managing psychosocial difficulties that arise in the context
of chronic illness, the presence and availability of integrated behavioral health
services vary. Further, in situations where concerns about social and emotional

functioning are brought to the attention of a provider, diagnosis and/or treatment may be deferred because the child does not meet full diagnostic criteria for a mental health condition (e.g., major depressive disorder), making access to treatment more difficult. School-based professionals with expertise in social, emotional, and academic functioning may be the first professionals to identify, address, and offer support for such difficulties. This emphasizes the importance of linking systems of care across school, community, and medical settings and addresses the role of school clinicians in facilitating collaboration with a multidisciplinary team to support behavioral and physical health for youth with chronic illnesses (Power, Shapiro, & DuPaul, 2003).

The school-based clinician serves a vital role not only in monitoring and identifying a student's psychosocial needs within the school environment, but also in coordinating services related to developing a plan to promote positive school adjustment. Youth with a chronic illness likely have many providers involved in their care, and school clinicians can serve to encourage communication among all parties. Supporting a student's psychological and social well-being has a direct influence on the child's ability to successfully transition back to school and reintegrate into academic and peer activities after extended absences due to illness. A well-developed and well-implemented plan can reduce the stress experienced by students, parents, and other school personnel during the school reintegration process (Kliebenstein & Broome, 2000).

Specific to the school experience for youth with chronic illness, there are two developmentally significant areas of functioning that may be interrupted: educational achievement and social interactions. These two areas of functioning are intertwined, and disrupted functioning in one may be a catalyst for disrupted functioning in the other. For example, a child who has deficits in academic performance related to prolonged school absences may experience difficulties with self-esteem that result in disengagement from educational or social experiences. To address school re-entry in a manner that integrates social and emotional needs, planning should occur at the earliest opportunity and should involve discussions with the student, parents, medical staff, and relevant school staff. Thus, it is extremely important for school clinicians to be familiar with social and emotional risk factors unique to the experiences of youth living with a chronic illness, to closely monitor functioning, and to provide appropriate interventions to support adaptive adjustment at school.

EMOTIONAL AND BEHAVIORAL FUNCTIONING

Mariah is an 11-year-old female who was recently diagnosed with juvenile idiopathic arthritis. She is a high-achieving student who enjoys school, and her previous teachers describe her as a pleasant student who is kind to classmates, participates in class, and completes all assignments. This school year, Mariah has experienced flare-ups in her arthritis. During flare-ups, she reports severe pain in her ankles, knees, hips, and wrists and has difficulty walking and doing things with her hands.

Mariah's teachers informed the clinician that Mariah has been lashing out at classmates, participating less, and seems to be absent every other week. Mariah also seems to become frustrated easily with assignments, and at times she cries in class and makes statements like "School is too hard," "I don't understand it!" or "I can't do this, I'm not smart enough."

The school clinician met with Mariah to inquire about school, and Mariah reported negative thoughts about school, how it was not fair that she had arthritis, and that she didn't want to come to school anymore because she "couldn't do any of the things she used to do." The clinician decided to schedule a meeting with Mariah's parents. At this meeting, the clinician and teachers shared observations about changes in behavior, and expressed concern in wanting to support Mariah. During this conference, Mariah's mother shared that Mariah receives infusions every other week as part of her medication regimen, and Mariah will have additional anticipated absences for physical therapy sessions. The clinician was also able to obtain a release of information from Mariah's mother, allowing the clinician to speak to Mariah's medical providers. The clinician was able to talk to the nurse in Mariah's rheumatology clinic and clarified recommendations about physical limitations, strategies for pain management, and side effects of a steroid medication that could affect school performance. The clinician determined that Mariah would benefit from a 504 plan that provided her additional time to transition between classes, permission to take notes and complete assignments on a computer, and modifications to her physical education activities. As a result of the meeting, the clinician offers to meet with Mariah to teach her skills for managing stress and frustration.

Comorbidity of Health Conditions with Mental Health Disorders

Whereas some studies have identified chronic health conditions as putting children at a higher risk for symptoms of depression (Bennett, 1994) and overall internalizing and externalizing problems (Barlow & Ellard, 2006; Karsdorp, Everaerd, Kindt, & Mulder, 2007; Mcquaid, Kopel, & Nassau, 2001; Pinquart & Shen, 2011; Rodenburg, Stams, Meijer, Aldenkamp, & Deković, 2005), other studies have reported that children with chronic health conditions are not at an elevated risk for psychosocial problems (Miller, 1993). While acknowledging these discrepancies, in their meta-analysis, Barlow and Ellard (2006) concluded that children with a chronic illness are at a greater risk of experiencing psychosocial difficulties than children without a chronic illness, although most youth do not meet the clinical threshold for diagnosis of a mental health disorder. Pinquart and Shen (2011) completed the first meta-analysis to suggest that psychosocial impairment extends beyond internalizing and externalizing problem behaviors, and they reported elevated levels of inattention and social difficulties among children with chronic illnesses. Although the prevalence of youth who may benefit from psychological intervention has not been identified, findings strongly suggest that

Table 2.1. COMMON BEHAVIORAL HEALTH CHALLENGES AMONG YOUTH
WITH CHRONIC ILLNESS

School Functioning	Social-Emotional	Health
Neurocognitive abilities: attention, memory, executive functioning, hyperactivity, processing speed, language	Peer relationships: delay in age-appropriate social skills, navigating intimate relationships, teasing, bullying	Sleep disturbances that affect mood, behavior, and cognitive performance
Delayed progress in academic curriculum and instruction	Self-esteem, body image	Physical growth and development: changes in appearance, delayed maturation
Attendance: medical appointments, hospitalizations, school avoidance	Restricted participation in activities	Physical symptoms: fatigue, pain, stomach aches, discomfort
Physical limitations to participation	Emotional and behavioral regulation: irritability, mood, worry, fear	Treatment adherence
	Increased stressors across settings: peers, school, family	

children with chronic illness should be screened for psychosocial difficulties in the areas of internalizing problems, externalizing problems, attention, and peer relations (see Table 2.1).

Stress and Coping

For youth with a chronic health condition, typical stressors related to childhood and adolescence are likely to be heightened due to factors associated with managing a chronic illness. Youth and their families report experiencing stress related to interruptions to daily routines, treatment, and uncertainty about the condition (Compas, Jaser, Dunn, & Rodriquez, 2012). When returning to the classroom after frequent and/or prolonged health-related absences, youth will have varying levels of need for accommodation. For example, academic achievement may be affected by school absences that result from doctor appointments, treatment, illness progression, and/or psychosocial problems with adjustment. Prior to returning to school, youth with chronic health conditions may experience anxiety about having to make up work and catch up to their peers. Additionally, these youth are more likely to have frequent school absences due to the perceived challenges of reintegrating into school (Chan, Piira, & Betts, 2005), a situation emphasizing the importance for youth to develop adaptive coping strategies for managing stress.

Much attention has been paid to how youth with chronic health conditions experience and respond to stress, and how to improve their response in a way that facilitates a normative course of development. The literature provides a variety of definitions of coping, but studies have indicated common elements of coping as it relates to youth with a chronic health condition. Compas and colleagues (2012) identified the following commonalities in models of coping for children and adolescents with a chronic health condition:

1. Primary copingstrategies that directly target changing the stressor or the emotional response to the stressor.
2. Secondary copingstrategies that alter internal responses to the stressor (e.g., thoughts, beliefs).
3. Disengagement coping—strategies that disengage the youth from the stressor or responding to the stressor.

Furthermore, when conceptualizing coping among youth with a chronic health condition, a central component of predicting the effectiveness of a coping strategy is the perceived controllability of the stressor (Rudolph, Dennig, & Weisz, 1995). That is, the degree to which the child/adolescent perceives he or she has control over the stressor affects overall coping. Therefore, the multidimensional approach to coping encompasses efforts that address emotion, cognition, behavior, and the environment.

There is consistent empirical evidence supporting the use of secondary coping as a means for enhancing adjustment to a chronic illness (Campbell et al., 2009; Dufton, Dunn, Slosky, & Compas, 2011; Edgar & Skinner, 2003; Hocking et al., 2011; Jaser & White, 2011; Thomsen et al., 2002; Walker et al., 1997). Some examples are diaphragmatic breathing, progressive muscle relaxation, positive self-talk, and adaptive distraction activities (e.g., engaging in an enjoyable activity). Handouts 2.1 and 2.2 contain strategies for teaching students such activities.

Findings were mixed regarding the use of primary coping to improve adjustment. Compas and colleagues (2012) hypothesized that primary coping strategies may be a better fit for some stressors than others. For example, primary coping strategies, such as training in problem-solving skills, may be particularly helpful with difficulties related to school absences or making up assignments; however, they may be less helpful for socialization issues with peers. Finally, passive approaches to coping (e.g., disengagement, denial, avoidance) have been found to be associated with higher levels of social and emotional distress among youth with a chronic health condition (Compas et al., 2006).

Recognizing Difficulties

Chronic health conditions are unique in the types of stressors and difficulties that they present for children and families. Children with chronic health issues, and their parents, report moderate to high levels of stress related to functioning in daily routines/tasks, medical treatment, and uncertainty about the medical condition (Rodriguez et al, 2011). Parents identified that stress related to managing normal daily routines (e.g., stress caused by school absences, make-up work, medical appointments, and activity restrictions) is the most significant for youth. Considering the varied acute and chronic stressors that families experience, LeBlanc, Goldsmith, and Patel (2003) discussed predictive factors for positive outcomes. Among the domains they identified, the following are those that school-based clinicians are able to monitor readily within the context of routine school-based activities: coping strategies, academic functioning, internalizing problems, and externalizing problems. Although clinicians may be able to easily screen informally for problems in these domains, it has been recommended that students with chronic health conditions should be formally assessed in the areas of learning, psychosocial function, and physical health upon returning to school from extended health-related absences (Lurie & Kaufman, 2001).

An important precursor to ensuring appropriate monitoring of psychosocial adjustment is establishing positive homeschool communication early on, as well as communication with other relevant healthcare providers to gather information about any concerns regarding adjustment or coping (Helms et al., 2016). Upon a clinician's first meeting with a student's family, the clinician should obtain written consent to meet with the student, as well as consent for release of information in order to talk with outside providers. Appropriate monitoring of emotional functioning requires routine check-ins with the identified student and relevant teaching staff, during which data regarding coping (behavioral observations, teacher report, student report), academic functioning (attendance, assignment completion, grades), and internalizing and externalizing behaviors (behavioral observation, teacher report, student report) are gathered and reviewed. Significant changes in the data can indicate difficulties in adjustment. Data about social and emotional functioning should be gathered from multiple sources. Table 2.2 provides a list of questions/prompts that can be used in clinical interviews with students to screen for behavioral health difficulties and to make a determination if further assessment is warranted for internalizing or externalizing problems.

If the data collected indicate of a pattern of avoidant coping behaviors or internalizing or externalizing symptoms, further assessment may be warranted (LeBlanc et al., 2003). Clinicians may supplement their interviews and observations by administering rating scales to measure emotional and behavioral functioning. Commonly used measures that have been validated with medical populations include the Achenbach Child Behavior Checklist (Achenbach & Edelbrock, 1991), the Revised Children's Manifest Anxiety Scale (Gerard & Reynolds, 1999), and the Children's Depression Inventory (Kovac, 2010). A referral for psychological services is appropriate when a clinician has evidence of the child's impaired functioning (LeBlanc et al., 2003). Schilling and Getch (2012) suggested that, in addition to undertaking an individualized assessment of the student's needs, school-based clinicians should hold regular multidisciplinary team meetings to review the student's progress and accommodations. Schilling and Getch (2012) provided the following questions to be assessed 1 week after a student returns

Table 2.2. STUDENT INTERVIEW PROMPTS AND QUESTIONS TO ASSESS FUNCTIONING

Domain	Prompts/Questions	Interpretation Comments
Managing academics	Tell me about your classes. How have you been managing schoolwork since returning? Have you been able to make up assignments/keep up with work? If not, which parts have been difficult?	Consider length of absence, potential neurocognitive effects of the condition, pre-existing learning differences, and academic performance prior to diagnosis.
School avoidance	How often do you miss school due to your condition? How often do you have bad feelings about coming to school because you are worried/afraid/embarrassed about something (peers, assignments, teacher)? How do you spend your days when you don't come to school?	Can provide information to determine if absences are due to school avoidance or medical appointments, while also potentially eliciting information about internalizing and externalizing behaviors symptoms and coping.
Adjustment to health condition	How have you been managing your [chronic health condition]?	Gather information about medication/regimen adherence and coping.
Sleep/Appetite	How do you sleep? Have you noticed any changes in your appetite?	May indicate internalizing difficulties.
Engagement in enjoyable activities	Tell me about the last thing you did for fun. Which school clubs are you interested in getting involved in?	May elicit information about social isolation and/or withdrawal.
Available supports	Who have you been going to when you need help?	May elicit information about coping styles and support system within school.
School accommodations	Has your 504 plan/IEP/school health plan been helpful in managing your condition?	May elicit information about helpfulness of school accommodations and additional needs.

Table 2.2. CONTINUED

Domain	Prompts/Questions	Interpretation Comments
Social interactions/ Social supports	Tell me about your friends. How often do spend time with them? Do any of your friends know about your [health condition]?	Provides information about protective factors.
Negative peer experiences	How do you get along with your classmates? How do you resolve disagreements with friends or classmates? Have you had to change any of your social activities because of your [health condition]? Have you ever been picked on or bullied?	Provides information about social experiences that may lead to difficulties with adjustment.

to school (however, these questions can also be addressed with students at other times). (1) Are the supports that have been put in place working? (2) Are all challenges currently being addressed? (3) Is the student able to make it through an entire day of school successfully? (4) Is the student making academic progress? (5) Is the student getting along with peers?

Addressing Difficulties

Once a student is identified as having emotional difficulties, the next step is to determine the appropriate level of support for addressing the student's needs. The clinician's role is to identify and collaborate with the relevant school personnel to determine whether the student's needs require a 504 plan (to allow appropriate access to the educational environment) or a psychoeducational evaluation for social and emotional problems that may be interfering with the student's educational process and therefore warrant an individualized education plan through special education services. For students having difficulty adjusting to school routine and managing academically related stressors, clinicians can provide direct support by helping students with areas like stress management, problem-solving, study skills, social skills, and coping with illness. See Handout 2.3 for an example of how a clinician may facilitate an activity on the topic of coping.

Social Relationships

*Jena is a 16-year-old female with cystic fibrosis (CF) who is a sophomore in high
school. She was diagnosed at age 4 years, and she has been relatively healthy; she was
hospitalized for the first time only this school year for a pulmonary infection. Jena is
an honor-roll student who has been involved in art club and the honor society. Since
her hospitalization, she has had difficulty adjusting to her new medical regimen,
which requires her to wake up early before school to complete breathing treatments
and a 45-minute chest physical therapy session with a vest, before eating breakfast and taking oral medications. Before lunch, she visits the nurse to take enzyme
supplements, and, in the evenings after school, she receives respiratory therapy. Jena
reports that the most difficult part of her new regimen is waking up earlier to complete treatments because it makes her feel tired in class. She also reports difficulty with
increased coughing episodes, and that during first and second period, her coughing
episodes are disruptive to the class, and she often leaves to go to the restroom.*

*Jena reports that her close friends know about her diagnosis, but most of her
classmates do not know. She often feels embarrassed and like she is a burden during
her coughing episodes, because students tend to look at her when she coughs. She has
also overheard classmates make comments about how "gross" her coughing sounds,
so she tries to suppress her coughs. A classmate even asked her if she was okay, because it sounded like she was going to "hack up a lung." Jena noticed that no one
wanted to be her partner during group work and she wondered if they knew she was
not contagious. Jena has started feeling like she is different than all other students
at her high school, and she has slowly stopped participating in art club. She also has
not been able to make meetings of the honor society, because they conflict with her
respiratory therapy appointments.*

*Jena's parents contacted her principal to discuss concerns about her decline in grades
and school participation, and he invited the clinician to a conference with Jena and
her parents. The clinician suggested that Jena educate her peers and teachers about
CF. He also suggested that a 504 plan be developed for Jena that accommodates
her completing assignments missed due to medical appointments and deadline
extensions due to her fatigue associated with her medical regimen. The clinician
invited the school nurse to work with him and Jena to find teacher resources and to
help deliver a presentation about CF to Jena's classmates.*

During childhood and adolescence, friendships and peer interactions become increasingly central to normative development and psychosocial adjustment. Peer
relationships are an important protective factor for psychosocial adjustment, but
youth with chronic health conditions are at a higher risk of experiencing difficulties
in peer relationships than youth without chronic illness (Pinquart & Teubert, 2011;
Reiter-Purtill, Waller, & Noll, 2009). The risk also varies according to illness type.
Children with cancer have reported experiencing higher levels of peer acceptance

compared to healthy peers (Noll et al., 1999). Children with chronic illnesses that are associated with intermittent symptoms that cause students to miss school frequently, cause physical deformities or limitations, and require ongoing parental assistance that conflicts with developmental stage may result in increased social isolation and peer difficulties (Sandstrom & Schanberg, 2004). The implications of these social and functional interruptions are that youth are likely to experience fewer positive peer interactions, are less likely to feel emotional support and belonging at school, and may be more likely to develop a negative self-concept.

Perceived Differences from Peers

For children and adolescents living with a chronic illness, the changes they experience related to their condition range in external visibility (e.g., cognitive/executive functioning impairments, physical distortions, academic difficulties, limitations in mobility, medical equipment) and these differences can make attending school more difficult. In adolescence, youth are in a developmental phase where exploring and beginning to define their identity among peers and family members are expected. During this time, being perceived as different from peers can have a lasting influence on identity development, and youth do not want to share information that will cause them to stand out from their peers. Appearance also becomes increasingly important for adolescents, bcause it is a defining characteristic for peer acceptance (Vannatta, Gartstein, Zeller, & Noll, 2009). Academic performance is another area where youth may feel singled out, or different from their peers. Some chronic health conditions and their medical treatments can result in changes in cognitive functioning (e.g., attention, concentration, memory) and wellness (e.g., nausea, fatigue, drowsiness) that negatively affect classroom performance.

It is particularly imperative for school-based clinicians to gain an understanding of characteristics that youth with chronic health conditions may identify as factors that negatively distinguish them from their peers. Youth with chronic health conditions want more than anything to be treated the same as their peers. Once a clinician has gathered information reflecting specifics about perceived factors that differentiate them from peers, and thereby present as a barrier to social engagement or school attendance, this information can be used to design targeted activities for building resiliency (e.g., skills training, role-playing, etc).

Peer Victimization and Bullying

Peer victimization occurs when there is an imbalance of power and the aggressor engages in aggressive acts toward the victim, who is the person with less power (Juvonen & Graham, 2013). When the aggressive acts, whether they are physical, verbal, relational, or cyber attacks, are repeated over time, the situation is considered to be bullying (Olweus, 1993). Youth with chronic health conditions are at an increased risk for experiencing peer victimization because they are more likely to encounter factors that increase their vulnerability than are their peers without a chronic illness (Faith et al., 2015; Sentenac et al., 2013). Because bullies target victims whom they perceive to be of lesser social status (Hodges & Perry, 1999; Olweus, 1993), children who present with noticeable physical and/or emotional or behavioral differences or who have few friends are unfortunately positioned to be the targets of the aggressive acts (Hodges, Bovin, Vitaro, & Bukowski, 1999; Sentenac et al., 2011). Thus, children with chronic health conditions have an increased risk of presenting with the physical abnormalities or limitations, impaired social functioning, and decreased academic performance that make them targets for peer victimization.

There has been limited research that suggests that peer victimization is differentiated according to the nature of the chronic illness, with conditions that affect physical features related to attractiveness (e.g., face, body shape) increasing the likelihood of being targeted (Pinquart, 2017). It is important for school-based clinicians to screen for incidents of bullying among youth with chronic illnesses, because being a victim of bullying has been reported to decrease adherence to self-management of medication protocols (Janicke et al., 2009; Storch et al., 2006), as well as to increase the prevalence of psychosocial problems (Reijntjes, Kamphuis, Prinzie, & Telch, 2010) and to adversely affect academic performance (Schwartz, Gorman, Nakamoto, & Toblin, 2005). Interventions for reducing victimization among youth with chronic illnesses include teaching strategies for managing emotions and developing supportive peer relationships, as well as programming to educate peers about the symptoms and difficulties related to the illness, with the overarching goal being to increase understanding and empathy in unaffected children.

Social Isolation

After the child experiences extended periods of illness-related absence from school parents can have problems enforcing compliance with school attendance because of unclear boundaries between allowing the child to stay home for reasons directly related to the illness (e.g., appointments, treatment, feeling unwell) and maintaining expectations for educational achievement. Not only is school attendance an important factor in academic achievement, but also returning to school promptly is an important protective factor against social isolation as well as a factor in full-time school reintegration. Frequent and sustained absences make it difficult to maintain relationships with peers and teachers. It is important for the clinician to support families in creating a plan that encourages school attendance. The clinician may be responsible for contributing to the development of an attendance plan. Important components to consider include school flexibility (e.g., allowing the student to attend part time vs. full time, support for managing the condition at school) and multidisciplinary collaboration among parents, the school nurse, the teachers, the mental health clinician, and the school administrator.

Once a student has transitioned back to school, he or she may still face challenges with developing a sense of belonging, because he or she may be more likely to be excluded or ignored by peers as a consequence of perceived differences. Youth who utilize passive coping styles to respond to such school social stressors, such as avoidant or socially isolating behaviors, are more likely to have poor psychosocial adjustment (Meijer et al., 2002). Isolating behaviors rooted in social anxiety or withdrawal not only can be indicative of an internalizing disorder, but also can inhibit normative stages of child and adolescent development. In childhood and adolescence, peer relationships are an increasingly important aspect of socialization and identity development. Additionally, peer social support plays a significant role in facilitating psychosocial adjustment (Meijer et al., 2002). Preventing and minimizing social isolation among youth with chronic health conditions can be addressed by assessing peer social interactions and by intervening when necessary to facilitate normative peer interactions that will enhance a sense of identity and belonging (e.g., social skills training, extracurricular activities, friendship groups).

Inconsistent peer relationships combined with academic difficulties may result in frustration and feelings of helplessness or hopelessness, and school clinicians should monitor the student for depression and anxiety. The increased risk for psychosocial difficulties emphasizes the importance of clinicians' developing a plan for social support in the school.

STRATEGIES FOR IDENTIFYING AND ADDRESSING DIFFICULTIES WITH SOCIAL RELATIONSHIPS

Assessing and understanding social relationships among youth is best understood when data are collected using a multimethod, multi-informant approach. Helgeson and Holmbeck (2014) reviewed literature about peer interactions in youth with chronic illnesses and discovered that findings varied dependent on who was reporting information (peers, youth, or parents) and methodology (e.g., observation, rating scale). Helgeson and Holmbeck hypothesized that parents may be more accurate reporters based on the breadth of their experiences, and that youth may have limited awareness of their social functioning. On the other hand, youth may be more accurate at depicting their peer relationships because parents may have a tendency to attribute their child's social difficulties to the chronic health condition. Thus, a comprehensive assessment of social relationships should involve input from multiple reporters and should include interview and observational data. See Table 2.2 for questions that clinicians can ask during student interviews to determine if social difficulties exist.

Information about social interactions can also be obtained from parents and teachers. Specifically, clinicians can ask parents about the names and ages of their children's friends and how often they get together. Additionally, they should ask questions about how the children get along with same-age peers, how they resolve disagreements with peers, and if they've ever talked about being teased or bullied. It is also important to obtain parental perceptions of how the child's health condition affects participation in social activities. Teachers can provide information about how the student gets along with other students, whether he or she seeks out peer interactions, and how he or she resolves disagreements with peers. The teacher may also be able to provide information about how the student's peers · perceive him or her and whether teasing or bullying has been a problem for the student.

Addressing Difficulties

RESPONDING TO PEER QUESTIONS

One way to support youth in building their self-esteem is to help them take an active approach in managing challenges related to talking to peers about their condition. Youth are in control of educating peers and teachers about their illness, and the student's role in the education of others can be varied.

Peer education is one strategy for supporting children with chronic illness in schools. This activity can be presented in various formats, with various levels of detail depending on the student and family's wishes and the developmental level of peers. Providers may need to work with youth to define what information they want peers to know. Topics that can be covered in the presentation may include facts about condition, perceived differences (e.g., why the child looks different, uses a particular device, etc.), how the condition affects daily activities, why they take medication, why they are absent sometimes, or helpful ways classmates can interact with the child. The child and family can have varying levels of involvement: some children want to be present, some children want to participate in or lead the discussion, and some students wish not to be present. Further, children may be selective about which peers they want to know about their diagnosis. In the school re-entry program described by Worchel-Prevatt and colleagues (1998), the authors identify four approaches to a school-based presentation about health conditions: (1) a hospital-based team with a nurse facilitates a discussion and allows questions and answers, (2) a nurse provides a demonstration of medical procedures, (3) the school offers a puppet show or interactive activities, or (4) the student discusses his or her experiences with the condition. The provider can also help the child find resources to use during the presentation (e.g., handouts, videos, equipment).

In addition to sharing educational information with peers, providers can work with children to prepare them to respond to difficult questions from peers. Common questions will vary depending on the illness, but providers can help children create a list of anticipated questions, or questions the child did not feel comfortable answering in the past. The child and provider can create a script of questions and answers (a sample script follows this paragraph). After generating a script, the provider should role-play with the child and provide feedback about the child's performance. Areas of feedback may include body language, tone, or volume, with the goal being to be comfortable answering questions from peers. The provider should allow the child to rehearse the script multiple times and should reflect with the child about how it went. The provider should continue to provide feedback, acknowledging strengths and encouraging rehearsal, until the student feels comfortable. Here is a sample script for a child with diabetes:

Q: "Why do you go to the nurse every day before lunch?"
A: *"I have diabetes, which means my body's sugar levels go up and down. I have to check my blood sugar before I eat meals."*
Q: "Does it hurt when you stick yourself to check your blood?"
A: *"Not anymore, at first it felt like a pinch."*
Q: "Did you get the disease from eating too much sugar?"
A: *"No, you don't get diabetes from eating too much sugar."*
Q: "How do we know if your sugar is too high or too low?"
A: *"The best way for me to know is by using my meter to check. Sometimes, if I'm low, I feel light-headed and shaky and my vision changes. When my sugar is high, I feel sick, sometimes I vomit, feel really tired, and use the restroom a lot."*
Q: "What should we do if we notice you acting differently?"
A: *"The most helpful thing you can do is let an adult know, and offer to walk to the nurse with me."*

Another strategy clinicians can employ to encourage positive peer interactions and psychosocial adjustment is facilitating development of a positive peer group. During adolescence, youth begin to progressively seek out peers for emotional comfort, in addition to their parents (Collins & Laursen, 2004). For youth with a chronic health condition, structured peer support reduces behavioral health symptoms (Kohut et al., 2014). The provider first needs to identify the type of needs to be addressed and then to use this finding to establish a group purpose. Next, it is important to decide which population of youth the group will target; groups can be facilitated strictly for youth with a health condition, or they can also include youth without a health condition. Finally, logistic details for the time, duration, frequency, and location of the group meetings need to be established.

In addition to benefitting from a peer support group, youth can also benefit from involvement in school-based activities and community-based extracurricular activities. The provider can facilitate the student's exploration of areas of interest, and if necessary help the student navigate any potential barriers to participation in activities. Participation in extracurricular activities can improve self-esteem (Feldman & Matjasko, 2005). Finally, providers can also explore options for activities that are specific to a chronic health condition. Youth attending camps specific to their condition tend to report short-term benefits of improved relationships with peers (Meltzer et al, 2018; Moola, Faulkner, White, & Kirsch, 2014).

CONCLUSION

Youth and families affected by chronic health conditions experience many challenges that begin during the phases of diagnosis and that extend into establishing a treatment regimen, and then into day-to-day treatment maintenance. These stressors, combined with normative childhood/adolescence difficulties, often put affected youth at an increased risk for social and emotional difficulties. The difficulties can manifest as disturbed social relationships, academic difficulties, and problems with management of routine daily tasks, and functioning in these areas is most predictive of global psychosocial adjustment. Although many medical clinics have behavioral health providers who collaborate in the identification and treatment of behavioral health difficulties, the availability of this resource widely varies, a condition that emphasizes the important role of school-based clinicians in facilitating collaborative treatment across systems of care.

The nature of the stressors associated with chronic health conditions makes the affected youth more likely than their healthy peers to experience internalizing and externalizing mental health symptoms, in addition to behavior difficulties. Coping style and peer support have been identified as two key components in positive outcomes for youth with a health condition. Specifically, youth who engage in active coping strategies, such as modifying thoughts or emotional responses, relaxation, or problem-solving, report less emotional distress than peers who use avoidant coping. Similarly, youth who have peer support and appropriate social interactions with peers report greater well-being. School-based clinicians are ideally positioned to assist in identifying, monitoring, and responding to the social and emotional needs of youth with a chronic health condition.

REFERENCES

Achenbach, T. M., & Edelbrock, C. (1991). *The Child Behavior Checklist manual.* Burlington: The University of Vermont.

Barlow, J., & Ellard, D. (2006). The psychosocial well-being of children with chronic disease, their parents and siblings: An overview of the research evidence base. *Child: Care, Health and Development, 32*(1), 19–31. doi:10.1111/j.1365-2214.2006.00591.x

Bennett, D. S. (1994). Depression among children with chronic medical problems: A meta-analysis. *Journal of Pediatric Psychology, 19*(2), 149–169. doi:10.1093/jpepsy/19.2.149

Bilfield, S., Wildman, B. G., & Karazsia, B. T. (2005). Brief report: The relationship between chronic illness and identification and management of psychosocial problems in pediatric primary care. *Journal of Pediatric Psychology, 31*(8), 813–817.

Campbell, L. K., Scaduto, M., Van Slyke, D., Niarhos, F., Whitlock, J. A., & Compas, B. E. (2009). Executive function, coping, and behavior in survivors of childhood acute lymphocytic leukemia. *Journal of Pediatric Psychology, 34*(3), 317–327. doi:10.1093/jpepsy/jsn080

Chan, E., Piira, T., & Betts, G. (2005). The school functioning of children with chronic and recurrent pain. *Pediatric Pain Letter, 7*(23), 11–16.

Collins, W. A., & Laursen, B. (2004). Changing relationships, changing youth: Interpersonal contexts of adolescent development. *The Journal of Early Adolescence, 24*(1), 55–62.

Compas, B. E., Boyer, M. C., Stanger, C., Colletti, R. B., Thomsen, A. H., Dufton, L. M., & Cole, D. A. (2006). Latent variable analysis of coping, anxiety/depression, and somatic symptoms in adolescents with chronic pain. *Journal of Consulting and Clinical Psychology, 74*(6), 1132–1142. doi:10.1037/0022-006X.74.6.1132

Compas, B. E., Jaser, S. S., Dunn, M. J., & Rodriguez, E. M. (2012). Coping with chronic illness in childhood and adolescence. *Annual Review of Clinical Psychology, 8*(1), 455–480. doi:10.1146/annurev-clinpsy-032511-143108

Dufton, L. M., Dunn, M. J., Slosky, L. S., & Compas, B. E. (2011). Self-reported and laboratory-based responses to stress in children with recurrent pain and anxiety. *Journal of Pediatric Psychology, 36*(1), 95–105. doi:10.1093/jpepsy/jsq070

Edgar, K., & Skinner, T. (2003). Illness representations and coping as predictors of emotional well-being in adolescents with type 1 diabetes. *Journal of Pediatric Psychology, 28*(7), 485–493.

Faith, M. A., Reed, G., Heppner, C. E., Hamill, L. C., Tarkenton, T. R., & Donewar, C. W. (2015). Bullying in medically fragile youth: A review of risks, protective factors, and recommendations for medical providers. *Journal of Developmental & Behavioral Pediatrics, 36*(4), 285–301. doi:10.1097/DBP.0000000000000155

Feldman, A. F., & Matjasko, J. L. (2005). The role of school-based extracurricular activities in adolescent development: A comprehensive review and future directions. *Review of Educational Research, 75*(2), 159–210.

Gerard, A. B., & Reynolds, C. R. (1999). Characteristics and applications of the Revised Children's Manifest Anxiety Scale (RCMAS). In M. E. Maruish (Ed.), *The use of psychological testing for treatment planning and outcomes assessment* (pp. 323–341). Mahwah, N.J.: Lawrence Erlbaum Associates Publishers.

Helgeson, V. S., & Holmbeck, G. N. (2014). An introduction to the special issue on peer relations in youth with chronic illness. *Journal of Pediatric Psychology, 40*(3), 267–271.

Helms, A. S., Schmiegelow, K., Brok, J., Johansen, C., Thorsteinsson, T., Simovska, V., & Larsen, H. B. (2016). Facilitation of school re-entry and peer acceptance of children with cancer: A review and meta-analysis of intervention studies. *European Journal of Cancer Care, 25*(1), 170–179.

Hocking, M. C., Barnes, M., Shaw, C., Lochman, J. E., Madan-Swain, A., & Saeed, S. (2011). Executive function and attention regulation as predictors of coping success in youth with functional abdominal pain. *Journal of Pediatric Psychology, 36*(1), 64–73. doi:10.1093/jpepsy/jsq056

Hodges, E. V., Boivin, M., Vitaro, F., & Bukowski, W. M. (1999). The power of friendship: Protection against an escalating cycle of peer victimization. *Developmental Psychology, 35*(1), 94.

Hodges, E. V., & Perry, D. G. (1999). Personal and interpersonal antecedents and consequences of victimization by peers. *Journal of Personality and Social Psychology, 76*(4), 677.

Janicke, D. M., Gray, W. N., Kahhan, N. A., Junger, F. W. K., Marciel, K. K., . . . Jolley, C. D. (2009). Brief report: The association between peer victimization, prosocial support, and treatment adherence in children and adolescents with inflammatory bowel disease. *Journal of Pediatric Psychology, 34*(7), 769–773. doi:10.1093/jpepsy/jsn116

Jaser, S. S., & White, L. E. (2011). Coping and resilience in adolescents with type 1 diabetes. *Child: Care, Health and Development, 37*(3), 335–342. doi:10.1111/j.1365-2214.2010.01184.x

Juster, R. P., McEwen, B. S., & Lupien, S. J. (2010). Allostatic load biomarkers of chronic stress and impact on health and cognition. *Neuroscience & Biobehavioral Reviews, 35*(1), 2–16.

Juvonen, J., & Graham, S. (2013). Bullying in schools: The power of bullies and the plight of victims. *Annual Review of Psychology, 65*(1), 159–185. doi:10.1146/annurev-psych-010213-115030

Karsdorp, P. A., Everaerd, W., Kindt, M., & Mulder, B. J. M. (2007). Psychological and cognitive functioning in children and adolescents with congenital heart disease: A meta-analysis. *Journal of Pediatric Psychology, 32*(5), 527–541. doi:10.1093/jpepsy/jsl047

Kliebenstein, M. A., & Broome, M. E. (2000). School re-entry for the child with chronic illness: Parent and school personnel perceptions. *Pediatric Nursing, 26*(6), 579.

Kohut, S. A., Stinson, J. N., Giosa, L., Luca, S., & van Wyk, M. (2014). Systematic review of peer support interventions for adolescents with chronic illness: A narrative analysis. *International Journal of Child Adolescent Health, 7*(3), 183–197.

Kovac, M. (2010). *Children's Depression Inventory 2™* (CDI 2). North Tonawanda, NY: Multi-Health Systems.

LeBlanc, L. A., Goldsmith, T., & Patel, D. R. (2003). Behavioral aspects of chronic illness in children and adolescents. *Pediatric Clinics of North America, 50*(4), 859–878.

Lemanek, K. L., Kamps, J., & Chung, N. B. (2001). Empirically supported treatments in pediatric psychology: Regimen adherence. *Journal of Pediatric Psychology, 26*(5), 253–275.

Lurie, M., & Kaufman, N. (2001). An initial reintegration treatment of children with acute lymphoblastic leukemia (ALL). *Research in the Schools, 8*(1), 29–43.

Mcquaid, E. L., Kopel, S. J., & Nassau, J. H. (2001). Behavioral adjustment in children with asthma: A meta-analysis. *Journal of Developmental & Behavioral Pediatrics, 22*(6), 430–439.

Meijer, S. A., Sinnema, G., Bijstra, J. O., Mellenbergh, G. J., & Wolters, W. H. (2002). Coping styles and locus of control as predictors for psychological adjustment of adolescents with a chronic illness. *Social Science & Medicine, 54*(9), 1453–1461.

Meltzer, L. J., Graham, D. M., Leija, S., Booster, G. D., Carroll, T., Seeger, B., & Bledsoe, M. (2018). Benefits of disease-specific summer camps: Results from quantitative and qualitative studies at Roundup River Ranch. *Children and Youth Services Review, 89*, 272–280.

Miller, J. J., III. (1993). Psychosocial factors related to rheumatic diseases in childhood. *The Journal of Rheumatology, 38*(Suppl.), 1–11.

Moola, F. J., Faulkner, G. E. J., White, L., & Kirsh, J. A. (2014). The psychological and social impact of camp for children with chronic illnesses: A systematic review update. *Child: Care, Health and Development, 40*(5), 615–631.

Noll, R., Gartstein, M., Vannatta, K., Correll, J., Bukowski, W., & Davies, W. (1999). Social, emotional, and behavioral functioning of children with cancer. *Pediatrics, 103*(1), 71–78. doi:10.1542/peds.103.1.71

Olweus, D. (1993). *Bullying at school: What we know and what we can do.* Oxford, UK: Blackwell Publishers.

Pinquart, M. (2017). Systematic review: Bullying involvement of children with and without chronic physical illness and/or physical/sensory disability—A meta-analytic comparison with healthy/nondisabled peers. *Journal of Pediatric Psychology, 42*(3), 245–259. doi:10.1093/jpepsy/jsw081

Pinquart, M., & Shen, Y. (2011). Behavior problems in children and adolescents with chronic physical illness: A meta-analysis. *Journal of Pediatric Psychology, 36*(9), 1003–1016. doi:10.1093/jpepsy/jsr042

Pinquart, M., & Teubert, D. (2011). Academic, physical, and social functioning of children and adolescents with chronic physical illness: A meta-analysis. *Journal of Pediatric Psychology, 37*(4), 376–389.

Power, T. J., Shapiro, E. S., & DuPaul, G. J. (2003). Preparing psychologists to link systems of care in managing and preventing children's health problems. *Journal of Pediatric Psychology, 28*(2), 147–155.

Reijntjes, A., Kamphuis, J. H., Prinzie, P., & Telch, M. J. (2010). Peer victimization and internalizing problems in children: A meta-analysis of longitudinal studies. *Child Abuse & Neglect, 34*(4), 244–252. doi:10.1016/j.chiabu.2009.07.009

Reiter-Purtill, J., Waller, J. M., & Noll, R. B. (2009). Empirical and theoretical perspectives on the peer relationships of children with chronic conditions. In M. C. Roberts & R. G. Steele (Eds.), *Handbook of Pediatric Psychology, Fourth Edition* (pp.672–688). New York, NY, US: The Guilford Press.

Rodenburg, R., Stams, G. J., Meijer, A. M., Aldenkamp, A. P., & Deković, M. (2005). Psychopathology in children with epilepsy: A meta-analysis. *Journal of Pediatric Psychology, 30*(6), 453–468. doi:10.1093/jpepsy/jsi071

Rodriguez, E. M., Dunn, M. J., Zuckerman, T., Vannatta, K., Gerhardt, C. A., & Compas, B. E. (2011). Cancer-related sources of stress for children with cancer and their parents. *Journal of Pediatric Psychology, 37*(2), 185–197.

Rudolph, K. D., Dennig, M. D., & Weisz, J. R. (1995). Determinants and consequences of children's coping in the medical setting: Conceptualization, review, and critique. *Psychological Bulletin, 118*(3), 328–357. doi:10.1037/0033-2909.118.3.328

Sandstrom, M. J., & Schanberg, L. E. (2004). Brief report: Peer rejection, social behavior, and psychological adjustment in children with juvenile rheumatic disease. *Journal of Pediatric Psychology, 29*(1), 29–34. doi:10.1093/jpepsy/jsh004

Schilling, E. J., & Getch, Y. Q. (2012). Getting my bearings, returning to school: Issues facing adolescents with traumatic brain injury. *Teaching Exceptional Children, 45*(1), 54–63.

Schwartz, D., Gorman, A. H., Nakamoto, J., & Toblin, R. L. (2005). Victimization in the peer group and children's academic functioning. *Journal of Educational Psychology, 97*(3), 425–435. doi:10.1037/0022-0663.97.3.425

Sentenac, M., Arnaud, C., Gavin, A., Molcho, M., Gabhainn, S. N., & Godeau, E. (2011). Peer victimization among school-aged children with chronic conditions. *Epidemiologic Reviews*, *34*(1), 120–128.

Sentenac, M., Gavin, A., Gabhainn, S. N., Molcho, M., Due, P., Ravens-Sieberer, U., . . . Godeau, E. (2013). Peer victimization and subjective health among students reporting disability or chronic illness in 11 Western countries. *European Journal of Public Health*, *23*(3), 421–426.

Storch, E. A., Heidgerken, A. D., Geffken, G. R., Lewin, A. B., Ohleyer, V., Freddo, M., & Silverstein, J. H. (2006). Bullying, regimen self-management, and metabolic control in youth with type I diabetes. *The Journal of Pediatrics*, *148*(6), 784–787. doi:10.1016/j.jpeds.2006.01.007

Thomsen, A. H., Compas, B. E., Colletti, R. B., Stanger, C., Boyer, M. C., & Konik, B. S. (2002). Parent reports of coping and stress responses in children with recurrent abdominal pain. *Journal of Pediatric Psychology*, *27*(3), 215–226.

Vannatta, K., Gartstein, M. A., Zeller, M., & Noll, R. B. (2009). Peer acceptance and social behavior during childhood and adolescence: How important are appearance, athleticism, and academic competence? *International Journal of Behavioral Development*, *33*(4), 303–311.

Walker, L. S., Smith, C. A., Garber, J., & Van Slyke, D. A. (1997). Development and validation of the Pain Response Inventory for children. *Psychological Assessment*, *9*(4), 392.

Wildman, B. G., Stancin, T., Golden, C., & Yerkey, T. (2004). Maternal distress, child behaviour, and disclosure of psychosocial concerns to a paediatrician. *Child: Care, Health and Development*, *30*(4), 385–394.

Wissow, L. S., van Ginneken, N., Chandna, J., & Rahman, A. (2016). Integrating children's mental health into primary care. *Pediatric Clinics*, *63*(1), 97–113.

Worchel-Prevatt, F. F., Heffer, R. W., Prevatt, B. C., Miner, J., Young-Saleme, T., Horgan, D., . . . Frankel, L. (1998). A school reentry program for chronically ill children. *Journal of School Psychology*, *36*(3), 261–279.

HANDOUT 2.1.

COPING WITH STRESS

For Things You Can Control	For Things OUTSIDE Your Control

• Problem-solving steps
  • Describe the problem.
  • Brainstorm different solutions.
  • What would happen if you chose each solution?
  • Choose a solution to try.
  • What happened? Need to try another solution?
• Identify your feelings
• Talk it through with a friend or trusted adult
	• Acceptance
	• Step away from the stressor
	• Notice thinking traps
	• Reword your thoughts
	• Relaxation strategies
	  • Deep breathing
	  • Imagine your favorite place
	  • Picture the people you care about
	  • Take a break
	• Mindfulness strategies
	  • Take a mindful walk
	  • Yoga
	  • Journal
	  • Meditation
	• Progressive muscle relaxation

HANDOUT 2.2.

CHANGING NEGATIVE THOUGHTS TO POSITIVE THOUGHTS

Identify the negative thoughts you tell yourself in difficult or stressful situations and brainstorm positive thoughts you can try to tell yourself instead.

Thoughts I have during _____.

Things I'm Thinking (Negative Thoughts)	Change My Thinking (Positive Thoughts)

Thoughts I have during _____.

Things I'm Thinking (Negative Thoughts)	Change My Thinking (Positive Thoughts)

Thoughts I have during _____.

Things I'm Thinking (Negative Thoughts)	Change My Thinking (Positive Thoughts)

WHAT I CAN AND CANNOT CONTROL

Helping students understand what they can and cannot control is important for both their academic success and for their emotional well-being. Trying to control things that are outside of their control can leave them feeling anxious, overwhelmed, and unable to focus on their schoolwork. This is a simple activity to use with students who need a visual reminder to conceptualize the things they can and cannot control.

1. Prompt the student write or draw the things that are in their control in the inner circle.
   Examples: my behavior, my ideas, the words I choose to say, the way I react to others, taking care of myself
2. Prompt the student to write or draw things that are not in their control in the outer circle.
   Examples: what people say, what people think, how other people feel, the past, my family, the weather
3. Discuss strategies the student can employ to cope with things that are not in their control.
   Examples: relaxation techniques, problem-solving strategies, labeling unhelpful thoughts and creating more helpful self-talk
4. Use the student's written items to coach them through problematic scenarios.
   Examples: I cannot control how other students speak to me. I can control how I think about the situation. I can control my actions. I can control my body.

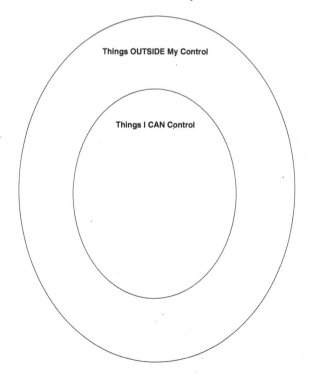

Academic Issues Related to Pediatric Health Conditions in Schools

CHRISTY M. WALCOTT AND SAYWARD E. HARRISON ■

In 1896, Lightner Witmer—an early American psychologist now largely credited with founding the field of clinical psychology—began to treat a child to whom he gave the pseudonym Charles Gilman. Young Charles was referred to Witmer's recently established psychological clinic—the first in the nation—by his grade-school teacher due to a host of learning difficulties (Witmer, 1907). As Witmer detailed in the seminal article "A Case of Chronic Bad Spelling," Charles displayed deficiencies in his reading and spelling despite being a boy of "fair intelligence and general information" (Witmer, 1907, p. 54). Charles was unable to correctly spell or read the most simple of English words.

> By questioning him and his teacher I learned that his spelling lesson was prepared at home with the help of his mother and sister. Although he spent hours in preparation, he would misspell more than half of the lesson when [words were] dictated to him the following day. When [he was] copying from the blackboard his teacher reported that he could never take down more than one syllable at a time, and his copy showed many blunders. Thus he would write *cone* for *come*, and *hone* for *home*—a blunder the significance of which I did not appreciate at that time. (Witmer, 1907, p. 55)

Careful inquiry and examination with both pupil and teacher yielded an answer: Charles needed glasses. In fact, Charles' diplopia (i.e., double vision) had gone unrecognized for many years, leading to significant academic delays (Witmer, 1907; Zenderland, 2001).

Physical health and school achievement are indelibly linked, as Witmer's case study demonstrates; yet, the relationship between them too often goes unrecognized by the healthcare providers, educators, and mental health professionals who are intimately involved in the care and treatment of children. Understanding the academic impacts of health conditions—whether an easily corrected case of diplopia or a more involved chronic condition, such as sickle cell disease—is critical for effective prevention and intervention. Psychologists and other school-based clinicians, with their expertise in consultation and collaboration, their ability to engage in direct (i.e., client-centered) and indirect (i.e., systems-level) services, and their emphasis on data-based decision-making and evidence-based practices, are in prime positions to take a lead in recognizing and remedying the academic effects of chronic pediatric health conditions (PHCs).

The past century has born witness to a remarkable shift in the epidemiology of childhood diseases. Advances in medical technology, improved systems of care, and expanding public health efforts (e.g., vaccination, improved sanitation) have significantly reduced the mortality rates previously associated with many medical conditions (Houtrow, Larson, Olson, Newacheck, & Halfon, 2014). However, the drop in mortality has corresponded with increased morbidity and decreased quality of life associated with a range of PHCs (Houtrow et al., 2014). In fact, the prevalence of chronic conditions has more than doubled in the past 30 years, likely due both to a broadening concept of health and disease (i.e., awareness and inclusion of many conditions not previously recognized), as well as a growing number of children who survive conditions like prematurity and childhood cancers that in earlier generations were fatal (Halfon & Newacheck, 2010; Van Cleave, Gortmaker, & Perrin, 2010).

Estimates of how many school-age children experience a PHC vary based on which conditions are included within a particular survey methodology. When mental health and learning disorders are included in prevalence studies, the number of children affected by PHCs is staggering, with approximately 23% of children in the United States having one or more chronic physical and mental health conditions that affect their daily life (U.S. Department of Health and Human Services, 2014). Despite the variation in the conditions that are included under the umbrella of "chronic illness," it is clear that millions of American children experience long-term challenges to their health that also often affect their academic, social-emotional, and/or behavioral functioning, requiring a strong system of support that extends beyond a student's medical home. Schools are an opportune setting in which to provide services to children with PHCs. Not only do a majority of children with medical conditions attend school, but also the school setting provides the opportunity to address any academic, social, and behavioral sequelae of the health condition.

EDUCATIONAL IMPACTS OF PHCS

The vast majority of children with PHCs in the United States attend public schools, and the schools are well equipped to offer an array of services to meet students' learning, psychosocial, and behavioral needs. School-based provision of care is also critical because children and adolescents with PHCs often perform more poorly than healthy peers on a wide range of educational outcomes, including receiving poorer grades, and they often report more dislike of school (Crump et al., 2013; Lum et al., 2017; Thies, 1999). Thus, services frequently must go beyond attending to the medical needs of students to also address the academic, social-emotional, and behavioral needs that are caused or exacerbated by their health conditions.

There are several reasons why students with PHCs may function more poorly than their healthy peers academically and socially. First, some conditions limit time spent at school or in contact with peers due to frequent doctor's visits, prolonged hospital stays, or chronic fatigue. The less time children have in contact with peers, the fewer opportunities they have to develop social skills (Merrell & Gimpel, 1998), and chronic school absences may impede academic success (Madan-Swain, Katz, & LaGory, 2004). Second, impairments in cognitive abilities (e.g., memory, attention, executive functioning, global intelligence) are associated with some PHCs, such as epilepsy and sickle cell disease, and with some treatments, such as cranial radiation (Mitby et al., 2003; Taras & Potts-Datema, 2005). The cognitive deficits can affect both academic learning and social problem-solving. Third, aggressive behavior or depressive symptoms associated with PHCs may affect social and academic functioning (Pinquart & Shen, 2011).

Longitudinal survey data, meta-analyses, and systematic review papers have all documented a link between PHCs and lower academic functioning (Lum et al., 2017; Martinez & Ercikan, 2009; Pinquart & Teubert, 2012). Based upon reviews of both disease-specific studies and those examining PHC status more broadly, children with identified chronic illnesses, on average, have lower academic outcomes than their healthy peers. However, all the review studies noted that the type of illness matters, with illnesses affecting central nervous system (CNS) functioning having a significantly stronger negative relationship with academic outcomes. For example, Pinquart and Teubert (2012) found that illness-specific effect sizes for poorer academic functioning were largest for cerebral palsy, spina bifida, and sickle cell disease. Lum and colleagues (2017) also found that more consistent and severe academic outcomes were associated with illnesses or treatments that involved cognitive functioning (e.g., brain tumors, epilepsy, chronic kidney disease).

As noted, there are several reasons why PHCs would be related to academic delays, with direct CNS impacts (e.g., stroke) and negative treatment effects (e.g., cranial radiation or medications that affect attention or executive functioning) being the most apparent culprits. However, academic achievement is also negatively impacted by the psychosocial ramifications of having a chronic illness as well as by school absences for medical appointments, hospitalizations, and treatments. The remainder of this chapter outlines major academic considerations for children with PHCs, with emphasis on cognitive and learning impacts, school absenteeism and refusal, and suggestions for individualized planning for school supports.

NEUROCOGNITIVE EFFECTS OF PHCS AND THEIR TREATMENTS

Many PHCs and their treatments yield neurocognitive effects that create a host of academic challenges. For some conditions, such as childhood cancers, neurocognitive effects are common, with recent studies indicating that up to 40% of children who survive cancer show long-term impairment in specific cognitive domains, including processing speed, attention, and memory (Moleski, 2000). Thus, recommendations for neurocognitive monitoring, evaluation, and intervention for this subset of children are well established and often are a routine aspect of their specialized medical care (Castellino, Ullrich, Whelen, & Lange; 2014; Krull et al., 2008). Other PHCs are associated with less well-known and rarer neurocognitive deficits, making it important for school-based practitioners to gather as much information as possible about potential cognitive effects of a particular health condition in order to plan, assess, and intervene effectively.

Neurocognitive effects associated with PHCs can be conceptualized as disease-related or treatment-related. The pathophysiology of a particular health condition will determine the mechanism through which the brain and subsequent neurological functioning is affected, with common mechanisms including disease-related processes that damage brain structures, organization, and development (e.g., tissue damage from brain tumor or stroke), deoxygenation of the brain (e.g., hypoxia from sickle cell disease), chronic inflammation of the CNS (e.g., inflammation from vasculitis), or faulty metabolic processes (e.g., impaired delivery of glucose to the brain in diabetes; Compas, Jaser, Reeslund, Patel, & Yarboi, 2017). Executive functioning (e.g., attention, planning, problem-solving, organization, working memory) are among the neurocognitive deficits associated with certain PHCs, such as sickle cell disease (Schatz & Roberts, 2007), chronic kidney disease (Gipson et al., 2006), and epilepsy (Parrish et al., 2007). Interestingly, a child's initial temperament and early levels of executive functioning may be important influences on adherence to treatment (e.g., ability to set goals and flexibility to adapt to treatment regimens). For example, McNally, Rohan, Pendley, Delamater, and Drotar (2010) found that executive functioning was related to adherence, which was in turn related to type 1 diabetes control.

Treatment-related effects, on the other hand, result not from the disease itself but from surgery, radiation therapy, chemotherapy, or other pharmacologic treatments of the health condition. For instance, corticosteroids—used to treat inflammation associated with a number of PHCs (e.g., asthma, cystic fibrosis, juvenile arthritis)—can cause a variety of side effects, including severe mood changes (e.g., mania, depression), psychosis, and cognitive or executive functioning impairments (e.g., inattention, memory deficits; Brown & Chandler, 2001). Treatments for brain tumors and acute lymphocytic leukemia, which include surgery, radiation therapy, and chemotherapy, often yield long-term cognitive impairments (i.e., "late effects") that may consist of lowered IQ scores, problems with memory and attention, poor eye–hand coordination, behavioral problems, and delayed development (American Cancer Society, 2016).

Children and adolescents are particularly vulnerable to neurocognitive insults from both diseases and their treatments because of the rapid brain development that occurs during infancy and childhood, including the growth of white matter (i.e., myelination) within the brain that is critical to cognitive development and learning (Compas et al., 2017; Nagy, Westerberg, & Klinberg, 2004). A thorough review of the specific neurocognitive deficits associated with each childhood PHC is beyond the scope of this chapter; however, the reader is directed to recent work by Compas and colleagues (2017) that provides a review of meta-analyses of neurocognitive effects of some of the most common PHCs, as summarized in Table 3.1.

Across the diverse group of PHCs examined by Compas and colleagues (2017), neurocognitive impacts were common, ranging from decreases in global intelligence to deficits in specific domains that have important implications for learning (e.g., attention, memory, processing speed). Such neurocognitive deficits contribute to the lower educational achievement of children with a variety of PHCs, including receiving poor grades and poorer performance on "end-of-grade" tests of reading and math (Crump et al., 2013; Thies, 1999). The range of neurocognitive deficits associated with PHCs makes it imperative that school-based personnel become informed about the risks associated with a particular condition and engage in close monitoring of the student's academic achievement, social-emotional skills, and behavior in order to intervene as early as possible should symptoms appear. Some children with PHCs will require comprehensive neuropsychological evaluations either because of the nature of their disorder (i.e., diagnosis of traumatic brain injury, routine evaluations for late effects of cancer treatment) or because difficulties emerge that may be related to their health condition. In such cases, traditional psychological evaluation may be insufficient to measure the subtle memory, attention, and processing deficits that often characterize the cognitive sequelae of various health disorders, and consultation and/or evaluation by a specialist, such as a clinical neuropsychologist or a pediatric school psychologist, may be warranted. If assessment is needed, the assessment battery should be comprehensive, in order to assess the student's cognitive strengths and weaknesses, and also should incorporate information from multiple sources and settings (e.g., home, school, healthcare provider). Given their familiarity with the child, school-based practitioners may be the first to notice neurocognitive changes that should alert parents and physicians to changes in the health status of the child (e.g., tumor growth, increased seizure activity).

SCHOOL ABSENTEEISM AND SCHOOL REFUSAL

One way that PHCs often interfere with the normal trajectory of schooling is through the accrual of student absences. In the United States, a student is typically considered chronically absent if 18 or more days are missed annually (an average of 2 days/month during an academic year). Frequent or prolonged school

Table 3.1. SUMMARY OF RECENT META-ANALYTIC FINDINGS OF NEUROCOGNITIVE
IMPACTS OF SIX COMMON CHRONIC PEDIATRIC HEALTH CONDITIONS AS IDENTIFIED
BY COMPAS ET AL. (2017)

Chronic Health Condition	Suggested Neurocognitive Effects and Corresponding Effect Sizes		Reference
Acute lymphocytic leukemia (ALL)	Medium effect sizes: Small to medium effect sizes:	Full-scale IQ Verbal IQ Nonverbal IQ Attention Information processing Executive functioning Visual spatial Verbal memory Visual memory	Campbell et al. (2007). Meta-analytic review of long-term neurocognitive effects of childhood ALL including 28 studies conducted between 1980 and 2004, with a total of 1,005 ALL patients in remission and 1,141 healthy controls.
Pediatric brain tumors	Large effect sizes: Medium to large effect sizes:	Attention Psychomotor Visual spatial Verbal memory Full-scale IQ Verbal IQ Nonverbal IQ Academic achievement	Robinson et al. (2010). Meta-analysis on long-term neurocognitive effects of pediatric brain tumors, including 39 studies published between 1992 and 2009, with data from 1,318 survivors of pediatric brain tumors.
Congenital heart disease (CHD)	Small effect size:	Overall cognitive ability*	Karsdorp, Everaerd, Kindt, & Mulder (2007). Meta-analysis of psychological and cognitive functioning among children and adolescents with CHD who had undergone surgery or interventional catheterization, with 25 studies providing data on cognitive functioning of 1,712 patients with CHD.
Sickle cell disease (SCD)	Small effect size:	Full-scale IQ	Schatz, Finke, Kellet, & Kramer (2002). Meta-analysis of cognitive impacts of SCD including 18 studies reporting data on 659 children with SCD but without history of cerebral infarction and 474 healthy controls.

Table 3.1. CONTINUED

Chronic Health Condition	Suggested Neurocognitive Effects and Corresponding Effect Sizes		Reference
Type 1 diabetes	Small effect sizes:	Full-scale IQ Verbal IQ Performance IQ Visual-spatial deficits Perceptual motor speed Sustained attention Reading and writing achievement	Naguib, Kulinskaya, Lomax, & Garralda (2009). Meta-analysis of neuropsychological functioning of youth with type 1 diabetes, including 24 studies with data on 894 patients and 758 healthy controls
Traumatic brain injury (TBI)** Mild TBI Moderate to Severe TBI	Small effect sizes[+]: Moderate to large effects:	Full-scale IQ Performance IQ Verbal IQ Full-scale IQ Verbal IQ Performance IQ	Babikian & Asarnow (2009). Meta-analytic review of neurocognitive effects of TBI, including 28 publications published from 1988 to 2007 documenting neurocognitive outcomes among pediatric patients with accidental TBI

*There is significant heterogeneity in effects associated with varying disease severity (e.g., there is a large effect on full-scale IQ for children with hypoplastic left heart syndrome but a small effect for those with transposition of the great arteries).
**Severity of TBI was a significant moderator of effects and thus findings are reported for mild, moderate, and severe TBI. [+]Nonsignificant.

absences occur for many reasons, some related to the illness itself and others to concomitant psychosocial issues (Emerson et al., 2016). In a recent retrospective cohort study of over 22,000 children with PHCs, Crump and colleagues (2013) found the absentee rate was 1.3 times greater for chronically ill children than for their healthy peers. This held true even after adjusting for covariates (age, gender, ethnicity, language, grade level, special education, parental education). Although frequency and duration of days absent varied dramatically by student and health condition, Newacheck and Halfon (1998) reported that children with PHCs missed an average of 6.2 days annually, although the range of absences was quite large, with some students missing up to 6 weeks of school annually. Students who are often absent from school may be targeted for educational intervention, grade retention, or placement in special education because of the large amount of missed instructional material and resulting academic delays. To complicate matters, parents may underestimate the significant negative impact of chronic school absenteeism and may fail to recognize the close links between absenteeism and a child's psychosocial functioning (Gottfried, 2014).

Following the experience of a medical incident or prolonged sickness, a child's social well-being can either promote or deter the return to school, and the child may show signs of school refusal or somatic complaints due to psychosocial stressors (e.g., bullying, marginalization/stigma, anxiety, depression; Shaw & McCabe, 2008). One useful resource for school personnel is the AbsencesAddUp. org website, which reviews the importance of school attendance and provides resources to encourage school attendance and to address issues that cause children to unnecessarily miss school. Of course, if school absences result from illness-related complications, then they may not be readily avoidable. Illness-related absences can result from symptoms (e.g., severe pain episodes), a compromised immune system (e.g., children undergoing chemotherapy), medical appointments or treatments during school hours, or hospitalizations. Clearly, different strategies are needed depending on the underlying cause of PHC-related absenteeism. Below and in Table 3.2, we present some decision-making criteria to guide intervention selection.

Interventions to Address Absenteeism

If the reason for school absenteeism is illness-related, then intervention will depend upon whether the absences are intermittent or long-term. For students who are unable to attend school for extended periods of time due to PHCs, educational services may be delivered via a hospital school or through homebound services. Medical homebound instruction may be provided for both special education and regular education students who cannot attend school for a medical reason. Each school district should have procedures to approve homebound instruction, which typically requires that a licensed physician certify the medical condition and the need for homebound services. The intent of medical homebound instruction is to connect students with PHCs to the regular curriculum until a return to the classroom setting is possible. Medically homebound students must be provided opportunities to participate in extracurricular activities with typical peers as deemed appropriate, and the ultimate goal is for the student to transition back into the regular school environment as soon as possible. Established school re-entry programs are available and provide models for supporting students and families through this process (e.g., Prevatt, Heffer, & Lowe, 2000; Shaw & McCabe, 2008).

For students with intermittent illness-related absences, individualized accommodation plans can outline ways to connect them with missed instruction, curriculum content, and extracurricular opportunities. For example, flexible school days can address limitations in vitality and pain-related crises. Technology can be used to allow students "virtual visits" with their classroom to share ideas and interact with peers. Online classroom tools or email can be used to send and receive schoolwork. Importantly, technology now makes available many opportunities to provide direct instruction via online lectures, online courses, or computer-assisted

Table 3.2. PROBLEM-SOLVING FRAMEWORK FOR STUDENTS WITH CHRONIC PEDIATRIC HEALTH CONDITIONS (PHCs)

Stage	Activities	Special considerations
I. Problem Identification	• Seek consent to exchange information among home, school, and healthcare providers • Collect data on PHC (e.g., etiology, symptoms, treatment, neurocognitive impacts) • Examine school records, including attendance • Gather information on learning and social-emotional and/or behavioral functioning • Consider student's ability to participate in daily school activities	If child is on medication or undergoing treatment (e.g., chemotherapy)→ assess for side effects that may affect school functioning
II. Problem Analysis	• Develop an individualized healthcare plan to address school-related health needs • Assess impact of PHC on student's school achievement • If significant → consider potential eligibility for special education • If not significant → consider whether accommodations (i.e., Section 504 plan) are needed	If child has significant absences, consider cause (e.g., symptoms, susceptibility to infection, fatigue, medical appointments, psychosocial reasons)
III. Treatment Implementation	• Implement healthcare plan for all students with PHCs • Implement special education services and/or accommodations as indicated • Ensure frequent communication among home, school, and healthcare providers to monitor symptoms and evaluate for changes in learning, social-emotional, and/or behavioral functioning	Remember that impact of PHC is likely to change over time, necessitating frequent modifications to services
IV. Treatment Evaluation	• Routinely assess symptoms and impact of PHC on school-related outcomes (i.e., progress monitoring) • Meet regularly to determine whether current services/accommodations are appropriate	School personnel may need to lead efforts to communicate with healthcare providers; up-to-date medical information is critical

instruction. Given the growing popularity of distance education and online coursework at the university level, there is surprisingly little research on the use of such methods at the K-12 level, particularly for students with PHCs. At the high-school level, more U.S. states are offering opportunities for virtual high schools or Internet-based courses. However, the availability of distance education at the elementary and middle-school levels remains fairly limited. Yet, computer-assisted programs can be helpful in supporting students with PHCs due to the ease of implementation, the standardized scope and sequence of curriculum, and the possibility of individualization through regular monitoring of progress paired with adaptive instruction.

In addition to the more obvious physical effects of illness, there is also a link between PHCs and psychosocial problems, and children living with PHCs may be at risk for a number of mental and behavioral health challenges relative to healthy peers (Pinquart & Teubert, 2012). Although the emotional stress of coping with a chronic illness is one obvious challenge for students, studies have documented that a number of other social and behavioral difficulties are also associated with chronic illness, such as experiencing anxiety and depression, feeling stigmatized or marginalized because of a health condition, and experiencing victimization by peers (Pinquart & Teubert, 2012). Shaw and McCabe (2008) recommended that schools specifically address issues of social support and affective adjustment for students with PHCs. Social support from same-age peers who are also living with chronic illnesses may be particularly valuable. Such opportunities are often available via summer camps and other special programming for children with PHCs. Schools will need to be flexible and creative in addressing the unique psychosocial needs of chronically ill students. Parents and schools should proactively address psychosocial stressors and the potential for school refusal by planning for peer education about the PHC, building mentorship and social supports into the school setting, and creating outlets for the student to discuss affective issues (e.g., access to mental health professionals). Furthermore, warm, responsive student–teacher relationships are important to promote academic and social functioning. Studies suggest that many students with PHCs want to continue their connection to school and learning, although teachers may believe that chronically ill students should be exempt from daily schoolwork obligations (Wilkie, 2012). Although reluctance by teachers to initiate contact or to academically engage students with PHCs may be well intentioned, reducing expectations for the student with a PHC can in fact marginalize the student and reduce opportunities for typical developmental experiences.

Students with PHCs may experience stress from managing complicated treatments and medical schedules, missing school, and feeling different from peers (Shaw & McCabe, 2008). Although some peer-related stress may be internalized as feelings of being "undesirably different" than others (Räty, Söderfeldt, Larsson, & Larsson, 2004), it is also the case that students with PHCs report higher rates of peer victimization and bullying (Sentenac et al., 2013). Thus, it is crucial for school personnel to assess for bullying and to build bullying prevention into curriculum and school activities. School personnel must work to engender positive and supportive learning environments for chronically ill students and their families, to support school attendance, and to identify and treat specific emotional and behavioral problems that arise.

SCHOOL PLANNING FOR STUDENTS WITH CHRONIC HEALTH CONDITIONS

Addressing the diverse challenges that are faced by students with PHCs requires collaboration across systems, including the home, school, and healthcare settings. However, collaboration is only possible with effective communication. As an initial step, parents or guardians must be willing to disclose health-related information and provide consent for a child's relevant medical information to be shared with the school system—including diagnoses, medical history, and medication regimens. Such information is critical to planning for supports in the school environment. However, communication should not stop there; consent for school and community providers to relay information about a student's academic, social-emotional, and behavioral performance back to the child's medical team is also critical. Noticeable changes in a child's functioning at school may often be the first indication of new or worsening symptoms that require prompt medical attention. For instance, up to 35% of children with sickle cell disease experience silent cerebral infarctions (i.e., "silent" strokes) that have no overt symptoms yet yield permanent injury to the brain and cause a variety of cognitive impairments (Dowling, Quinn, Rogers, & Buchanan, 2010). School personnel may be the first individuals to notice changes in the child's executive functioning—including inattention and memory deficits—that frequently signal a recent silent infarct. Thus teachers and other personnel who interact on a daily basis with the child with a PHC should be aware of the risks posed by the health condition and should be able to communicate quickly with parents or guardians and healthcare providers if such symptoms are noted. Because there is significant stigma attached to sickle cell disease—and many other PHCs—schools must create climates of trust and support with families in order for open and effective lines of communication to be maintained.

Once school personnel are aware of a student's PHC, frequent communication is needed to keep the school abreast of any changes in the child's health. Depending upon the course of the illness and the treatments involved, symptoms and daily functioning may vary tremendously. Communication among the family, healthcare provider, and school is key, and early efforts should delineate who the primary contacts are for each system, what method will be used for communication (e.g., in-person meetings, phone contact, email), how frequently communication should occur, and what the limits are to confidentiality of the information that is shared.

Individualized Healthcare Plans

A number of options are typically available to support students with PHCs in the school environment. The National Association of School Nurses (NASN) promotes the use of an individualized healthcare plan for any student whose healthcare needs may affect their potential to achieve safe and optimal school attendance and academic performance (NASN, 2013). The individualized healthcare plan serves to document a student's medical condition(s) and all related needs. Guided by the nursing process model, school nurses are trained to review medical records and to complete assessment or diagnosis of student needs, to outline required school-based services and intervention, and to document expected outcomes of care (NASN, 2013). Typically, school nurses draft individualized healthcare plans in collaboration with the student, parents, a multidisciplinary team of school staff, and the student's primary or specialty healthcare providers. Although the format varies by state and by school district, most have common elements, including specific documentation of the roles and responsibilities of the student, family, and school. For example, an individualized healthcare plan may delineate what medications will be provided during the school day, the dosage, how medication will be administered, who will administer it, and possible side effects. If necessary, a plan for staff training may be included to educate school personnel and to prepare them to be involved in the student's care. Such plans must be revisited regularly (typically at least once per year) and altered as health and/or treatments change. In addition, an emergency care plan may also be developed that provides clear action steps to be taken by school faculty and staff in case the student experiences a medical emergency or health crisis while on school grounds (NASN, 2013).

Individualized Accommodations

Some students with PHCs require additional supports in order to allow the student to participate fully in the school environment and to ensure that the school is in compliance with state and federal laws. Most notably, students with PHCs may be eligible for services under Section 504 of the Rehabilitation Act of 1973. Amended in 2008, Section 504 is a federal law designed to protect the rights of individuals with disabilities in programs and activities that receive federal funds, including public schools. Students who have physical or mental impairments that significantly limit major life activities may be eligible for a Section 504 Accommodation Plan. Major life activities include many aspects of daily functioning, such as caring for one's self, walking, seeing, hearing, speaking, and learning. Limitations to major bodily functions (e.g., immune system, bowel and bladder functions, neurological functioning, etc.) are also included in the eligibility criteria (U.S. Department of Education, 2015).

Public schools must determine whether a students with such impairments requires individualized accommodations in order to have their educational needs met to the same extent as "nondisabled" peers. If so, a Section 504 plan may be developed that outlines any accommodations that are necessary for the student. For example, a student who experiences fatigue due to congenital heart disease may require a number of accommodations that are not needed by his healthy peers. He may need assistance when changing classes or he may require late passes because it takes him longer than his healthy peers to walk from one classroom to another. The student may need frequent breaks and close monitoring during periods of physical activity. He may require rest breaks built into the school day or he may need multiple sets of books so that he does not have to carry heavy books between classes. Best practices dictate that school personnel work collaboratively with families, healthcare providers, and relevant agencies to design individuals support plans that are likely to help the student's academic performance and overall school functioning (Power & Bradley-Klug, 2012).

Individualized Interventions

For a proportion of children with PHCs, illness will significantly and negatively impact their academic achievement. Schools should be aware of the neurocognitive risks associated with a child's specific health condition, put academic interventions into place as early as possible, and closely monitor the student's academic progress. If such supports are insufficient to remedy the academic deficits or if the child needs more support than regular education can provide, a referral for special education may be necessary. In such cases, a multidisciplinary team, including parents, administrators, regular education teachers, and special education teachers, may wish to consider the child's eligibility for special education under the disability category of other health impairment—a disability category for students with medical conditions that negatively affect their learning to the extent that special education is required:

> Other health impairment means having limited strength, vitality, or alertness, including a heightened alertness to environmental stimuli, that results in limited alertness with respect to the educational environment, [and] that—(i) is due to chronic or acute health problems such as asthma, attention deficit disorder or attention deficit hyperactivity disorder, diabetes, epilepsy, a heart condition, hemophilia, lead poisoning, leukemia, nephritis, rheumatic fever, sickle cell anemia, and Tourette syndrome, and (ii) adversely affects a child's educational performance. (Individuals with Disabilities Education Act, 2004)

Merely having one of the listed health conditions does not alone convey the need or eligibility for special education. Rather, there must be evidence that the student's health condition is significantly and negatively affecting the student's educational performance and that the student requires specially designed instruction outside of what can be provided in the general education curriculum. Students who are found eligible for special education must be provided with an individualized education plan (IEP) that is developed collaboratively with the multidisciplinary team. The plan outlines a student's present levels of performance, specifies measurable short-term and long-term goals for all areas of need, and details the special education services that will be provided to the student in order to attain those goals. Teams must work to ensure that students are educated in the least restrictive environment possible, and mandated reviews of the IEP allow for services to be modified as needed. Importantly, having an IEP or a Section 504 plan does not make a student ineligible for an individualized healthcare plan, and students with PHCs may benefit from having the school nurse involved in any collaborative team meetings to offer insight on specific needs related to their health condition.

CONCLUSION

In conclusion, children with PHCs may face a number of challenges in the school environment that can best be anticipated, recognized, and treated when systems that often operate in "silos" come together to engage in student-centered problem-solving. Families, school personnel, and healthcare providers must be willing to partner on all steps of a problem-solving process—from initially sharing information about a student's chronic illness to implementing and monitoring a treatment plan that is sufficiently broad to address any academic, social-emotional, and behavioral needs that may arise in the school setting. Collaboration and flexibility are critical for this process to be successful, and, above all, schools should work to ensure that the individual needs of the child—rather than any particular diagnosis or prognosis—are foremost in determining the services and supports that are put into place for the student.

REFERENCES

American Cancer Society. (2016). *Children diagnosed with cancer: Late effects of cancer treatment.* Retrieved from https://www.cancer.org

Babikian, T., & Asarnow, R. (2009). Neurocognitive outcomes and recovery after pediatric TBI: Meta-analytic review of the literature. *Neuropsychology, 23,* 283–296. doi:10.1037/a0015268

Brown, E. S., & Chandler, P. A. (2001). Mood and cognitive changes during systemic corticosteroid therapy. *Primary Care Companion Journal of Clinical Psychiatry, 3*(1), 17–21.

Campbell, L. K., Scaduto, M., Sharp, W., Dufton, L., Van Slyke, D., Whitlock, J. A., & Compas, B. (2007). A meta-analysis of the neurocognitive sequelae of treatment for childhood acute lymphocytic leukemia. *Pediatric Blood & Cancer, 49,* 65–73. doi:10.1002/pbc.20860

Castellino, S. M., Ullrich, N. J., Whelen, M. J., & Lange, B. J. (2014). Developing interventions for cancer-related cognitive dysfunction in childhood cancer survivors. *Journal of the National Cancer Institute, 106*(8), 1–16. doi:10.1093/jnci/dju186

Compas, B. E., Jaser, S. S., Reeslund, K., Patel, N., & Yarboi, J. (2017). Neurocognitive deficits in children with chronic health conditions. *American Psychologist, 72*(4), 326–338. doi:10.1037/amp0000042.

Crump, C., Rivera, D., London, R., Landau, M., Erlendson, B., & Rodriguez, E. (2013). Chronic health conditions and school performance among children and youth. *Annals of Epidemiology, 23*, 179–184. doi:10.1016/j.annepidem.2013.01.001

Dowling, M. M., Quinn, C. T., Rogers, Z. R., & Buchanan, G. R. (2010). Acute silent cerebral infarction in children with sickle cell anemia. *Pediatric Blood & Cancer, 54*(3), 461–464. doi:10.1002/pbc.22242

Emerson, N. D., Distelberg, B., Morrell, H. E. R., Williams-Reade, J., Tapanes, D., & Montgomery, S. (2016). Quality of life and school absenteeism in children with chronic illness. *The Journal of School Nursing, 32*(4), 258–266. doi:10.1177/1059840515615401

Gipson, D. S., Hooper, S. R., Duquette, P. J., Wetherington, C. E., Stellwagen, K. K., Jenkins, T. L., & Ferris, M. E. (2006). Memory and executive functions in pediatric chronic kidney disease. *Child Neuropsychology, 12*, 391–405. doi:10.1080/09297040600876311

Gottfried, M. A. (2014). Chronic absenteeism and its effects on students' academic and socioemotional outcomes. *Journal of Education for Students Placed at Risk* (JESPAR), *19*, 53–75. doi:10.1080/10824669.2014.962696

Halfon, N., & Newacheck, P. W. (2010). Evolving notions of childhood chronic illness. *JAMA, 303*(7), 665–666. doi:10.1001/jama.2010.130

Houtrow, A. J., Larson, K., Olson, L. M., Newacheck, P. W., & Halfon, N. (2014). Changing trends of childhood disability, 2001–2011. *Pediatrics, 134*(3), 530–538. doi:10.1542/peds.2014-0594

Karsdorp, P. A., Everaerd, W., Kindt, M., & Mulder, B. J. (2007). Psychological and cognitive functioning in children and adolescents with congenital heart disease: A meta-analysis. *Journal of Pediatric Psychology, 32*, 527–541. doi.10.1093/jpepsy/jsl047

Krull, K. R., Okcu, M. F., Potter, B., Jain, N., Dreyer, Z., Kamdar, K., & Brouwers, P. (2008). Screening for neurocognitive impairment in pediatric cancer long-term survivors. *Journal of Clinical Oncology, 26*, 4138–4143. doi:10.1200/JCO.2008.16.8864

Lum, A., Wakefield, C. E., Donnan, B., Burns, M. A., Fardell, J. E., & Marshall, G. M. (2017). Understanding the school experiences of children and adolescents with serious chronic illness: A systematic meta-review. *Child: Care, Health and Development, 43*, 645–662. doi:10.1111/cch.12475

Madan- Swain, A., Katz, E. R., & LaGory, J. (2004). School and social reintegration after a serious illness or injury. In R. T. Brown (Ed.), *Handbook of pediatric psychology in school settings* (pp. 637–655). Mahwah, NJ: Lawrence Erlbaum Associates.

Martinez, Y. J., & Ercikan, K. (2009). Chronic illnesses in Canadian children: What is the effect of illness on academic achievement, and anxiety and emotional disorders? *Child: Care, Health and Development, 35*, 391–401. doi:10.1111/j.1365-2214.2008.00916.x

McNally, K., Rohan, J., Pendley, J. S., Delamater, A., & Drotar, D. (2010). Executive functioning, treatment adherence, and glycemic control in children with type 1 diabetes. *Diabetes Care, 33*, 1159–1162. doi:10.2337/dc09-2116

Merrell, K. W., & Gimpel, G. (1998). *Social skills of children and adolescents: Conceptualization, assessment, treatment.* Mahwah, NJ: Lawrence Erlbaum Associates.

Mitby, P. A., Robison, L. L., Whitton, J. A., Zevon, M. A., Gibbs, I. C., Tersak, J. M., . . . Mertens, A. C. (2003). Utilization of special education services and educational attainment among long-term survivors of childhood cancer: A report from the Childhood Cancer Survivor Study. *Cancer, 97,* 1115–1126. doi:10.1002/cncr.11117

Moleski, M. (2000). Neuropsychological, neuroanatomical, and neurophysiological consequences of CNS chemotherapy for acute lymphoblastic leukemia. *Archives of Clinical Neuropsychology, 15,* 603–630. doi:10.1016/S0887-6177(99)00050-5

Naguib, J. M., Kulinskaya, E., Lomax, C. L., & Garralda, M. E. (2009). Neuro-cognitive performance in children with type 1 diabetes—A meta-analysis. *Journal of Pediatric Psychology, 34,* 271–282. doi:10.1093/jpepsy/jsn074.

Nagy, Z., Westerberg, H., & Klingberg, T. (2004). Maturation of white matter is associated with the development of cognitive functions during childhood. *Journal of Cognitive Neuroscience, 16,* 1227–1233. doi:10.1162/0898929041920441

National Association of School Nurses. (2013). *Position statement: Individualized healthcare plans, the role of the school nurse.* Retrieved from https://schoolnursenet.nasn.org/nasn/advocacy/professional-practice-documents/position-statements

Newacheck, P. W., & Halfon, N. (1998). Prevalence and impact of disabling chronic conditions in childhood. *American Journal of Public Health, 88,* 610–617.

Parrish, J., Geary, E., Jones, J., Seth, R., Hermann, B., & Seidenberg, M. (2007). Executive functioning in childhood epilepsy: Parent-report and cognitive assessment. *Developmental Medicine & Child Neurology, 49,* 412–416. doi:10.1111/j.1469-8749.2007.00412.x

Pinquart, M., & Shen, Y. (2011). Behavior problems in children and adolescents with chronic physical illness: A meta-analysis. *Journal of Pediatric Psychology, 36,* 1003–1016. doi:10.1093/jpepsy/jsr042

Pinquart, M., & Teubert, D. (2012). Academic, physical, and social functioning of children and adolescents with chronic physical illness: A meta-analysis. *Journal of Pediatric Psychology, 37*(4), 376–389. doi:10.1093/jpepsy/jsr106.

Power, T. J., & Bradley-Klug, K. L. (2012). *Pediatric school psychology: Conceptualizations, applications, and strategies for leadership development.* New York, NY: Routledge.

Prevatt, F. F., Heffer, R. W., & Lowe, P. A. (2000). A review of school reintegration programs for children with cancer. *Journal of School Psychology, 38,* 447–467. doi:10.1016/S0022-4405(00)00046-7

Räty, L. K. A., Söderfeldt, B. A., Larsson, G., & Larsson, B. M. W. (2004). The relationship between illness severity, sociodemographic factors, general self-concept, and illness-specific attitude in Swedish adolescents with epilepsy. *Seizure, 13,* 375–382. doi:10.1016/j.seizure.2003.09.011

Robinson, K. E., Kuttesch, J. F., Champion, J. E., Andreotti, C. F., Hipp, D. W., Bettis, A., . . . Compas, B. E. (2010). A quantitative metaanalysis of neurocognitive sequelae in survivors of pediatric brain tumors. *Pediatric Blood & Cancer, 55,* 525–531. doi:10.1017/S1355617712000987

Schatz, J., Finke, R. L., Kellett, J. M., & Kramer, J. H. (2002). Cognitive functioning in children with sickle cell disease: A meta-analysis. *Journal of Pediatric Psychology, 27,* 739–748. doi:10.1093/jpepsy/27.8.739

Schatz, J., & Roberts, C. W. (2007). Neurobehavioral impact of sickle cell disease in early childhood. *Journal of the International Neuropsychological Society: JINS, 13*, 933–943. doi:10.1017/S1355617707071196

Sentenac, M., Gavin, A., Gabhainn, S. N., Molcho, M., Due, P., Ravens-Sieberer, U., . . . Godeau, E. (2013). Peer victimization and subjective health among students reporting disability or chronic illness in 11 Western countries. *European Journal of Public Health, 23*(3), 421–426. doi:10.1093/eurpub/cks073

Shaw, S. R., & McCabe, P. (2008). Hospital-to-school transition for children with chronic illness: Meeting the new challenges of an evolving health care system. *Psychology in the Schools, 45*, 74–87. doi:10.1002/pits.20280

Taras, H., & Potts-Datema, W. (2005). Chronic health conditions and student performance at school. *Journal of School Health, 75*, 255–266. doi:10.1111/j.1746-1561.2005.00034.x

Thies, K. M. (1999). Identifying the educational implications of chronic illness in school children. *Journal of School Health, 69*, 392–397.

U.S. Department of Education. (2015). *Protecting students with disabilities.* Retrieved from https://www2.ed.gov/about/offices/list/ocr/504faq.html

U.S. Department of Health and Human Services, Health Resources and Services Administration, Maternal and Child Health Bureau. (2014). *The health and well-being of children: A portrait of states and the nation, 2011–2012.* Rockville, MD: U.S. Department of Health and Human Services.

Van Cleave, J., Gortmaker, S. L., & Perrin, J. M. (2010). Dynamics of obesity and chronic health conditions among children and youth. *JAMA, 303*, 623–630. doi:10.1001/jama.2010.104

Wilkie, K. J. (2012). Absence makes the heart grow fonder: Students with chronic illness seeking academic continuity through interaction with teachers at school. *Australasian Journal of Special Education, 36*, 1–20.

Witmer, L. (1907). A case of chronic bad spelling—Amnesia visualis verbalis, due to arrest of post-natal development. *The Psychological Clinic, 1*(2), 53.

Zenderland, L. (2001). *Measuring minds: Henry Herbert Goddard and the origins of American intelligence testing.* Cambridge, UK: Cambridge University Press.

4

Role of the School-Based Professional in Linking Systems of Care

MILENA A. KELLER-MARGULIS, SARAH OCHS, KERRI P. NOWELL, AND SARAH S. MIRE ■

School-based professionals, including school psychologists and other educational specialists, have an important role in connecting the systems that serve children and families (Power, DuPaul, Shapiro, & Kazak, 2003; Power, Shapiro, & DuPaul, 2003). Children exist in, and interact with, numerous settings, including the home, school, and community. When significant health concerns are present, children bring their needs with them to all settings. To provide adequate support to children in schools, school-based professionals must recognize the various systems in which children exist, understand the effect that a pediatric health condition (PHC) may have across systems, and take an active role in connecting the systems.

The numerous systems with which children with PHCs interact include the school, family, community, and the medical system (e.g., institutions employing pediatricians, family doctors, psychologists, psychiatrists, and various other medical specialists for children with PHCs). Models of service delivery in which interdisciplinary teams work to provide services to children in a single setting, such as integrated care clinics or integrated school-based health centers exist, but they are less common than the scenario where care is obtained from several disconnected systems. In addition, as Power, DuPaul, et al. (2003) pointed out, individual symptoms and systems of the body may be addressed by specialists in a focused way because of how the medical system is structured. The emotional and behavioral issues that a child or family may experience as a result of a PHC, in contrast, are more pervasive and general in their effect. Given that children spend a substantial amount of time in school, school-based professionals are in an ideal position to facilitate communication among the school and outside settings and to serve as coordinators, ensuring necessary information is shared among stakeholders (Canto, Chesire, Buckley, Andrews, & Roehrig, 2014; Nastasi, 2004; Power, Shapiro, et al., 2003). The school psychologist may serve in a leadership role, coordinating services and communication, but the leader could also be the school nurse, counselor, or other designated case manager. This chapter provides a rationale for school-based professionals to work across systems to serve children with PHCs and the chapter outlines practical considerations involved. Engaging stakeholders across systems allows for improved service delivery and ultimately improved outcomes for children.

THEORETICAL FRAMEWORK

The need for school-based professionals to work across the various systems that may affect children is grounded in theory. Ecological systems theory (Bronfenbrenner, 1979; Bronfenbrenner & Morris, 2006) posits that children exist within many systems simultaneously and that children are affected by the various systems or contexts with which they interact. The model is often visually depicted by a series of concentric circles, with the child at the center and the various levels of influence or systems in which the child exists as the outer rings. This perspective has been suggested to be an important framework for understanding children with PHCs (Kazak, Alderfer, & Reader, 2017). The systems closest to the child are those that the child engages with most often and most directly, and they are referred to as microsystems in Bronfenbrenner's theory. These systems include the family, school, and, for children with PHCs, medical settings and service providers. The influence and interaction of these systems are most critical to understand when working to provide services to children with PHCs (Kazak et al., 2017). Ecological systems theory is the primary lens through which we understand the role of the school-based professional as central to connecting and collaborating with the systems that affect the child with a PHC.

DEVELOPING PARTNERSHIPS ACROSS SYSTEMS

Models for System Collaboration

Given the complexity of interprofessional collaboration, the use of a structured process in collaboration is a valuable way to ensure that outcomes are effective (Grier & Bradley-Klug, 2011; Ritzema, Sladeczek, Manay-Quian, Ghosh, & Karagiannakis, 2014). Various approaches to interprofessional collaboration exist, and conjoint behavioral consultation (CBC; Sheridan et al., 2009) is the model that is widely applicable and well aligned with ecological systems theory. Evidence supports the use of CBC, a model for solving problems collaboratively, as one approach to effectively working with outside professionals (Sheridan et al., 2009). Typically, the CBC process involves collaboration among teachers, parents, and a consultant, who work together on a common goal of behavior change for a student (Sheridan, Ryoo, Garbacz, Kunz, & Chumney, 2013). There is great value in this framework for children with PHC, either with or without behavioral needs. The CBC approach recognizes the cooperative, bidirectional process of planning and service provision. We present the CBC model as an ideal framework to structure the collaborative process and to highlight that, in order to achieve the best outcomes for students, school-based professionals should actively engage all parties involved with the child to facilitate a team approach to planning and service provision.

Legal Considerations When Working Across Systems

Before delving into important issues related to communication across systems, it is necessary to mention that legal parameters exist that protect students' privacy. Specifically, two federal laws pertain to cross-systems communication regarding students with PHCs: the Family Educational Rights and Privacy Act (FERPA) and the Health Insurance Portability and Accountability Act of 1996 (HIPAA). These laws are covered in greater detail in Chapter 5 of this volume ("Legal and Policy Issues Relevant to Working with Students with Pediatric Health Conditions"). Generally speaking, schools are required to adhere to FERPA, whereas healthcare providers (including institutions) operate under HIPAA. Both laws regulate disclosure of a child's information, although the privacy considerations are central to FERPA and only a component of HIPAA (i.e., HIPAA Privacy Rule). For this reason, school-based professionals and their non-school-based collaborators must be aware of legal regulations applicable to their communications.

FERPA (34 CFR Part 99) applies to schools or other educational agencies and institutions that receive any money from the U.S. Department of Education. Under FERPA, student "education records"—which include health records maintained by a school or school employee—may not be shared without parental (or legal guardian's) consent (the few exceptions to this are beyond the scope of this chapter). The HIPAA Privacy Rule requires that "covered entities" (i.e., healthcare providers, including healthcare institutions) have safeguards in place to protect patient health information, as well as to set limits and conditions on how the information can be used and disclosed without the patient's (or caregiver's) authorization. The intersection of these laws can create considerable confusion about which is applicable and under what circumstances. School-based personnel should be aware of the legal parameters in place to protect student information and how different laws are applicable to different systems of care. Having at least a basic working knowledge of similarities in FERPA and HIPAA can allow for knowledgeable discussions with families.

Additionally, school-based professionals must be aware of the policies and procedures of their district and school for implementing privacy laws. Specifically, issues pertaining to obtaining the written consent of parents to communicate about student health information could include knowing which forms to use (which should include language and details consistent with the applicable law), how to complete the forms, when to obtain parent signatures, and which school-based team members are designated to do so. Beyond these legal and procedural considerations, however, are pertinent practical issues that contribute to successfully linking systems of care. For example, while obtaining signatures is a legal requirement and using district-approved forms is a procedural responsibility, carefully explaining the reason for the release of information (i.e., to be able to talk directly with the hospital-based specialist who oversees their child's care so that school-based professionals can ask questions and for help implementing care procedures) and the purpose of the release (i.e., protecting the child's and family's privacy) is critical communication that can both facilitate rapport-building with families and engender parents' trust of the school. Strong relationships with families, along with knowledge of the relevant legal parameters, provide the foundation for effectively working across systems of care. This is facilitated by fostering strong communication across systems, a necessary but often challenging task.

Potential Barriers to Communication

Effective collaboration across settings requires effective communication. Although caregivers, providers, and trainers of providers agree about the importance of communication across settings, evidence suggests that such communication does not occur regularly (Canto et al., 2014; Greene, Ward-Zimmerman, & Foster, 2015). Potential barriers to effective communication among multiple stakeholders include relying on parents to communicate needs to relevant providers, the need to include multiple outside professionals, collaboration with health providers who have been educated to frame their clients' difficulties from the perspective of their specific discipline (D'Amour, Ferrada-Videla, Roriguez, & Beualiey, 2005), and other organizational constraints. School-based professionals and outside providers are constrained by time factors; allocating sufficient time to address multiple needs is challenging, particularly when ongoing collaboration is required to meet a student's needs. Furthermore, medical needs may be underidentified in the school setting as a result of a lack of disclosure by parents, failure to acknowledge implications of medical or mental health needs in the educational setting, and limited training of educational staff (Canto et al., 2014). Professionals across settings may use different terminology, have varying definitions of criteria for service eligibilities, and may lack knowledge about service availability in other settings or about the roles of the various providers. For example, a medical provider might give parents a written prescription for the child to receive special education services. The parent may then erroneously believe that this is sufficient for their child to qualify for services in the school setting. Although a prescription is often the pathway to services in the medical setting, eligibility for special education is determined very differently. These significant differences across systems may result in unproductive relationships (Shaw & Paez, 2002). The subsequent sections of this chapter detail key considerations for the school-based professional in collaborating with families, outside service providers, and other educators, in order to work across system differences and meet the needs of children with PHC.

COMMUNICATING AND COLLABORATING WITH FAMILIES

Communication between school-based professionals and parents is critical to facilitating students' success. There are many reasons that school-based professionals should collaborate with parents, particularly those whose children have PHCs, and two topics are essential points of collaboration: (1) the influence of the medical condition and related symptoms on the child's functioning in school and (2) the coordination of support and implementation of interventions to meet the academic, behavioral, and medical needs of students.

Effect of the Health Condition on School Functioning

One of the first steps a school-based professional can and should take when working with a child with a PHC and his or her family is to understand the child's condition and its potential adverse effects on school functioning. School-based professionals are not expected to have knowledge about all PHCs that may affect children; rather, they should be prepared with general knowledge about how health concerns may affect school-based functioning, as well as how and where to find information specific to various health concerns. It is the responsibility of the school-based professional to investigate, as needed, the potential effects of health conditions experienced by the children they serve.

Depending on the health condition, the child may experience any number of symptoms, sometimes intermittent, that may affect readiness to learn in the school setting. A PHC can affect academics, behavior, and interpersonal or social functioning (for an overview, see DuPaul, Power, & Shapiro, 2017). In addition to the direct effects that symptoms have on functioning, missed instructional time due to medical appointments, sick days, or time spent engaged in medical care/ management may further adversely affect school functioning. One notable issue to discuss with families is the potential for changes in cognitive functioning that may affect learning. For example, children who undergo cancer treatment may experience cognitive functioning changes that affect their learning and behavior (Gurney et al., 2009). It is important to note that even children with the same PHC may have very different needs in the school setting. When professionals communicate with parents about the potential effect of a PHC on school functioning, parents should be made aware of the options they have for formalizing supports that their child may require. A child with a PHC may be eligible for special education in the school setting as a child with a disability under the federal legislations known as the Individuals with Disabilities Education Improvement Act (IDEIA), which would offer an individualized education plan to support their medical and educational needs. Extensive discussion of this topic is beyond the scope of this chapter, but Chapter 5 of this volume covers additional details.

Coordinating and Supporting Intervention

In addition to ensuring that parents understand the potential effect of their child's PHC on school functioning, another critical role for school-based professionals working with parents is in the coordination and support of intervention implementation. This can take many different forms, including supporting medication management or treatment adherence, as well as addressing mental health or behavioral needs related to the primary condition (DuPaul et al., 2017). For example, school-based professionals may work with a psychiatrist treating a child for attention deficit hyperactivity disorder (ADHD) to collect data regarding time on task or other attention-related variables before and after the start of a new medication regimen to determine whether the treatment is having the desired effect on behavior. As another example, a child with diabetes may be taught decreased reliance on prompts from school personnel to check blood glucose levels as she learns to self-monitor levels at school. In either of the examples, school-based professionals may also coordinate data collection and sharing of information with stakeholders.

Supporting interventions may also include providing support to the parents and siblings of the child experiencing the health condition. Caring for a child with a PHC may be a source of stress for the family system, including siblings, who often are affected by having a sibling with a PHC (Sharpe & Rossiter, 2002). The school-based professional may need to serve as a resource for families, connecting them with outside therapeutic services for the family system. For example, consider a case in which a child is being treated for cancer. It is common for the family system to be disrupted by this type of diagnosis and the subsequent treatment (Alderfer et al., 2010). As a result, the ill child's sibling(s) may experience emotional or behavioral concerns, which also are likely to emerge in the school setting. It is the responsibility of the school-based professional to recognize that it is possible for the sibling(s) to be affected by the disruption to the family system and to communicate with the family should this occur. School-based services, such as counseling or mentoring to support the sibling, can be provided, particularly if acute issues emerge.

Although not discussed in detail here, communication with families may also include coordination of services to support reintegration of the child to school after an absence due to illness or hospitalization. In such circumstances, it is critical to develop a transition plan with the child and those involved with the child's care, to communicate with parents and across other relevant systems, and to coordinate implementation of necessary interventions or supports for the student.

COMMUNICATING AND COLLABORATING WITH OUTSIDE PROVIDERS

To effectively provide services to children with mental or physical health conditions, school-based professionals must coordinate with any professionals serving the child and family outside of the school setting. Ecological systems theory emphasizes the reciprocal relationship between children and the various systems in which they exist and highlights the need to understand how that relationship affects both the child and the system (Grier & Bradley-Klug, 2011; Kubiszyn, 1999; Nabors & Lehmkul, 2004; Nastasi, 2004; Power, Shapiro, et al., 2003). Consistent with this, medical providers are also encouraged to collaborate with school-based professionals to ensure that the patient's needs are met effectively (Council on Children with Disabilities and Medical Home Implementation Project Advisory Committee, 2014). In addition, parents place a high value on interdisciplinary communication (Greene et al., 2015). Children with PHCs often present with highly complex needs and receive services through multiple systems of care. Many times, those services are not organized in a way that facilitates transfer of information, often resulting in fragmented services. Importantly, school-based professionals can play a key role in communicating with outside providers to facilitate the identification and acquisition of necessary information, to assess and prioritize a student's needs, and to develop and monitor interventions.

As noted previously, communication across providers is an essential component of interdisciplinary collaboration and has the potential to improve outcomes of students with medical and mental health difficulties. For example, school-based professionals need to communicate with outside mental health providers to avoid replication of services (e.g., counseling, behavior plans), to ensure that school interventions are not counterproductive to outside therapies, to provide opportunities for generalization of strategies and skills, and to facilitate the provision of intensive therapies that may not be feasible to implement in school or clinical settings alone (Villarreal & Castro-Villarreal, 2016). There is also evidence that collaboration across providers results in improved outcomes and is potentially a cost-effective method of providing effective care for students with PHCs (Villarreal & Castro-Villarreal, 2016; Yu, Kolko, & Torres, 2017). However, while there is widespread consensus that communication across settings is important (Greene et al., 2015; Kubszyn, 1999; Nabors & Lehmkuhl, 2004; Nastasi, 2004; Power, Shapiro, et al., 2003), there is also recognition that the process is complex (Shaw & McGabe, 2008; Villarreal & Castro-Villarreal, 2016). In many instances, the school-based professional will need to establish strong working relationships to ensure that effective, ongoing collaboration can occur. For example, meeting the needs of students with diabetes is multifaceted, and requires an ongoing, collaborative, multidisciplinary approach (Wyckoff, Hanchon, & Gregg, 2015). For students transitioning from hospital to school, school-based professionals are key at each stage. Establishing and maintaining effective relationships to achieve common goals requires planning and, potentially, skill development.

General Processes

Effective collaboration requires that school-based professionals recognize and be prepared to navigate the potential barriers that exist. Beyond the general theoretical approaches to collaboration, there has been a call for a standardized, efficient method of collaborative communication (Greene et al., 2015). Prior to communicating with outside professionals, it is important for school-based professionals to invest time identifying points of contact and collaboration goals. The school-based professional should ensure that a full team of professionals is included in the collaborative process so that no essential data are overlooked. Initially, the family may be able to identify key professionals with whom they are in contact and who provide ongoing care for their child. However, depending on a families' situation, it may be necessary to develop and review an exhaustive checklist of possible types of providers to ensure that specific providers who may have the potential to provide essential information are not inadvertently forgotten. Depending on the complexity of the health issues, the student may visit several different outpatient providers across various clinics. In some instances, outside providers may rely on parents to communicate health related needs to the school (Canto et al., 2014) and the school-based professional may need to form a team to facilitate sharing information among relevant stakeholders. Identifying potential collaborators will involve working closely with caregivers to identify outside care providers, acquiring necessary releases, and identifying points of contact.

Developing structured agendas, specific goals, and measures toward collaborative objectives can ensure face-to-face communication is focused on client goals (Sulkowski, Jordan, & Nguyen, 2009; Villarreal & Castro-Villarreal, 2016). It is highly likely that time constraints will interfere with opportunities to engage in face-to-face communication, so the school-based professional should be prepared to offer a variety of communication methods. For example, videoconferencing avoids the need for finding physical meeting space, and using secure, online file-storage programs can protect confidentiality while also facilitating communication. Depending on the unique needs of the child, points of contact may occur at various times and at varying rates. At a minimum, however, communication should occur during the initial information-gathering phase, as well as prior to, or during, key decision-making meetings (such as Section 504 or IEP planning meetings).

Like school-based professionals, providers outside of the school system are constrained by time factors; thus, clearly identifying the type of information needed to develop an appropriate plan for the child with a PHC is important. In addition, recognizing system-specific differences and working collaboratively to minimize misunderstandings surrounding the differences (e.g., medical vs. school-based terminology, educational classification vs. medical/clinical diagnoses) may facilitate interprofessional collaboration. When school-based professionals review literature regarding an unfamiliar medical condition, they may be able to maximize consultation time without relying solely on the outside provider for education about a particular condition (Shaw & McGabe, 2008). Depending on the child's needs, various types of information may need to be collected. For example, information about any medical conditions, comorbid complications, potential for future procedures, medical orders, side effects of medications, and potential for pain-related complications might be important data to collect. When consulting with outside providers, it is appropriate to discuss information about the goals of treatment, the theoretical orientation of the treatment approach, progress, and unmet needs. Communication across providers is bidirectional. In addition to acquiring specific information about the child and condition, the school professional will need to communicate essential information about the child and his or her functioning within the school environment to the provider. Information regarding the school's lay-out, school scheduling, and methods of progress monitoring (e.g., behavior charts, medication adherence, etc.) may be important for planning across settings.

COMMUNICATING AND COLLABORATING WITH EDUCATORS AND SCHOOL PERSONNEL

Many school-based professionals can both design and provide direct services to support the emotional, behavioral, and physical health needs of students, as well as communicate health information to others and collaborate to promote school success. Although families or health providers may be hesitant to disclose student health information, studies demonstrate that teachers and students benefit from sharing information about a diagnosed health condition (Cunningham & Wodrich, 2006, 2012; Wodrich, 2005). For example, one study showed that when a teacher received diagnosis-specific health information in a child's cumulative folder, the teachers more accurately attributed student problems (e.g., poor handwriting) to the child's health condition and implemented classroom-level accommodations to promote individual student learning (Wodrich, 2005). Sharing relevant health information among key staff can assist school personnel in providing an optimal educational experience for all students. Communication should first focus on maximizing access to the curriculum and identifying the student's strengths. This can help educator feel empowered to serve students with diverse health conditions by identifying available resources and maximizing their own capacity.

Managing Dissemination of Information

Though some families may be reluctant to share information with the school, other families may share a great deal of information with school-based professionals, beyond what is vital to educational programming. School-based professionals are then faced with the often-difficult task of sharing only relevant and necessary information with other school personnel. Although schools are only one part of a child's network of care, school-based providers have the unique challenge of communicating relevant health information across multiple subsystems (e.g., classroom teachers, administrators, bus drivers, nurses, or food-service workers). Throughout any given school day, students interface with a vastly different array of individuals across unique settings. School-based professionals may be charged with communicating different information to different stakeholders while determining what information is essential.

When deciding what information to share in schools, professionals should ask themselves three main questions. First: Is this information directly germane to student functioning at school? Information about a student's health condition may be important to share if it affects academic functioning or is essential to implement or support school-based services necessary for success. Many of the children who attend school every day may be living with a diagnosed health condition that is well managed and fails to affect school functioning, making it unnecessary to disseminate health-related information. Second: Does the individual to whom I am considering disclosing the information provide direct services to the student? In most cases, only members of the school community who directly interface with the student will need to be made aware of any health-related information. Third: Why am I sharing this information—what are my motivations? It can be helpful to pause and critically analyze the reasons for sharing student health information. General guidelines for sharing health-related information are listed in Table 4.1. Often, individuals working in schools care deeply about students and are highly invested in their lives and success. However, care should be taken to manage personal feelings or reactions regarding a student to avoid unnecessary sharing of private health information.

For students with existing health conditions, level of impairment may range significantly, and along with that, so may the needed frequency of communication with relevant school personnel. Some students may have minimal functional impairment throughout the school day but will require frequent visits with specialists, increasing their number of absences. In this case, qualified school-based providers may need to communicate with teachers to inform them of the

Table 4.1. Guidelines for Sharing Health-Related Information in the Schools

DO	DO NOT
• Inform guardian(s) about what information has been communicated and to whom • Document what information was shared, who received the information, when, and any follow-up required • Follow all relevant ethical and legal guidelines for maintenance of privacy and confidentiality • Communicate accurate, factual information in a compassionate way	• Share information that is not pertinent to the individual or setting • Gossip • Add your own interpretation of information or recommendations • Share information by insecure means (e.g., texting, email, social media) • Talk about student health information in public spaces (e.g., hallways, offices with open doors)

reason for absences and support any modifications to instructional delivery. In contrast, a student with a severe food allergy may require formal written plans outlining care and emergency procedures, as well as communication with food-service staff, teachers, bus drivers, field trip chaperones, or other students. Schools must have procedural safeguards, and frequent checks, in place to ensure that all parties, even substitute staff, are aware of, and closely adhere to, these plans.

School-based professionals should use their expertise to assist in the development, implementation, and evaluation of school-based interventions and accommodations. This may include disseminating information and providing support to school staff directly involved with implementation (e.g., 504 or special education coordinator). It may be necessary for staff to receive additional training or to complete documentation, such as an emergency medication provision record or a disease-specific emergency plan (e.g., how to handle a seizure). Trained staff may support student health needs by communicating the importance of evaluating and modifying interventions, and by recommending evidence-based assessment and intervention options.

Many teachers may feel overwhelmed or anxious when learning that a member of their class or school community has a chronic health condition, but with clear and consistent communication, reliance on available resources, and a detailed, documented plan, school staff can successfully provide an optimal and inclusive educational experience for all students, including those with PHCs. When sharing information, trained school-based professionals can support other school staff by providing education, helping to alleviate any fears, correcting any erroneous preconceived ideas, and accurately communicating expectations for functioning and achievement. School staff may subscribe to negative stereotypes about conditions (e.g., human immunodeficiency virus infection) or be unaware of the school-based manifestations of a health condition.

Other Types of Communication in Schools

Communication within schools may also reach beyond school staff to include talking to students. When appropriate, general information about a PHC may be used to educate students and to make them aware of any necessary precautions. For instance, teachers as well as classmates may benefit from learning how to respond if a peer with epilepsy experiences a seizure in school. School staff members need to decide, in collaboration with parents/guardians, the appropriate level of peer disclosure. Separately, but importantly, school-based professionals can also advocate for comprehensive health services and policies at their school. This type of communication may focus on health-inclusive policy at the district level (e.g., obtaining health history information for all new or entering students) or at the local, state, or national level. While being mindful about adhering to employer policies regarding political activities in the workplace, school-based staff can educate other personnel about relevant legislation affecting education or, more specifically, services to support student health needs in schools.

SCHOOL-BASED INTEGRATED CARE CLINICS

Integrated care clinics housed in school settings are the gold standard approach for service provision and offer great promise for facilitating the connection of the various systems that simultaneously serve students. School-based health centers (SBHCs) have many different names (e.g., teen or mobile clinic, integrated care clinic) but share the same approach to the delivery of health services in schools. Commonly a partnership among schools and community agencies or providers, SBHCs employ an integrated team of health providers to address the myriad health needs of children, including medical, dental, behavioral, and vision, in a safe, convenient location. Although not all SBHCs follow the integrated approach, over half do employ an extended services team with specialists across areas of health (School-Based Health Alliance [SBHA], 2016).

SBHCs may extend the system of care for youth or provide a medical home when care is not accessed elsewhere, which is particularly true for children of low socioeconomic status or without health insurance. Projections indicate that the percentage of white students enrolled in public school will continue to decline through 2025, and enrollment of Hispanic students will increase (Kena et al., 2016), indicating the rapidly changing demographics of schoolchildren. The growing percentage of ethnic minorities makes directly addressing health equity a priority. Youth with a racial or ethnic minority status or who come from a low-income home are more likely to experience chronic health conditions but are less likely to receive care (Bloom & Simpson, 2015).

SBHCs are a mechanism for addressing disproportionality in health care by placing critical health services in the place where all school-aged youth have access. Therefore, the Community Preventive Services Task Force (2016), established by the U.S. Department of Health and Human Services, recommended "the implementation and maintenance of SBHCs in low-income communities to improve educational outcomes." Additionally, there is a clear relationship between health and educational performance and attainment. Health problems like poor vision, obesity, ADHD, and asthma, as well as risk-taking behaviors, such as unhealthy eating or substance use, continue to be associated with poor academic performance (Bradley & Greene, 2013; Ickovics et al., 2014; McCord, Klein, Foy, & Fothergill, 1993). School-based clinics emphasize early intervention and detection of health risk for all students, including those of traditionally underserved populations. For example, over three quarters (76.5%) of SBHCs were located in schools in which the majority of the students were eligible for free or reduced lunch, and the SBHCs often served the larger community (SBHA, 2016). In addition, 83.4% of SBHCs reported providing individual chronic disease management. Families with a child with a chronic health condition living outside of a major metropolitan area can face challenges in accessing care. SBHCs are an ideal model for addressing barriers to quality care in rural areas. In fact, rural SBHCs are increasing more rapidly than those in other areas and accounted for approximately 60% of newly established SBHCs since 2011 (SBHA, 2016).

Services Available

SBHCs can provide a range of services. Most SBHCs employ a staffing model, which includes a primary care provider and behavioral health specialist. Over 70% of SBHCs screen for depression and anxiety, and more than 67% screen for ADHD and other social-emotional-behavioral concerns (SBHA, 2016) that can affect a child's functioning in school and beyond. This service is critical, given the estimates that one of every five youth has a diagnosable behavioral, emotional, or mental health disorder (Kessler et al., 2005). SBHCs also provide preventative services, including immunizations. Many facilities carry vaccines against influenza, diphtheria/tetanus/acellular pertussis, hepatitis B, varicella, and polio (SBHA, 2016). Students with access to a SBHC were more likely to attend more than three primary care visits (52% vs. 34%) and to have received an influenza or hepatitis B vaccine (Allison et al., 2007).

Much of the research on SBHCs focuses on reproductive health, mental health, access, or academic outcomes. Although some findings were mixed, a review of the literature suggests that SBHCs with four or more services or that are accessible beyond school hours were associated with the greatest reduction in visits to the emergency department (Knopf et al., 2016). When students have access to a range of healthcare services in schools, they may miss less instructional time for appointments, and guardians do not need time off from work to take their child to a separate facility (SBHA, 2016). Despite the potential benefit and positive effect of SBHCs, particularly for students with a PHC, less than 2% of schools have a SBHC (SBHA, 2016; U.S. Department of Education, National Center for Education Statistics, 2016).

School-based integrated care clinics permit more frequent and more convenient communication among school-based and healthcare providers than may achievable otherwise. When providers from different domains (e.g., physical health, mental health, education) work in the same building, there are fewer barriers to communication. It is important to note that, in most cases, health records maintained by a SBHC are considered educational records and are therefore subject to FERPA and are generally exempt from the HIPAA Privacy Rule (45 CFR 160.103). Although FERPA prohibits school personnel from sharing student educational records (including health information) without written parental consent, exceptions allow information disclosure to other school employees without written consent, if there is a "legitimate educational interest" (34 CFR 99.31). Providing services under one legal umbrella allows more efficient transfer of information among all the relevant parties providing an array of services to a student within one system: the school.

CONCLUSION

For children with a PHC, their health needs have the potential to affect them across all the systems in which they exist, including the family, school, and community.

Outside of the family system, children spend most of their time in schools. For this reason, it is critical that school-based professionals not only are informed of the child's needs, but also are prepared to serve as leaders in linking the systems that provide services to the child. Although SBHCs may offer the most efficient and effective way to provide services to children and families, they are not a very prevalent means of service delivery at this time. However, school personnel working in traditional school settings can use best practices in providing services to children by initiating and maintaining purposeful communication across systems and by adopting collaborative monitoring and intervention approaches.

REFERENCES

Alderfer, M. A., Long, K. A., Lown, E. A., Marsland, A. L., Ostrowski, N. L., Hock, J. M., & Ewing, L. J. (2010). Psychosocial adjustment of siblings of children with cancer: A systematic review. *Psycho-Oncology, 19*(8), 789–805.

Allison, M. A., Crane, L. A., Beaty, B. L., Davidson, A. J., Melinkovich, P., & Kempe, A. (2007). School-based health centers: Improving access and quality for low-income adolescents. *Pediatrics, 120*(4), 887–894. doi:10.1542/peds.2006-2314

Bloom, B., & Simpson, J. L. (2016). *Tables of summary health statistics for U.S. children: 2015 National Health Interview Survey.* Atlanta, GA: National Health Center Statistics. Retrieved from http://www.cdc.gov/nchs/nhis/SHS/tables.htm

Bradley, B. J., & Greene, A. C. (2013). Do health and education agencies in the United States share responsibility for academic achievement and health? A review of 25 years of evidence about the relationship of adolescents' academic achievement and health behavior. *Journal of Adolescent Health, 52*(5), 523–532. doi:10.1016/j.jadohealth.2013.01.008

Bronfenbrenner, U. (1979). *The ecology of human development.* Cambridge, MA: Harvard University Press.

Bronfenbrenner, U., & Morris, P. A. (2006). The biological model of human development. In R. M. Lerner & W. Damon (Eds.), *Handbook of child psychology: Theoretical models of human development, Volume 1* (6th ed., pp. 793–828). Hoboken, NJ: John Wiley & Sons.

Canto, A. I., Chesire, D. J., Buckley, V. A., Andrews, T. W., & Roehrig, A. D. (2014). Barriers to meeting the needs of students with traumatic brain injury. *Educational Psychology in Practice, 30*(1), 88–103.

Community Preventive Services Task Force. (2016). *Promoting health equity through education programs and policies: School-based health centers.* Retrieved from https://www.thecommunityguide.org/sites/default/files/assets/Health-Equity-School-Based-Health-Centers_1.pdf

Council on Children with Disabilities and Medical Home Implementation Project Advisory Committee. (2014). Patient- and family-centered care coordination: A framework for integrating care for children and youth across multiple systems. *Pediatrics, 133*, e1451–e1460. http://dx.doi.org/10.1542/peds.2014-0318

Cunningham, M. M., & Wodrich, D. L. (2006). The effect of sharing health information on teachers' production of classroom accommodations. *Psychology in the Schools, 43*(5), 553–564. doi:10.1002/pits.20166

Cunningham, M. M., & Wodrich, D. L. (2012). Teachers' academic appraisals and referral decisions: The effect of sharing health information when diabetes is presented. *Psychology in the Schools, 49*(9), 852–863.

D'Amour, D., Ferrada-Videla, M., San Martin Rodriguez, L., & Beaulieu, M. (2005). The conceptual basis for interprofessional collaboration: Core concepts and theoretical frameworks. *Journal of Interprofessional Care, 19,* 116–131. doi:10.1080/13561820500082529

DuPaul, G. J., Power, T. J., & Shapiro, E. S. (2017). Schools and reintegration into schools. In M. C. Roberts & R. G. Steele (Eds.), *The handbook of pediatric psychology* (5th ed., pp. 580–593). New York, NY: Guilford Press.

Greene, C. A., Ward-Zimmerman, B., & Foster, D. (2015). Please break the silence: Parents' views on communication between pediatric primary care and mental health providers. *Families, Systems, & Health, 2,* 155. doi:10.1037/fsh0000117

Grier, B. C., & Bradley-Klug, K. L. (2011). Collaborative consultation to support children with pediatric health issues: A review of the biopsychoeducational model. *Journal of Educational & Psychological Consultation, 21*(2), 88–105.

Gurney, J. G., Krull, K. R., Kadan-Lottick, N., Nicholson, H. S., Nathan, P. C., Zebrack, B., . . . Ness, K. K. (2009). Social outcomes in the childhood cancer survivor study cohort. *Journal of Clinical Oncology, 27*(14), 2390–2395.

Ickovics, J. R., Carroll-Scott, A., Peters, S. M., Schwartz, M., Gilstad-Hayden, K., & McCaslin, C. (2014). Health and academic achievement: Cumulative effects of health assets on standardized test scores among urban youth in the United States. *Journal of School Health, 84*(1), 40–48.

Kazak, A. E., Alderfer, M. A., & Reader, S. K. (2017). Families and other systems in pediatric psychology. In M. C. Roberts & R. G. Steele (Eds.), *The handbook of pediatric psychology* (5th ed., pp. 566–579). New York, NY: Guilford Press.

Kena, G., Hussar W., McFarland J., de Brey C., Musu-Gillette, L., Wang, X., . . . Dunlop Velez, E. (2016). *The condition of education 2016* (NCES 2016-144). Washington, DC: U.S. Department of Education, National Center for Education Statistics. Retrieved from https://nces.ed.gov/pubs2016/2016144.pdf

Kessler, R. C., Berglund, P., Demler, O., Jin, R., Merikangas, K. R., & Walters, E. E. (2005). Lifetime prevalence and age-of-onset distributions of DSM-IV disorders in the National Comorbidity Survey replication. *Archives of General Psychiatry, 62*(7), 593–602. doi:10.1001/archpsych.62.6.593

Knopf, J. A., Finnie, R. K. C., Peng, Y., Hahn, R. A., Truman, B. I., Vernon-Smiley, M., . . . Fullilove, M. T. (2016). School-based health centers to advance health equity: A community guide systematic review. *American Journal of Preventive Medicine, 51*(1), 114–126.

Kubiszyn, T. (1999). Integrating health and mental health services in schools: Psychologists collaborating with primary care providers. *Clinical Psychology Review, 19*(2), 179–198.

McCord, M. T., Klein, J. D., Foy, J. M., & Fothergill, K. (1993). School-based clinic use and school performance. *Journal of Adolescent Health, 14,* 91–98.

Nabors, L., & Lehmkuhl, H. (2004). Children with chronic medical conditions: Recommendations for school mental health clinicians. *Journal of Developmental and Physical Disabilities, 16*(1), 1–15.

Nastasi, B. (2004). Meeting the challenges of the future: Integrating public health and public education for mental health promotion. *Journal of Educational and Psychological Consultation, 15*(3–4), 295–312.

Power, T., Shapiro, E., & DuPaul, G. (2003). Preparing psychologists to link systems of care in managing and preventing children's health problems. *Journal of Pediatric Psychology, 28*(2), 147–155. doi:10.1093/jpepsy/28.2.147

Power, T. J., DuPaul, G. J., Shapiro, E. S., & Kazak, A. E. (2003). *Promoting children's health: Integrating school, family, and community.* New York, NY: Guilford Press.

Ritzema, A., Sladeczek, I., Manay-Quian, N., Ghosh, S., & Karagiannakis, A. (2014). Improving outcomes for children with developmental disabilities through enhanced communication and collaboration between school psychologists and physicians. *Canadian Journal of School Psychology, 29*(4), 317–337. doi:10.1177/0829573514536529

School-Based Health Alliance (SBHA). (2016). *2013–2014 digital census report.* Washington, DC: Author. Retrieved from http://censusreport.sbh4all.org

Sharpe, D., & Rossiter, L. (2002). Siblings of children with a chronic illness: A meta-analysis. *Journal of Pediatric Psychology, 27*(8), 699–710.

Shaw, S. R., & McCabe, P. C. (2008). Hospital-to-school transition for children with chronic illness: Meeting the new challenges of an evolving health care system. *Psychology in the Schools, 45*(1), 74–87.

Shaw, S. R., & Páez, D. (2002). Best practices in interdisciplinary service delivery to children with chronic medical issues. In A. Thomas & J. Grimes (Eds.), *Best practices in school psychology IV* (pp. 1473–1483). Washington, DC: National Association of School Psychologists.

Sheridan, S. M., Ryoo, J. H., Garbacz, S. A., Kunz, G. M., & Chumney, F. L. (2013). The efficacy of conjoint behavioral consultation on parents and children in the home setting: Results of a randomized controlled trial. *Journal of School Psychology, 51*(6), 717–733.

Sheridan, S. M., Warnes, E. D., Woods, K. E., Blevins, C. A., Magee, K. L., & Ellis, C. (2009). An exploratory evaluation of conjoint behavioral consultation to promote collaboration among family, school, and pediatric systems: A role for pediatric school psychologists. *Journal of Educational and Psychological Consultation, 19*, 106–129.

Sulkowski, M., Jordan, C., & Nguyen, M. (2009). Current practices and future directions in psychopharmacological training and collaboration in school psychology. *Canadian Journal of School Psychology, 24*(3), 237–244. doi:10.1177/0829573509338616

U.S. Department of Education, National Center for Education Statistics. (2016). *Digest of education statistics, 2015.* Retrieved from https://nces.ed.gov/fastfacts/display.asp?id=84

Villarreal, V., & Castro-Villarreal, F. (2016). Collaboration with community mental health service providers: A necessity in contemporary schools. *Intervention in School and Clinic, 52*(2), 108–114.

Wodrich, D. L. (2005). Disclosing information about epilepsy and type 1 diabetes mellitus: The effect on teachers' understanding of classroom behavior. *School Psychology Quarterly, 20*(3), 288–303. doi:10.1521/scpq.2005.20.3.288

Wyckoff, L., Hanchon, T., & Gregg, S. R. (2015). Psychological, behavioral, and educational considerations for children with classified disabilities and diabetes within the school setting. *Psychology in the Schools*, *52*(7), 672–682.

Yu, H., Kolko, D. J., & Torres, E. (2017). Collaborative mental health care for pediatric behavior disorders in primary care: Does it reduce mental health care costs? *Families, Systems, & Health*, *35*(1), 46–57. doi:10.1037/fsh0000251

5

Legal and Policy Issues Relevant to Working with Students with Pediatric Health Conditions

SARAH S. MIRE, KIMBERLY D. SCHOGER,
AND ASHLEY N. RAMCLAM ■

Jonnie is a 10-year-old boy in fourth grade who has asthma, a pediatric health condition (PHC). To manage his asthma, Jonnie requires frequent doctor's appointments, preventative and acute medication access, and alterations to some of his school-based activities (i.e., PE) and environments (e.g., construction/dusty areas, science labs). Jonnie has more absences from school than do his peers without a PHC. He makes several emergency department visits every year, and he even requires occasional hospitalizations.

In many ways, the special considerations necessary for successful management of Jonnie's asthma are similar to those relevant to other PHCs. School personnel involvement with Jonnie's care during the school day is critical, and this involvement has many legal and policy-related considerations. Throughout this chapter, we return to Jonnie's case as we consider various laws and policies that are relevant to working with students with PHCs in schools. Readers are urged to view the case example of Jonnie only as a starting point for consideration of working with their own students, in that state-to-state laws and regulations and district-to-district policies and procedures vary widely, and laws and policies intersect with the individuality of students served.

Knowledge of laws and policies affecting school-based services for students with PHCs is critical for school-based providers, including school psychologists, counselors, social workers, and nurses, as well as other school professionals with whom they work. Because school-based programming and service provision are designed by teams—which include both parents and the multiple professionals outside of schools who also serve students with PHCs—it is necessary that all concerned parties have awareness of the legal parameters under which schools are required to operate.

Laws relevant to the focus of this chapter, first and foremost, are designed for the protection of students with PHCs and their families. Because there are several professionals within multiple systems who are likely to be involved in the care of students with PHCs, knowledge of the school-based legal parameters applicable to this special population has several purposes and benefits. First, legal provisions are helpful because they increase the accountability of the school-based providers who serve these students by ensuring that all involved are adhering to the required legal safeguards. Second, school-based providers' familiarity with legal issues decreases the likelihood of their inadvertently doing something unlawful or not doing something lawfully required, which mitigates legal risk for the school and district. Finally, following relevant legal and policy requirements ultimately and ideally enhances service provision to students with PHCs because students' unique health-related circumstances are considered in terms of both the impact of the PHCs on school-based performance and the needs of individual students in their school based endeavors. The goal of this chapter is to provide a brief overview of current (at time of publication) laws and policies that are most relevant to working with students with PHCs.

Some laws, such as the Individuals with Disabilities Education Improvement Act (IDEIA; 2004) or the Americans with Disabilities Act (ADA; 1990), are applicable throughout the United States because they are federal laws and therefore require adherence regardless of the state or district in which a student resides. However, legal standards vary from state to state due to different state and local laws. More specifically, although each state is required to adhere to the federal law in order to receive federal funding, states are able to make their own laws about how to apply federal laws in their state. Importantly, however, state laws and state regulations must not contradict federal legislation and must provide at least what is required under the federal law. School-based personnel must understand—and be able to communicate to families—that state laws and state implementation of federal laws can differ if families move to a different state. Although it is certainly beyond the scope of this chapter to overview every state's laws guiding school-based services for students with PHCs, the chapter provides links that may help school-based providers access their states' laws and implementation regulations (see Table 5.3).

Federal, state, and local laws may be updated or changed in response to court proceedings. With case law, for example, legal precedents and authority emanate from the outcomes of court rulings, judicial decisions, and administrative findings or rulings. Although legal precedents set by case law typically are jurisdiction specific (i.e., limited to a specific state or specific district), they may influence interpretations of issues in other jurisdictions. For cases decided at the federal level, however, the outcomes affect all states. A striking example of this is that in March 2017, the U.S. Supreme Court unanimously expanded the rights of students with disabilities, including many students with PHCs, when they revisited the "free and appropriate public education" (FAPE) provision of the IDEIA (*Endrew F. v. Douglas County School District RE-1*, 2017). Importantly, this Supreme Court decision eschewed the standard that minimal educational benefit from an IEP is sufficient under IDEIA. Instead, the court held that students with disabilities should be provided the chance to make "appropriately ambitious" progress. This new standard sets the stage for districts' taking responsibility for designing more ambitious IEPs, implementing corresponding services, and providing clear and measurable evidence of progress. The effects of this case on school-based service implementation for students with PHCs may take several years to be fully manifest, but one implication of this case outcome is that district personnel will be held accountable for striving to meet the unique needs of students with PHCs. Certainly, the effects of the Endrew case ruling may differ from state to state and even from district to district, but the case represents a prime example of why school-based professionals must remain current in their knowledge of educational legislation and court decisions.

In addition to legal variations from state to state, policies and procedures can vary among school districts in the same state. For example, districts may adopt policies and procedures for convening student problem-solving teams that may lead to decisions regarding implementation of multitiered systems of support (MTSS) for struggling students and assessing students' progress in interventions implemented to address academic or behavioral difficulties (i.e., response to intervention [RtI]). Considering such differences, it is important that school-based providers commit to learning and staying up to date with school- and district-level policies, state laws and regulations, and federal laws and regulations. Several websites are included at the end of this chapter to assist school-based providers in identifying Internet-based resources for staying up to date with federal and state laws and policies. To maintain current knowledge about campus- and district-level policies and procedures, school-based providers are urged to utilize their campus and district administrators and their district legal advisors as resources. In addition, state and national organizations relevant to various school-based providers are often excellent resources for legal and policy updates regarding service provision for students with PHCs. Clearly, the current chapter is not (and cannot be) an exhaustive stand-alone resource. Rather, the chapter aims both to help school-based providers increase their awareness of legal parameters that affect various aspects of their jobs and to prompt them to seek out additional information on their own.

FEDERAL LEGISLATION

Students with PHCs often need, and are eligible for, school-based supports and services, and a number of federal laws provide parameters for these. There are also laws that apply to the sharing of information about the students among providers. Although families may not consider their child's PHC to be a "disability," this term is used in the laws to describe a condition that may require school-based assistance. Three federal laws discussed in this chapter are the laws most relevant to students with PHCs: the ADA, Section 504 of the Rehabilitation Act of 1973 (Section 504), and IDEIA. Also described are two federal laws regulating the disclosure of information about students with PHCs: the Family Educational Rights and Privacy Act of 1974 (FERPA) and the Privacy Rule of the Health Insurance Portability and Accountability Act of 1996 (HIPAA), which is part of the HIPAA Administrative Simplification Rules (45 CFR Parts 160, 162, and 164). Tables 5.1 and 5.2 summarize similarities and differences among the laws governing service provision and disclosure, respectively.

ADA

Jonnie, the fourth grader with asthma who was introduced in the case example at the beginning of this chapter, has legal protections under the ADA, which, for example, prevent him from being "benched" from the Friday afternoon kickball game to avoid the risk of his having an asthma attack on school property. The ADA is a civil rights law, and it guarantees equal opportunities for all students attending schools that receive federal or private funding (i.e., public and private schools). The law also prohibits discrimination against students with disabilities. Under the ADA, a person is considered to have a disability if one of three conditions is met: "the individual must have (A) a physical or mental impairment that substantially limits one or more of the major life activities of such individual, (B) a record of such an impairment, or (C) being regarded as having such an impairment" (42 U.S. Code § 12102; 28 CFR 35.108). The Americans with Disabilities Amendments Act (ADA AA) of 2008 further noted that "extensive analysis" is not necessary to determine an individual's disability status [42 U.S.C. § 12102(4)(A)], so that parent report of a PHC would be sufficient under ADA.

The U.S. Department of Education's Office of Civil Rights assists the Department of Justice in regulating school-based implementation of the ADA. Importantly, the legal obligations of the ADA apply to all schools, regardless of funding. This means that, as already stated, schools that receive federal funding and schools that receive funding from private sources all must abide by ADA regulations. Therefore, students with disabilities in both public and private schools are guaranteed equal opportunity to receive educational services, to access school buildings, and to participate in school-related activities.

Section 504

Like the ADA, Section 504 prevents discrimination against students, including those with PHCs. Unlike the ADA, however, Section 504 is applicable only to entities receiving federal funds (i.e., public schools). The implementation of Section 504 in K-12 and postsecondary schools is regulated by the Department of Education's Office of Civil Rights. Section 504 legally ensures that schools

Table 5.1. IDEIA[a] COMPARED TO SECTION 504[b]

	IDEIA	Section 504
Overseen by:	Department of Education's Office of Special Education and Rehabilitative Services, Office of Special Education Programs	Department of Education's Office of Civil Rights and the Department of Justice
Applicability:	Part B covers ages 3 to 21, for students attending public schools (although Child Find applies to students living within a school's jurisdiction even if they attend private school or home school)	Public preschool, elementary, secondary, and postsecondary schools.
To qualify for services/protections:	Student must have a disability according to the IDEIA definition and need specialized instruction as a result of the disability	Student must have a physical or mental impairment that substantially limits one or more of the child's major life activities
Disability defined by:	Thirteen disability categories are outlined in IDEIA and most students with PHCs are likely to qualify under the Other Health Impairment (OHI) category, if they are found to be eligible under IDEIA	One of three conditions is met: 1. A physical or mental impairment 2. A history of disability 3. Is regarded as having a disability Intended to provide broad coverage and protections for individuals with disabilities.
Timeline for an evaluation:	Sixty (60) calendar days (unless state law says differently)	No legal timeline provided. Best practice is to remain consistent with IDEIA timeline.
Evaluation components:	Multiple sources of data. Data must be gathered in all areas of suspected disability to determine presence of disabling condition and related educational need. A medical provider's evaluation may be included (and in some states may be required for designation under OHI).	Multiple sources of data. A team decides on the data needed to determine presence of a disability. A medical provider's evaluation may be included (and in some states may be required).

[a] Individuals with Disabilities Education Improvement Act, 20 U.S.C. § 1400 (2004).

[b] Rehabilitation Act of 1973, Pub. L. No. 93-112, § 504, 87 Stat. 355 (1973).

Table 5.2. FERPA[a] Compared to HIPAA Privacy Rule[b]

	FERPA	HIPAA Privacy Rule
BOTH	• **Apply to confidentiality of records**	
	• **Jurisdiction: federal**	
Overseen by:	U.S. Department of Education (US DOE)	U.S. Department of Health & Human Services
Record covered:	Educational	Medical
Who is subject:	Schools that receive any money from a program administered by the US DOE (i.e., public schools)	Covered entities (i.e., healthcare industry; providers who collect and store patient information electronically or otherwise)
What is protected:	The personally identifiable information (PII) contained in students' education records (academic report cards, transcripts, class schedules, disciplinary records, contact information, family information) and school health records maintained by school employees (considered part of the education record).	The protected health information (PHI) contained in a record created or received by a healthcare provider that relates to past, present, or future physical or mental health of any individual that identifies an individual; note that PHI explicitly excludes education records covered by FERPA.
Required for disclosures:	Written authorization from parent (or student age 18+). Exceptions when elementary and secondary schools are permitted but not required to disclose without consent: to school officials (including teachers) who have a "legitimate educational interest"; to new school for enrollment purposes; for directory information (e.g., name, address, DOB, etc.). Note that only "pertinent and necessary" information should be disclosed.	Written authorization from parent (or patient age 18+). Exceptions when covered entities are permitted but not required to disclose without consent: to the individual patient; for treatment payment/reimbursement purposes; public health (i.e., communicable diseases). Note that only the "minimum necessary" information should be disclosed.

[a] Family Educational Rights and Privacy Act of 1974, 20 U.S.C. § 1232 (1974).

[b] Health Insurance Portability and Accountability Act of 1996 Administrative Simplification Rules, 45 C.F.R. pts. 160, 162, and 164 (1996).

provide access to FAPE and also requires schools to provide certain protections for students with disabilities. Specifically, students with disabilities are granted equal access to educational programs and activities (i.e., they cannot be denied or excluded) and they are entitled to a school environment free of disability-based discrimination and harassment. Additionally, Section 504 mandates equal opportunity to access and engage in sports and extracurricular activities. The impact a disability has on a major life activity or bodily function is determined on a case-by-case basis; no educational need or adverse effect on educational progress caused by the disability is required.

Additionally, Section 504 legislation requires schools that receive federal funding to extend procedural safeguards to students with disabilities and their families. This means educational agencies must inform parents of evaluations and placement decisions, must allow parents to review school-based records, and must provide the opportunity for an impartial hearing. It is the expectation under Section 504 that schools will inform parents of these rights and will abide by the requirements accordingly. A clear understanding of Section 504 ensures that public elementary and secondary schools will provide students with PHCs a schooling experience free from discrimination or exclusion.

Initiating the process of determining eligibility for, and accessing, services under Section 504 may vary depending on a student's district, but the law requires both an evaluation and service availability. Each campus must have a 504 coordinator, and school-based providers should know who to seek out for district-specific information about Section 504 processes. In general, the process for a student like Jonnie could be somewhat like the following:

> Jonnie's mother, concerned about Jonnie's asthma-related needs, learned about Section 504 from Jonnie's pediatrician when he was diagnosed with asthma. She contacted his elementary school and learned that the role of Section 504 Coordinator on that campus was fulfilled by the school counselor. The counselor convened a meeting with Jonnie's mother, his teacher, and the school nurse to discuss Jonnie's needs. Thus, the team was comprised of people who knew Jonnie well, and, after obtaining Jonnie's mother's consent, the team worked together to decide how much information would be required to determine that Jonnie's needs constituted a "disability" and to complete a Section 504 evaluation. For Jonnie, the team used the pediatrician's note documenting the asthma diagnosis, the school nurse's documentation of Jonnie's clinic visits during the time he had been a student, Jonnie's attendance record (which indicated multiple asthma-related absences), and a brief interview from his parent and his teacher that provided information about their observations of asthma-related impacts and needs in Jonnie's life. The team noted that, taken together, the information they reviewed demonstrated that the asthma created a "substantial limitation on [Jonnie's] ability to learn", as well as to interact socially with his peers, another "major life activity."

Though Section 504 does not legally require a written plan, districts typically have policies and procedures for creating and implementing a 504 plan, as was the case with Jonnie's district. A Section 504 student accommodation plan might include information about the nature of the concern, the basis for determining the disabling condition and how it affects a major life activity, and the accommodations needed. In Jonnie's case, accommodations the team determined were necessary included that the nurse would work with the physical education (PE) teacher to develop an adaptive but inclusive class experience, that the school nurse would help with inhaler administration, that the teacher would develop a "missed class work plan" for absences, and that the school nurse would work with teachers to identify signs of an asthma crisis and with Jonnie to review his crisis plan.

IDEIA

Like Section 504, IDEIA provides guidelines for access to FAPE for students with disabilities, but IDEIA provides more procedural safeguards to students and families than does Section 504. IDEIA, a federal law, outlines services that fall under the Office of Special Education Program in the U.S. Department of Education. Importantly, many (though not all) students with PHCs may be eligible for special education (i.e., IDEIA) services in public schools. Under IDEIA, special education services must be delivered in the least restrictive environment needed to serve a child. To be eligible for services under IDEIA, a child must have a disability and as a result of that disability must need special education services in order to benefit from educational programming and to make more than minimal progress in school.

The most salient part of IDEIA for children with PHCs is Part B, which explains the requirements for public schoolchildren ages 3 to 21. Part B explains that all public schools receiving IDEIA funding must provide a FAPE to students with disabilities in the following categories: autism, orthopedic impairment, emotional disturbance, visual impairment, hearing impairment, specific learning disability, intellectual disability, multiple disabilities, deaf-blindness, traumatic brain injury, speech and language impairment, and other health impairment. Notably, specific disability categories may vary from state to state. Regardless of the category of disability under which a child is served, every child who qualifies for special education services under IDEIA must have a written individualized education plan (IEP) that outlines the student's current levels of performance, appropriate goals and objectives, methods to track progress, and individualized accommodations and modifications that will aid in the student's success. It is helpful to think of IEPs as legal contracts of service, and they must be updated annually to review progress, to make changes to ensure continued progress, and to create goals for the upcoming year that are appropriately challenging. Under IDEIA, the IEP must be thoughtfully and carefully implemented, and any member of the team (including parents) may request that the team meet and consider revisions at any time.

Many children with PHCs are served under an other health impairment (OHI) eligibility. The criteria for an OHI eligibility are threefold (IDEA, 2004). The first criterion is that the student exhibits limited strength, vitality, or alertness, including a heightened alertness to environmental stimuli that results in compromised attention. The second criterion is that the limitations are due to chronic or acute health problems, and examples may include (but are not limited to) asthma, attention deficit hyperactivity disorder (ADHD), epilepsy, cardiac conditions, hemophilia, lead poisoning, fetal alcohol syndrome (FAS), leukemia, nephritis, rheumatic fever, and sickle cell anemia. Importantly, this is a not an exhaustive list of OHI-qualifying conditions, and the list is often updated (Grice, 2002) and may vary from state to state or district to district; therefore, close attention to changing IDEIA court rulings is certainly warranted. The third criterion that must be met is that the child's condition adversely affects educational performance—and this is a key difference between eligibility under IDEIA vs. Section 504 (Table 5.1).

It is important to remember that a child who meets the above criteria may qualify under the OHI category with any acute or chronic health condition. Determination of OHI eligibility must be made on a case-by-case basis. Each student meeting eligibility for an OHI under IDEIA must have a completed eligibility report that documents that the child meets the three criteria. The form must be completed by a licensed healthcare provider. Perhaps most salient to this discussion, schools are required to provide school-based health services as a related special education service to students with chronic health conditions who are served under IDEIA. School-based health services may involve nursing services, social work services in schools, and parent counseling and training.

As described in the previous section, Section 504 may be applicable to Jonnie due to his disabling condition of asthma. It is also possible that Jonnie may need services under IDEIA. This is a decision that requires careful consideration. However, the key distinction is whether Jonnie's asthma "adversely affects educational performance." An example of a flow chart used to guide this process was created by personnel from Cincinnati Children's Hospital Medical Center (n.d.). In Jonnie's case, school personnel considered Jonnie's excellent academic performance, his positive peer relationships, and the lack of concerns about emotional or behavioral impact as indicators that his educational performance was not adversely affected by his asthma. Therefore, they determined accommodations through Section 504 would meet his needs at that time.

FERPA

Due to the myriad of possible medical conditions and the variability of school-based services students with PHCs may need, informed and thoughtful input from people who know the student well is crucial to positive outcomes. This requires communication among members of the decision-making team, which for students with PHCs is likely to include professionals inside and outside the schools. For Jonnie, the input may include communication by his pediatrician, pulmonologist, parents, and school-based providers. FERPA is the federal law that provides guidance for the protection of school-based information belonging to students with PHCs.

School-based providers typically must comply with FERPA, which applies to schools receiving any funds from the U.S. Department of Education (34 CFR Part 99). FERPA regulates disclosure of a student's educational records. The law mandates that the information contained in the records be released only with written parent (or legal guardian) consent or in an emergency situation. After the student is 18 years old, the records may only be released with the written permission of the student (or assigned custodian). Moreover, the law allows parents to inspect and to review educational records, including the health and medical information maintained by the school. Within the school and district, teachers and other school personnel may access the records without need for parental consent when they have "legitimate educational interests."

HIPAA's Privacy Rule

Whereas FERPA applies to educational records, HIPAA applies to medical records. HIPAA's Privacy Rule requires that covered entities (i.e., healthcare providers who maintain healthcare records) develop and maintain safeguards to protect patient health information (Table 5.2). Similar to FERPA, HIPAA provides guidelines for disclosure of an individual's information. Unlike FERPA, HIPAA's Privacy Rule does not typically apply to schools because schools are not generally considered HIPAA-covered entities, although there are exceptions (e.g., when primary care clinics are offered in conjunction with the school). In these unique situations, the clinics must adhere to HIPAA Transactions and Code Sets and Identifier Rules and HIPAA's Privacy Rule if medical records are kept separate from the educational records. However, the majority of school-based providers who deliver some form of healthcare (e.g., school psychologists, counselors, audiologists, nurses) do not undertake covered transactions (i.e., billing a health plan electronically for services rendered) and so their documentation is stored in the student's educational record and is thereby protected under FERPA.

It is important for school-based providers to be aware that HIPAA's Privacy Rule does apply to many of those with whom they may wish (and need) to collaborate on behalf of students with PHCs. Under the Privacy Rule of HIPAA, professionals working in "covered entities" (i.e., hospitals, clinics, physician's offices) may not share medical information with school-based providers without the written authorization of the patient (or, for minor students, their parent/guardian). Parental authorization is not required for those working in HIPAA-covered entities to share information about a student's health condition, medication regimen, and other aspects of the treatment plan with school-based providers attending to students' healthcare needs (i.e., the school nurse). Nevertheless, many providers will seek patient/parent consent before such communications. In Jonnie's case, this would mean that providers outside of the school would request that his parents sign a HIPAA-compliant consent for communication with his school-based team.

THE RELATIONSHIP BETWEEN LAW AND CODES OF ETHICS

Laws affect aspects of school-based personnel's interactions with children in terms of what they must (legally) do, or what they cannot (legally) do. However, the law does not cover all aspects of service provision; both discipline-specific codes of ethics and individual students' needs must be considered as well. Codes of ethics provide guidance for professional conduct, and school-based providers working with students with PHCs have codes of ethics to which they must adhere. It is acknowledged that codes of ethics vary somewhat depending on a providers' specific discipline (e.g., school psychology, school counseling, school social work, school nursing, school-based speech-language pathologists) and each should be thoroughly familiar with the code of ethics for their respective field. Though differences do exist, there are overarching domains of similarity. Websites that include codes of ethics for various school-based providers are included in Table 5.3.

For example, ethical standards on confidentiality and disclosure overlap across fields. The collaborative nature of the school setting and the need for cooperative networks of care for students with PHCs both contribute to the need for sharing information across disciplines and settings, as this increases the quality of services provided for a student. The act of disclosing, or sharing a student's personal information, must be done in a way that adheres to both legal and ethical guidelines. Regardless of discipline-specific codes of ethics, legal limits to confidentiality exist when issues of immediate safety arise, in which case providers are legally mandated or legally permitted to disclose information—although nuances of such disclosure vary among states. Outside of immediate safety issues outlined by federal and state laws, providers must obtain appropriate consent to release confidential information necessary for service provision that is in accordance with federal and state laws, and they must ensure that authorization adheres to privacy laws (e.g., FERPA, HIPAA). Further, when student-specific information is disclosed, ethics codes guide school-based providers to share only information pertinent and necessary for the particular situation. Information that is considered pertinent is likely to vary depending on the provider's role and student's needs at the time, and therefore it will change on an individual basis. In Jonnie's case, the nurse's code of ethics may be particularly important since the accommodations provided under Section 504 would rely heavily upon the nurse's role as the primary liaison among parents, teachers (e.g., PE teacher, classroom teacher), and private providers (e.g., pulmonologist).

Ethical decision-making can be complicated, and providers may find that models that provide a framework for approaching challenging situations in conscientious

Table 5.3. ONLINE RESOURCES FOR ADDITIONAL INFORMATION

Special Education Information by State	• The National Children's Cancer Society, special education information by state: http://www.thenccs.org/special-education-list?gclid=CjwKEAjwl9DIBRCG_e3DwsKsizsSJADMmJ11jsM_IByQGKxcx_8wfaCy9lh9H83eZA6dMxkJsC-SthoCfuzw_wcB) • Wrightslaw Directory of State Departments of Education: http://www.yellowpagesforkids.com/help/seas.htm) • National Association of State Boards of Education's State School Health Policy Database: http://www.nasbe.org/healthy_schools/hs/bytopics.php?topicid=4100
Education Law	• http://www.wrightslaw.com/
Discipline-Specific Ethics Codes	• School counselors: https://www.schoolcounselor.org/asca/media/asca/Ethics/EthicalStandards2016.pdf • School nurses: https://www.nasn.org/nasn-resources/professional-topics/codeofethics • School psychologists: https://www.nasponline.org/standards-and-certification/professional-ethics; http://www.apa.org/ethics/code/ • School social workers: https://www.socialworkers.org/LinkClick.aspx?fileticket=ms_ArtLqzeI%3d&portalid=0 • School speech-language pathologists: http://asha.org/Code-of-Ethics/
ADA	• https://www.ada.gov/ada_intro.htm • https://www.ada.gov/pubs/adastatute08.htm#12101b
Section 504	• https://www2.ed.gov/about/offices/list/ocr/504faq.html • https://www2.ed.gov/about/offices/list/ocr/docs/edlite-FAPE504.html • https://www2.ed.gov/about/offices/list/ocr/docs/504-resource-guide-201612.pdf
IDEIA	• https://sites.ed.gov/idea/?src=feature • http://www.wrightslaw.com/idea/law.htm
FERPA	• https://ed.gov/policy/gen/guid/fpco/ferpa/index.html
FERPA and HIPAA	• The overlap between FERPA and HIPAA: https://www2.ed.gov/policy/gen/guid/fpco/doc/ferpa-hipaa-guidance.pdf • Joint Guidance on the Application of the Family Educational Rights and Privacy Act (FERPA) and the Health Insurance Portability and Accountability Act of 1996 (HIPAA) to Student Health Records: https://www2.ed.gov/policy/gen/guid/fpco/doc/ferpa-hipaa-guidance.pdf

ways are helpful in these situations (Knapp, VandeCreek, & Fingerhut, Pope & Vasquez, 2016). While a comprehensive review of ethical decision-making models is beyond the scope of the current chapter, references both of the afore-mentioned books are included at the end of the chapter. In brief, however, core tenets present across many ethical decision-making models include: (1) determining the problem, (2) identifying all possible solutions, (3) evaluating the alternative outcomes with consideration for those involved, sociocultural factors, and the need for consultation, (4) taking action, and (5) assessing the results. It is also recognized that there are instances where laws or policies may contradict codes of ethics. In such cases, most disciplines provide guidelines for situations in which an ethical dictum directly conflicts with the law. Typically, codes of ethics hold professionals to higher standards than the law does, in which case providers should adhere to the higher standard.

Beyond discipline-specific codes of ethics, each student's individual needs must also be considered in conjunction with the legal parameters guiding school-based providers' work with students with PHCs. Other chapters in this volume include information about specific chronic health conditions, and we encourage readers to familiarize themselves thoroughly with diagnoses impacting students with whom they work. For example, Jonnie's school-based team should gain a working knowledge about the symptoms and effects of asthma, signals of an asthmatic crisis, and a plan for addressing a crisis. For the purposes of the current chapter, we raise the consideration of individual needs simply to remind readers that although legal, ethical, and policy parameters are critical, each student's situation is unique. Simply put, the intersection of all of these issues is complex, and even when students have the "same" PHC, each student's' strengths and needs with regard to school-based progress and service provision will vary. The way that Jonnie's asthma affects him at school may be different from symptom manifestation in another child with asthma, and the plan to address Jonnie's needs is unique to him (i.e., one cannot assume that all students with asthma will follow the same plans). School-based providers must concurrently strive to serve students' individual needs while operating within the parameters of federal and state law, their discipline-specific ethics codes, and local policies and procedures. Additionally, it is important to recognize that, as students matriculate from preschool through high school, the implications or applications of some aspects of the law may vary. Rather than providing an exhaustive discussion of these implications/applications, this chapter is a starting point for school-based providers in further investigation of the nuances of the law for students of different ages (e.g., legal guidelines for transition into public schools as a young child and out of public schools as an adult).

APPLICATION OF LAW TO SPECIFIC CONCERNS

This section addresses concerns that may arise about the application of laws and policies from school-based providers who serve students with PHCs. Although the list of questions is not exhaustive, it highlights examples of common questions asked by school-based professionals about the laws and policies governing education of children with PHCs. Within the response to each question, Jonnie's case is briefly considered as an example.

Does a Child with a PHC Automatically Qualify for Special Services in the School Setting?

The federal legislation of the ADA protects anyone with a disability in both public and private schools, as well as almost everywhere else. Although the ADA requires "reasonable accommodations" and prohibits discrimination against anyone who has a disability (or even anyone who is regarded as having a disability, such as by a teacher), the ADA does not specify what is needed. For many students with PHCs, public schools often do have a legal obligation to provide supports and/or services, though it does not happen automatically. That is, there must be a formalized pro-cedure for documenting the need and specific accommodations/interventions the child will receive. In Jonnie's case, although the ADA protects him from discrim-ination, processes and procedures must be initiated so that his unique needs can be met in the school setting. Specifically, there are two ways students with PHCs may qualify for special services from their school: IDEIA or Section 504. (Students served under IDEIA are automatically covered by Section 504—i.e., discrimina-tion on basis of disability is prohibited—but those with plans under Section 504 do not necessarily qualify for IDEIA services.) The decision tree in Figure 5.1 is one example of guidance that may be useful to the reader who is considering whether a student will be better served under Section 504 or through IDEIA. As noted al-ready, when the school-based team considered all the information gathered about Jonnie's asthma-related needs and the effect that they had on his schooling, they determined that Section 504 was the best framework for meeting his current needs.

Does a Child's Actual Diagnosis Matter in Terms of Directing School-Based Service?

Students with PHCs often have a medical diagnosis from outside providers, and the diagnosis should certainly be considered when the school is conducting an evalu-ation. However, in many cases, medical diagnoses are neither necessary nor suffi-cient for a student to become IDEIA eligible. This is because it is incumbent upon the school-based evaluation team to determine whether a student has a disabling condition according to IDEIA, and whether that condition necessitates specially designed instruction for accessing FAPE. Although Jonnie's school-based team did not identify an educational need related to his asthma, other children with the same diagnosis may indeed require IDEIA services if there is an educational need. Determination of "educational need" is sometimes vague, but schools' considera-tion of such need should extend beyond academics only. For example, if a student has excessive anxiety related to the possibility of an asthma attack that prevents him from work completion or results in self-isolation from peers or others, such circumstances could cause school-based providers and parents to identify an ed-ucational related to the PHC. Consultation with providers in the medical setting can assist in understanding a student's particular PHC and the unique needs and symptoms associated with it that may prevent a child from accessing instruction and participating in the school day. While a student's diagnosis can be important, the specifics of the individual child's needs are paramount in determining needed school-based services and accommodations, if any. Students with PHCs who are determined by the school-based evaluation team not to have an educational need (i.e., not to require special education and related services) can still access protections under Section 504, as in Jonnie's case.

What Is the Process for Determining the Specific Needs of a Child with a PHC in the School Setting?

IDEIA includes a mandate called "Child Find." Under this requirement, schools must identify, locate, and evaluate students with disabilities—even if the district is not providing special education services to that child (i.e., the child is found to be ineligible, or parents decline services). This means parents of any children (3–21 years old)—even if they are attending a private school and regardless of the severity of their disabling condition—are entitled to request a Full and Individual Evaluation (FIE) from their local public school district, because public school districts are required to evaluate students suspected—by anyone—of needing special assistance in order to access FAPE. Parents who notify the school of a student's health condition and request an evaluation must receive a written response from the school district regarding their intent to evaluate—or denial of this evaluation, although schools must undertake a refusal to evaluate with much care. School personnel should advise families of their right to request an evaluation and the need for the request to be put in writing.

During a school-based FIE, which must be completed within state-specified time limits, a team of assessment staff is assembled who are qualified to determine the presence of a disability and the extent to which a disability limits a student's access to FAPE. It is important to note that there is no "formula" for completing the FIE; rather, the IEP team determines what and how much information is sufficient for determination of a child's eligibility status. However, IDEIA does specify that the evaluation should be multidisciplinary (i.e., including data from professionals both in and outside the school, to the extent appropriate) and multimethod (e.g., observations, interviews, consultations with professionals serving the child). The data are used by the decision-making team to decide what (if any) accommodations or modifications are necessary to ensure the child receives a FAPE. If the child is IDEIA-eligible, the IEP team must determine specific goals and objectives that will help the student be successful in school, each year.

Does the School Have an Obligation to Follow Outside Providers' Recommendations for School-Based Services?

The school is not legally obligated to follow an outside provider's recommendations for school-based services, although it is strongly advised that the recommendations be considered. Often, specialized providers caring for students with PHCs have expertise beyond what most school-based providers possess regarding a particular condition; ignoring recommendations could adversely affect the students' health and well-being. Moreover, schools that do not take into account outside providers' recommendations may be in a legally indefensible position if the child's health suffers at school as a result. For example, Jonnie's pulmonologist has specialized knowledge about the PHC asthma, in general, and how it affects Jonnie specifically. The school-based team is likely to benefit from integrating— or at least considering—this specialized knowledge into their own school-based plans for Jonnie. When working together across settings, school-based teams (including parents) have a better understanding of individual needs and the best way to meet them, and outside providers may contribute enhanced understanding of educational implications of children's health conditions. In some cases, some recommendations may not be completely feasible or in accordance with school-based legal and ethical obligations or district policy and procedures. Ultimately, although the district may not follow all recommendations made by an outside provider, they should all be reviewed and considered. Not only does this provide an additional perspective regarding the child's PHC-related needs, school-based consideration of outside recommendations represents a point of potential follow-up consultation across systems in order to reach the most appropriate solution for the child.

Who Should the School-Based Team Communicate with to Best Serve Students with PHCs, and How?

Communication among schools, parents, and non-school-based providers is key for ensuring that students with PHCs receive the needed services and accommodations. As children with PHCs often have multiple adults striving to work on their behalf, each professional (as well as parent) has a different perspective to offer and brings differing expertise and knowledge about the child. It is critical to remember that federal privacy laws govern the disclosure of information about students, with schools usually subject to FERPA and providers outside of school bound by HIPAA. Thus, written consent from the parent for two-way communication will likely be needed. For a student like Jonnie, parents may be asked by school personnel to sign FERPA-compliant consent for communication with outside providers, as well as be asked by the pulmonologist or pediatrician to sign HIPAA-compliant consent. Although the consents may seem redundant to his parents, Jonnie's outcomes are maximized when across-setting communication is a priority to all involved, and this is facilitated by provision of requested authorizations.

It is also important to note that the laws were not designed to create barriers for teams with interest in helping a student but to protect a student's information and interests. Requesting permission from parents to converse with a specialist treating a student with a PHC has the potential to strengthen the individualization of their school-based services and also to bolster across-setting relationships. Face-to-face interactions between school-based providers and non-school-based providers are another form of communication.

IDEIA requires that parents be included in the development of school-based plans; under Section 504, parents are not legally required to participate in the meeting but must be provided the opportunity and informed of decisions made per the Section 504 Procedural Safeguards. (Note that parents must sign consent for evaluation under either IDEIA or Section 504.) Under IDEIA, school-based teams must meet at least once per year, although parents do have the right to request more frequent meetings. IDEIA requires that, in addition to parents, an IEP team include both a regular and special education teacher, a representative of the local education agency (i.e., administrator or someone with administrative authority), someone who can interpret evaluation results (such as the school psychologist or speech-language pathologist), others who have knowledge or expertise about a child, and the child him- or herself (when appropriate). This means that persons outside of the school may be IEP team members; parents may invite whomever they wish, including private providers (such as physicians or specialists).

What Are the Obligations of the School if Specialized Medical Services Are Needed During the School Day?

Some students with PHCs require medical services during the school day. "School health services" (such as catheterization or monitoring a child on the schoolbus, etc.) also should be listed in the IEP for a student who is IDEIA-eligible, and the school is responsible for ensuring that the services are provided without charge to the family. The IDEIA regulations note that "medical services" are a "related service" that must be provided, although the term *medical service* is defined as being provided by a licensed physician for the purpose of determining a child's medically related disability. An example provided in the nursing-oriented document *The Medically Fragile Child* (American Federation of Teachers, 2009) states that "Under IDEA, the school is not responsible for the replacement of a surgically implanted device the child may need to survive—but it is responsible for making sure that the device is monitored and maintained correctly while the child is being transported to and from school, or while he or she is at school."

What Is the School's Responsibility When a Student with a PHC Cannot Attend School?

If an IDEIA-eligible student is out of school for extended periods of time, the school is required to work with parents to decide how the student will receive assignments and how much in-home teaching time the student needs. This has to be included in the IEP. For a child like Jonnie, who is served under Section 504, accommodation of his health needs is a requirement, and the school-based team should ensure that his Section 504 plan includes strategies to address issues that could lead to absences. For example, the plan could include accommodations in PE class to help Jonnie avoid overexertion that could result in asthma-related illness, as well as a plan with the classroom teacher for helping Jonnie catch up with missed work and an adequate timeline for turning in make-up work.

What Is the School's Responsibility When a Student with a PHC Is in the Hospital?

When a student with an IEP is in the hospital, specially designed instruction also can be provided, although a student's ability to learn during hospitalizations must be taken into account as well. When it is possible, school-based teams can plan in advance of upcoming hospitalizations to determine how the student will receive work and create a plan for the student's reintegration into the school setting. Regardless of whether the child is at home or in the hospital, it is important for schools to work with parents and healthcare providers to determine what the student can reasonably complete during absences. Depending on individual needs and circumstances, school-based teams may need to plan for a steady increase or decrease in "school time" vs. homebound services. Homebound instruction allows for the provision of educational services in the home setting, and the details regarding time and length of these services are determined by the school-based committee.

When Students Are Receiving Services in a Setting Outside the School, How Does This Affect School-Based Service Delivery?

Services provided in addition to school-based services are likely to benefit the child, and whether the student receives additional services (i.e., outside the school) has no bearing on eligibility for school-based services. This is because school-based services are provided in order to help the child access FAPE, either under IDEIA or Section 504. Regardless of other services, schools must continue to provide the necessary services determined by the school committee. School-based committees determine what the child needs to access the same opportunities afforded to students without disabilities. If the student is IDEIA-eligible, the school-based team provides accommodations or modifications outlined in the student's IEP so that the child makes educational progress. Schools are required to provide IEP-designated services, either through the schools' current resources, through acquisition of new resources (at no cost to the parent), or through outside means.

How Are Student Transitions From School to School Handled?

As students matriculate, communication between professionals in various settings is important for continuity of services to ensure access to FAPE. Best practices in facilitating smooth transitions include that personnel involved in the planning of the student's educational plan (e.g., Section 504 planning team or IEP team) communicate with the new school; this includes traveling to the new school whenever feasible to ensure the new school has a clear understanding of accommodations or modifications deemed necessary for the student's progress, including medical services. It is the responsibility of the previous school to provide high-quality documentation (plans with thorough explanations of student needs, accommodations, modifications, and supports) so personnel in the new school can easily implement the plan and avoid denying FAPE. Moreover, schools are encouraged to work with parents when notified of an upcoming transition to a new school. It is up to a student's new school to determine if a current plan is sufficient (particularly with regard to differences in district policies or state laws and in response to grade and school-level changes). The new school may conduct its own evaluation and make changes to a student's current plan as deemed appropriate.

Where Can One Find More Information About Other Questions That Might Arise?

In addition to links included throughout this chapter and the resources at the end of this chapter, readers are urged to consult their state- and district-specific materials, as well as their discipline-specific ethics codes. Finally, consultation with other professionals both within and outside of the immediate school-based team is recommended.

SCHOOL-BASED PROVIDERS' ROLES AND RESPONSIBILITIES

As school-based providers work together with outside professionals to serve students with PHCs, multiple factors must be taken into account. Federal and state laws, discipline-specific ethical codes, district- and school-specific policies, and individual student concerns are relevant in providing services for students with PHCs. The following are broad recommendations for school-based providers:

- Be knowledgeable about the multiple legal parameters that exist for the protection of your students with PHCs.
- Commit to learning about, and staying up to date with, legal requirements and changes in the law. Subscribing to newsletters and

listservs from organizations like Wrightslaw (http://www.wrightslaw.com/) may be particularly helpful for busy professionals.

- School districts often have districtwide protocols for children with PHCs, and the protocols describe guidelines for the training and coordinated efforts of the practitioners involved. Be sure to inquire about the protocols with district administration and consult with others who have experience implementing district procedures.
- Become familiar with information about PHCs affecting students you serve, as a means of facilitating across-setting and interdisciplinary communication, which is an ethical responsibility. However, also note that the communication is also subject to legal parameters (such as those of HIPAA and FERPA).
- For specific PHCs affecting students you serve, be aware of special considerations related to the health condition (i.e., medical needs during the school day, frequent absenteeism or hospitalization, end-of-life issues), which may require more information and nuanced applications of the law.
- Help parents better understand the laws and policies applicable to their child's school-based services in order to facilitate better home–school–medical provider relationships. Remember that the law exists to protect students and their families. Remember also that parents are members of the school-based decision-making team, and they have perspectives on, and knowledge of, the students' needs and strengths that can be helpful for school-based providers.
- Relatedly, recognize the limits of your knowledge about laws and policies pertaining to school-based provision of services, and know who within your district is a good resource for assistance. Remember that you are a representative of the school-based team, and you must be appropriately cautious about promising services or accommodations before an IEP has been established, about denying services without appropriate data to support a denial, and about interpreting data without considering your own areas of professional competence, the child's unique background, and knowledge of health concerns.

CONCLUSIONS

As overviewed in this chapter, multiple federal and state laws, ethical guidelines, and district- and school-level policies are relevant to serving students with PHCs in schools. The laws and policies exist to protect students and to ensure that they will receive the education to which they are entitled. This brief overview is aimed not only to inform the reader about major legislative parameters that currently apply but also to describe the applicability of laws to some of the specific and major concerns facing students with PHCs. Given the complex needs of students with PHCs, school personnel have key roles to play in facilitating the collaborative relationships between families and schools in order to promote positive outcomes for all students.

REFERENCES

American Federation of Teachers. (2009). *The medically fragile child: Caring for children with special healthcare needs in the school setting.* Washington, DC: Author. Retrieved from https://www.aft.org/sites/default/files/medicallyfragilechild_2009.pdf

Americans With Disabilities Act of 1990, Pub. L. No. 101-336, 104 Stat. 328 (1990).

Americans with Disabilities Amendments Act of 2008, Pub. L. No. 110–325, § 2, 122 Stat. 3553 (2009).

Cincinnati Children's Hospital Medical Center. (n.d.). *IDEA/Section 504 decision chart.* Retrieved from https://www.cincinnatichildrens.org/-/media/cincinnati%20childrens/home/patients/child/special-needs/education/school/legislation/special-ed-legislation-504-flowchart-pdf.pdf?la=en

Endrew F., a Minor, by and Through His Parents and Next Friends, Joseph F. et al. v. Douglas County School District RE–1, 64 IDELR 38, (D., Co. 2014), 580 U.S. __ __ (2017).

Family Educational Rights and Privacy Act of 1974, 20 U.S.C. § 1232 (1974).

Grice, K. (2002). Eligibility under IDEA for other health impaired children. *Summer Law Bulletin.* Retrieved from http://www.iog.unc.edu/pubs/electronicversions/slb/slbsum02/article2.pdf

Health Insurance Portability and Accountability Act of 1996 Administrative Simplification Rules, 45 C.F.R. pts. 160, 162, and 164 (1996).

Individuals with Disabilities Education Improvement Act, 20 U.S.C. § 1400 (2004).

Knapp, S. J., VandeCreek, L. D., & Fingerhut, R. (2017). *Practical ethics for psychologists: A positive approach* (3rd ed.). Washington, DC: American Psychological Association.

Pope, K. S., & Vasquez, M. J. T. (2016). *Ethics in psychotherapy and counseling: A practical guide* (5th ed.). Hoboken, NJ: John Wiley & Sons.

Rehabilitation Act of 1973, Pub. L. No. 93-112, § 504, 87 Stat. 355 (1973).

6

Alternative Education Settings

PUJA G. PATEL, SASHA D. JAQUEZ, AND THEA L. QUINTON ■

Epidemiologic studies suggest that, in the United States, one out of every four children age 17 years or younger (approximately 15 to 18 million youth) suffers from a chronic health condition (Van Cleave, Gortmaker, & Perrin, 2010; Van der Lee, Mokkink, Grootenhuis, Heymans, & Offringa, 2007). A chronic health condition is defined as an illness with a biological, psychological, or cognitive basis that is expected to last for a significant duration (at least 3 months), that is expected to persist for 1 year, and that has more than one of the following sequelae: (1) the limitation of physical, cognitive, emotional, and social functioning; (2) dependency on medical interventions and accommodations (i.e., medications, special diet, medical technology, assistive device, or personal assistance); (3) the need for medical care or related services at home and school that exceed normative expectations for the child's age (Stein, Bauman, Westbrook, Coupey, & Irey, 1993; Stein & Silver, 1999).

Due to advances in medical treatment, children with cancer, HIV/AIDS, cystic fibrosis, and other severe chronic illnesses are living longer and have more functional skills (Weller, Minkwovitz, & Anderson, 2003). Children with a chronic health condition are at higher risk for cognitive and emotional impairments due to their illness or treatment-related effects, including sedation, restlessness, irritability, fatigue, difficulty focusing, pain, nausea, emotional lability, tremors, and limitations in coordination (Mukherjee, Lightfoot, & Sloper, 2000), which can alter or hinder school performance or engagement in learning (Madan-Swain, Katz, & LaGory, 2004). Additionally, children with a chronic illness are at higher risk for adverse educational outcomes, including reduced educational attainment (Champaloux & Young, 2015; Lancashire et al., 2010; Maslow, Haydon, McRee, & Halpern, 2012), lower quality peer and teacher relationships (Hokkanen, Eriksson, Ahonen, & Salantera, 2004; Martinez, Carter, & Legato, 2011; Moody, Eaden, & Mayberry, 1999; Sentenac et al., 2013), lower levels of student engagement and school motivation (Forrest, Bevans, Riley, Crespo, & Louis, 2011), and higher rates of grade repetition (Gerhardt et al., 2007). Thus, students with a chronic illness require additional support to promote academic resiliency.

For children with a chronic illness, a traditional academic path may not be possible due to increased absenteeism. Children with chronic illnesses are absent at least 50% more days than their healthy classmates due to medical appointments, hospitalizations, and feeling ill (A'Bear, 2014). Ultimately, medically related absences limit a child's participation, pose many challenges for a student's academic attainment, and place an additional strain on teachers. Additionally, it can be unsafe for students with compromised immune systems, either due to a medical condition or related to treatment, to attend school. Thus, depending on their clinical course and presentation, students with chronic health conditions often need an alternative educational setting.

LEGAL SUPPORT FOR SCHOOL-BASED SERVICES AND ACCOMMODATIONS

Section 504 of the Rehabilitation Act of 1973 requires schools to provide equal educational opportunities for all students with physical or mental impairments that substantiality limit major life activities, such as walking, seeing, hearing, speaking, breathing, learning, working, and caring for oneself. All students with chronic and acute health conditions may be appropriately considered eligible for 504 services because they require accommodations, but not necessarily specialized instruction. Not only can students qualify for 504 services when they are experiencing physical distress due to their medical condition, but also they can qualify when their chronic illness is in remission, episodic in nature, or mitigated by treatments. Another significant benefit of a 504 plan for students with a chronic illness is that it ensures the opportunity for support even when the students are doing well academically. Students with chronic illnesses may not always need to rely on their accommodations, but it is still important to have accommodations in place because of the unexpected nature of chronic health conditions and related side effects. A 504 plan can reduce the student's risk of falling further behind academically, as well as minimize anxiety about returning to school following a health-related absence. In order for an eligible child to receive formal services at school through a 504 plan, the child's parent must request (in writing) that a 504 plan be identified and implemented.

The Individuals with Disabilities Education Act of 1997 (IDEA) and the revised Individuals with Disabilities Education Improvement Act (IDEIA) of 2004 provide legal grounds for free and appropriate education delivered to children with disabilities in the least restrictive environment with the implementation of an individualized education plan (IEP). To qualify for services under IDEA, the disability must adversely affect a student's educational performance and in turn create the need for special education services. The law recognizes 13 different areas of impairment, including intellectual disability, hearing impairment, speech/language disability, vision impairment, co-occurring deafness/blindness, emotional disability, orthopedic impairment, autism spectrum disorder, traumatic brain injury, other health impairment (OHI), specific learning disability, developmental delay, and multiple disabilities. Research indicates that IEPs for students with chronic illness should include information regarding learning/curriculum outcomes as well as the physical, psychological, and social health and functioning needs of the student (O'Connor, Howell-Meurs, Kvalsvig, & Goldfeld, 2015).

National laws only guide broad school-based services and accommodations; they do not specifically address the issue of alternative educational placements. Individual states and school districts are responsible for determining which students are eligible for specific alternative educational settings, where such services can take place, and the length and duration of such services. The goals of an alternative educational setting are to ensure that children with chronic illness experience maximal educational attainment and to promote academic, cognitive, psychological, and social development (Boonen & Petry, 2011), as well as health.

TYPES OF ALTERNATIVE EDUCATIONAL SETTINGS

Hospital-Based Schooling

Children with chronic medical conditions may need to be hospitalized for necessary medical care. Severe chronic illnesses, such as cancer, sickle cell disease, and HIV/AIDS, can require particularly lengthy hospitalizations. Hospital-based schools have been established to address the academic needs of students with chronic illnesses during their medical treatment (Wilkie, 2011). Children's hospitals typically have a diverse range of educational services available to patients. Some hospitals utilize licensed teaching staff through local school districts, whereas others have their own teachers. Hospital-based teachers are licensed teachers certified in a variety of subjects. The criteria for hospital-based schooling vary depending on the hospital. It is important for educators to contact the hospital to learn about the specific criteria for their area.

Most frequently, hospital-based schooling is initiated by the medical team (i.e., with physician clearance). The eligibility for hospital-based schooling is dependent on particular hospital qualifications. For instance, some hospitals require that a child must have an inpatient admission for a duration of a certain number of days (e.g., 10 days or more) to qualify for hospital-based schooling. Other hospitals may initiate school services directly after a child's admission regardless of the planned length of stay. Additionally, some hospitals require children to enroll in the school district of the hospital-based school, while others allow children to continue to be enrolled in their own school district and coordinate academic work accordingly.

The objective of hospital-based schooling is to maintain acquired academic skills as well as deliver current grade-level instruction. Traditionally, hospital-based schooling can be delivered at bedside or in a classroom in the hospital. Bedside schooling involves a teacher's visiting with the patient in the patient's hospital room. This is a good option for children who are too ill to leave their rooms or who have weakened immune systems. In classroom schooling, a small group of patients meet with a teacher in a hospital classroom. Often, students in a hospital-based classroom will vary in age and grade. Thus students will often be doing independent self-paced work with individualized support from the classroom teacher.

There are several benefits to hospital-based schooling. It provides increased structure for patients within the medical setting while remaining flexible. Lessons can be scheduled around medical procedures and therapies, and at times of the day that maximize the patient's energy and strength. Students who can participate in classroom schooling have the opportunity for peer socialization. Schooling also gives children an opportunity for distraction from their illness and instills hope of being able to rejoin their usual activities after the hospitalization.

The challenge of hospital-based instruction is supporting the student in making adequate progress and receiving the appropriate curriculum for transition back to school. When children do not feel physically well, it is difficult to encourage academic functioning. Educators may consider focusing on building mastery of existing skills to help promote positive self-esteem and the routine of learning until the student's health improves. It is also beneficial to prioritize academic concepts and to limit the child's workload. Since each child responds differently to learning while ill, it is essential for long-term academic success to maintain ongoing communication between school personnel and the student's hospital-based teacher (Hay, Nabors, Sullivan, & Zygmund, 2015).

Homebound Instruction

Due to advances in healthcare, some children with chronic medical conditions may be able to be predominately treated in an outpatient setting, allowing them to remain in the safety and comfort of their own homes (Weller et al., 2003). Students with medical conditions that result in necessary confinement for at least four consecutive or cumulative weeks during the school year are eligible to receive homebound instruction from their school district. It is important to reiterate that, for the child to qualify for homebound instruction, a 504 plan must be officially requested by the child's parents, and a 504 plan must be in place. School 504 committees assist in the implementation of homebound services as well as the transition back to school. For this alternative educational placement, documentation from a physician indicating the type and severity of the condition, as well as the anticipated length of confinement at home, is required. Physician permission is also required in order for the child to return to school.

Homebound services are considered short-term solutions. The major goal is to maintain the child's academic level by providing lessons in core subjects (such as mathematics and language) and by testing the knowledge obtained. Homebound instruction is provided by a certified teacher, who is not necessarily the student's classroom teacher, but the classroom teacher provides the lesson plans and tests while the homebound teacher provides instruction. Thus, an important factor in homebound instruction is maintaining clear and effective communication among teachers, parents, and medical providers (American Academy of Pediatrics, Committee on School Health, 2000).

Although it can vary across school districts, generally 1 hour of homebound instruction is considered to be equivalent to a full school day (Rowland, 2014). Approximately 5 hours of instruction are provided each week during homebound service, usually with the teacher visiting the student twice a week. Thus, an immediate challenge of homebound instruction often is attempting to meet the academic demand of a full school day within condensed instructional time (Bessell, 2001). Success in a homebound setting often requires increased parent involvement, but it can be especially challenging when children with chronic illness have low motivation (Shaw & McCabe, 2008). Additionally, research has found that teachers tend to place lower than necessary expectations on chronically ill students and seek to avoid burdening the student with missed work, because it may add to the family's stress in dealing with the child's chronic illness (Nevile & Roberts, 1999).

Students receiving homebound services are at increased risk for social isolation and lack of connectedness to the school (Searle, Askins, & Bleyer, 2003). Bessell (2001) reported that students with chronic illness felt that homebound instruction was not an adequate substitute for attending school. In order to increase connectedness and to bolster social engagement, and in conjunction with homebound instruction, it can be helpful to allow patients to attend school, when it is medically safe for them to do so (for more information, see the section "Flexible Instruction"). Additionally, the homebound teacher has the unique opportunity to be a liaison between the child at home and classmates at school. For example, the homebound teacher can organize visits or the delivery of letters, postcards, and drawings from classmates.

A great resource for children with chronic illness is technology-based intervention, which connects students with their schools, teachers, and classmates from a laptop. Some hospitals and medical clinics have access to robotlike portable videoconferencing systems that can be remotely controlled by the student from home or the hospital. This allows patients to participate in interactive classroom discussions as well as to share in the social aspects of locker-side chats, lunch period, and moving from class to class. Some schools also support the use of general videoconferencing with a laptop or tablet to increase the ill child's classroom "presence" and to maintain social and educational links to the classroom with positive success (Weiss, Whiteley, Treviranus, & Fels, 2001).

Flexible Instruction

Flexible instruction employs nontraditional methods of instruction to provide academic continuity in the context of the individualized needs of a student with a chronic illness (American Academic of Pediatrics, Committee on School Health, 1993). To optimize on periods of wellness, flexible instruction promotes coordination of educational requirements with the medical and emotional needs of the student. The possibilities for flexible instruction are variable. A common form of flexible instruction is adjustment of school hours (such as half a day, late start, or early release) for a designated portion of time (Frieman & Settel, 1994). For instance, students who are medically fragile and transitioning back into the classroom environment may attend a modified day of school until they rebuild their stamina and confidence. Flexible instruction can also include alterations in the curriculum requirements. For instance, some schools may choose to allow outpatient physical therapy to fulfill a physical education requirement, thus reducing the overall burden on the student. Finally, flexible instruction encompasses differentiated instruction, allowing the teacher to adapt the instructional content, process, product, or learning environment based on the student's needs that day (Broderick, Mehta-Parekh, & Reid, 2005).

Another important consideration for students with frequent school absences is the heighted stress of keeping up with academic demands. The experience of stress can lead to school avoidance as well as adverse health effects (such as headaches, heightened pain, or anxiety). When a child has regular or extended absences from school, it may be beneficial for teachers to consider a reducing the child's workload. As a result, the child can continue to learn and practice concepts without becoming overwhelmed by a quantity of work that he or she may not be well enough to complete. Since research shows that school refusal may be five times greater in students who have a chronic illness (Vila et al., 2003), flexible instruction can allow for the modification of academic demands to create manageable expectations or a reduced workload in the context of a chronic illness. For some students, summer programs can supplement the curriculum so that they continue to meet the academic requirements but they experience reduced pressure from managing both their health and school demands.

The greatest challenge of flexible instruction can be the coordination required to provide the individualized flexibility needed for this type of plan (Tate, 2000). For instance, being prepared to provide homebound services on one day, one-half day of school the next, and a full day of school on the third day requires a significant amount of coordination (Clay, Cortina, Harper, Cocco, & Drotar, 2004). However, research shows that increasing flexibility in order to meet the individualized needs of the child with a chronic illness promotes optimal academic outcomes for the student (Shaw & McCabe, 2008). To make this type of instruction successful for a child, a school-based coordinator (e.g., counselor or classroom teacher) must be identified and must have clear and consistent communication with the parent to know when the child is feeling physically well enough to participate in the various levels of flexible instruction.

Technology and Online School Programs

Due to the advent of the Internet and advances in technology, opportunities for education and communication have grown exponentially. Use of technology can be an innovative method of increasing instructional flexibility as well as enhancing connectedness to the classroom and peers. Telephone consultation, e-mail, fax, instant messaging, text messaging, and delivery of assignments via e-mail can increase communication among parents, students, and the school (Shaw & Brown, 2011). Sending and receiving assignments and instruction via e-mail can allow interaction between student and teacher without the teacher's having to be physically present. Technology can also allow teachers to offer support to families by calling students to remind them of their schedules and to make themselves available to answer questions students may have.

Another way technology can be used to provide an alternative educational setting that meets the needs of students with chronic illnesses is through online school programs. These programs utilize multimedia formats to provide formal educational resources. They have the capability to support both real-time and asynchronous communication among teachers and students, and among students (Means, Toyama, Murphy, Bakia, & Jones, 2010). The online instructional approach provides the opportunity to reach students who may otherwise be unable to attend classes, such as children with compromised immune systems, those receiving treatment for a chronic illness, or those who experience side effects of medication or treatment that do not allow them to physically attend school.

Many types of technology and tools are used for online teaching. Asynchronous communication tools, such as e-mail and threaded discussions, allow students to contribute to the class at their convenience, at any time throughout the day. Synchronous technology, such as webcasts, chat rooms, and audiovisual technology, is used to approximate face-to-face interactions, such as delivering lectures or holding group meetings (Means et al., 2010). Synchronous technology also allows students who are not in the classroom to participate more actively and even to attend class in real time. Recently, online programs have started combining various forms of asynchronous and synchronous technology for more complete and comprehensive online learning opportunities.

At the time this chapter was being written, few rigorous studies existed showing the effectiveness of online learning for K-12 students (Means et al., 2010). However, research does suggest there may be certain advantages to online schooling, including increasing motivation, focused use of learning strategies, honing of problem-solving and number skills, and opportunities to explore patterns and relationships (Condie & Munro, 2007). Whereas these general benefits are valued, advantages have not been documented in all subject areas. Condie and Munro (2007) found that the most obvious benefits in individual subject areas have been observed in foreign language, history, geography, the sciences, physical education, and the creative arts. Unfortunately, this means online opportunities may not be as beneficial for core subjects, such as mathematics and language arts. Wilkie (2011) noted that students and teachers have highlighted both the need for, and desire for, interactions with others in effective learning of mathematics. Although online schooling may provide more flexibility to children who are chronically ill, care should also be given to ensure that the child is able to effectively learn necessary concepts for each class needing to be completed.

Social interactions should also be a consideration when deciding if online schooling is appropriate for a child with a chronic illness. Research suggests that interaction and discussion are fundamental to the process of learning (Wenger, 1998), and many children with chronic illness state that wanting to see friends is a primary reason for wanting to return to school after a prolonged absence. Furthermore, it has been cautioned that online learning at the elementary and secondary levels should be used only as a supplement or to enhance conventional lessons, due to the critical social and emotional development that takes place during those years (Gadanidis, Graham, McDougall, & Roulet, 2002). Although extant research supporting the advantages of online schools may be limited, the concept of online school is appealing and logistically sound for children with chronic illness. However, many considerations should be weighed, and depending on the age of the child, online schooling may be more (or less) appropriate as an educational alternative.

To assist in determining if online school is an appropriate alternative, the National Education Association, in collaboration with multiple other partners, put out the *Guide to Online High School Courses* (2002), which addressed how to assess online high school courses. It also provided questions that constituents, including policymakers, teachers, managers, administrators, parents/guardians, and students, should ask when evaluating online classes. The document noted that, to be an effective replacement for face-to-face courses, online courses should meet the highest possible standards of design and instruction. Finally, the National Education Association (2002) suggested that the quality of online course offerings should be considered in terms of the criteria presented in Table 6.1.

CASE EXAMPLES

Below are two case examples of children who should be considered for alternative education settings due to chronic illness. Each case example includes a worksheet designed to summarize relevant information that can be taken into consideration to assist in deciding the most appropriate alternative education setting.

Case Example 1

Sally is a 16-year-old female who recently completed treatment for an osteosarcoma (bone cancer). Her treatment included surgery to remove her tumor, followed by chemotherapy and localized radiation to her neck and shoulder. Due to the intensity of her medical treatment and her compromised immune system, Sally was unable to attend regular school, and she received homebound services during her sophomore year of high school. Prior to being diagnosed with cancer, Sally was a straight-A student and enjoyed school. As she faced reintegration into high school, she felt overwhelmed.

Table 6.1. Guide to Evaluating Online Programs

Key Feature	Description	Sample Questions to Consider
Curriculum	Should be challenging, relevant, and aligned with appropriate national, state, and/or district standards for student learning.	1. Does the curriculum meet graduation requirements? 2. Does the curriculum content (for grade level) match state/district requirements? 3. Is the curriculum able to meet needs where public school left off?
Instructional Design	Should be informed by, and reflect, the most current research on learning theory. Should take advantage of the special circumstances, requirements, and opportunities of the online learning environment and support the development of 21st century learning skills.	1. Does the design take into consideration multiple learning modalities (e.g., visual, auditory, kinesthetic, tactile, group learning)? 2. Does the design account for any special academic needs (such as specific learning disabilities)?
Teacher Quality	Should be skilled in the subject matter, learning theory, technologies, and pedagogies appropriate for the content area and the online environment.	1. Is the teacher appropriately qualified to teach the course? 2. Does the student have access to, and know how to communicate directly with, the teacher?
Student Roles	Student should be actively engaged in the learning process and interact on a regular basis with the teacher and online classmates in the course.	1. Is the student medically stable enough to appropriately participate in online school? 2. Is the student internally motivated to participate in online schooling?
Assessment	Should be authentic, formative, and regular, providing opportunities for students to reflect on their own learning and work quality during the course. End-of-course assessments should give students the opportunity to demonstrate appropriate skills and understandings that reflect mastery of the course content.	1. Are expectations of success in classes made clear to the student and teachers (e.g., course syllabus/rubric)? 2. Does the online teacher provide ongoing and timely feedback regarding students' work?
Technological Infrastructure	Infrastructure supporting the online course should provide the necessary tools for instruction and interactivity. The technology behind the course should work reliably, simply, and economically. Technical assistance should be available whenever needed by students or teachers (National Education Association, 2002).	1. Does the student have access to everything needed to engage in online school (e.g., consistent/accessible Internet connection, appropriate hardware/software)? 2. Is there appropriate technical assistance available for the student?

Following the completion of treatment, Sally continued to struggle with neck stiffness and shoulder pain, for which she received physical therapy and took pain medication. Although the medicine was helpful, it also made her feel drowsy, which was difficult because she was accustomed to being energetic. Additionally, her neuropsychological testing revealed attentional weaknesses and slower processing speed secondary to her cancer and cancer treatment. Recommendations resulting from the testing included that Sally receive extra time on assignments and tests, preferential seating, and a copy of class notes so that she could keep up with the pace of classroom instruction.

Additionally, Sally was hesitant to return to school for several reasons. Her peer relationships had become strained while she was undergoing cancer treatment and she thought it was difficult to connect with her friends. She reported that she could no longer relate to her friends when they talked about romantic relationships, hair and makeup, and social events because of the intensity of her experience with a life-threatening illness. She also expressed insecurity about the changes in her physical appearance (hair loss and reduced weight), which were slowly resolving. Finally, her identity as an athlete (all-star softball player) had shifted. Although she was medically cleared to play sports noncompetitively, her neck range of motion had not completely returned, altering her ability to play competitively. Given all of these changes and the trauma of battling cancer, Sally wanted to move on to the next stage of life and start college as soon as possible. She wanted to pursue a career in medicine, because she was very passionate about helping other sick kids with cancer. She had asked her parents to let her attend school online so that she could graduate early and make up for her lost time being sick. Her parents were concerned about her not returning to traditional school and they encouraged her to start individual therapy.

Table 6.2 contains a summary of the relevant aspects to consider in determining the most appropriate placement for Sally.

Case Example 2

Knox was a 10-year-old male in fifth grade who began experiencing seizures and was subsequently diagnosed with epilepsy. Due to multiple neurology appointments and inpatient EEGs, Knox missed a substantial amount of school. His neurology team determined that Knox's seizures appeared to be originating in the left frontal lobe of his brain. Knox began taking anti-epileptic medication, but his seizures remained poorly controlled.

Knox experienced almost nightly seizures, which caused confusion and sleepiness and often left him feeling groggy the next morning. He was generally able to become fully alert around 11:00 AM. He also experienced auras and suspected absence seizures throughout the day. Academically, Knox fell behind: his homework completion suffered due to his needing additional sleep in the morning and the frequent

Table 6.2. CONSIDERATIONS FOR SALLY

Name: Sally	Age: 16 years old Grade Level: 10th	Medical History: Osteosarcoma— in remission Age at diagnosis: 15 years old
Current Symptoms	Treatment	Side Effects
• Pain • Limited range of motion	• Medication—Lyrica • Weekly physical therapy • Follow-up oncology visits • Cancer monitoring	• Drowsiness • School absence • Potential anxiety/school absence

PHYSICAL CONCERNS	PHYSICAL RESILIENCY FACTORS
• Neck and shoulder pain • Low energy/fatigue • Can lift only less than 10 lbs • Ongoing medical appointments	• Able to be independent • Getting adequate sleep at night • Able to use rolling backpack
COGNITIVE CONCERNS	COGNITIVE RESILIENCY FACTORS
• Mild neurocognitive disorder (attention weakness & slower processing speed)	• Good academic standing • Motivated to complete school/go to college
EMOTIONAL CONCERNS	EMOTIONAL RESILIENCY
• Low self-esteem due to physical changes • Difficulty connecting with peers	• Started individual therapy • Insightful

CONSIDERATIONS FOR ACADEMIC PLACEMENTS	
Hospital-based school	*Does not qualify based on medical need*
Homebound services	*Does not qualify based on medical need*
Flexible instruction	*Good option to consider with areas of support* — Peer integration (involvement in athletics as team manager) — Academic support of 504 accommodations for attention weakness and extra time — Plan for when Sally misses school for medical appointments or when she has increased pain or drowsiness due to medication
Online school	*Good option to consider due to age* — Motivated to complete schoolwork and to graduate with good academic background — Consider alternative social engagement — Self-paced instruction could be beneficial due to need for extra time

need for him to leave school early because of the suspected absence seizures. He began to withdraw socially and he stated that he feared having a seizure around his friends and making them scared and not want to hang out with him anymore. He also stopped wanting to play basketball with his family and friends when he felt well.

Knox was referred for neuropsychological testing, which revealed difficulties with sustained attention, difficulties with initial focus, and a tendency to become overwhelmed with too much information. Recommendations included the implementation of a 504 plan at school to offer him additional time on assignments and tests, a decreased workload (with enough work to show mastery), and a distraction-free environment. While Knox's neurology team continued to pursue the best medication for controlling his epilepsy, his neurology nurse and the school advocate at the local children's hospital decided to set up a meeting with Knox, his parents, and his school counselor to determine the best plan for his academic and social success moving forward. Collectively, it was decided that Knox would initially complete one month of homebound school, which was signed off on by his neurologist. Knox would have a homebound teacher come to his house for 1 hour each day to work on homework, to be available to explain new concepts, and to help Knox work toward mastery of current skills. Homebound school also allowed the flexibility for Knox to attend his numerous medical appointments and to engage in therapy, given his social withdrawal and recently noted anhedonia. When Knox felt up to it, Knox's teacher suggested that he video conference with his regular class to hear lessons in real time. This also allowed Knox a chance to stay connected with his peers. His teacher completed a plan to have Knox's peers compose pages in a "We Miss You" book for Knox, which was delivered to him by his homebound teacher. Once the month of homebound school was finished, Knox began flexible instruction and Knox's medical/school team monitored his ability to tolerate school with increasing medical stability.

A summary of the relevant aspects to consider in determining the most appropriate placement for Knox is shown in Table 6.3.

Table 6.3. Considerations for Knox

Name: Knox	Age: 10 years old Grade Level: 5th	Medical History: Epilepsy—poorly controlled Age at diagnosis: 9 years old
Current Symptoms	**Treatment**	**Side Effects**
• Auras • Seizures • Staring spells	• Medication—Keppra • Follow-up neurology visits • Recommended weekly therapy	• Emotional lability • Missing class • Social withdrawal

Table 6.3. CONTINUED

PHYSICAL CONCERNS	PHYSICAL RESILIENCY FACTORS
• Safety from falls (protect head) • Unsteady on feet during auras	• Extra time between classes/elevator pass
• Limited physical activity	• Peer escort
	• Able to use rolling backpack
COGNITIVE CONCERNS	**COGNITIVE RESILIENCY FACTORS**
• Inattention • Difficulties with initial focus • Tendency to become overwhelmed • Observed decrease in academic functioning	• Additional time to complete assignments • Decreased workload • Present assignments in small, manageable chunks • Previously high achieving • Cognitive ability consistent with achievement
EMOTIONAL CONCERNS	**EMOTIONAL RESILIENCY**
• Emotional lability • Not coping well with illness and side effects • Social withdrawal	• Start individual therapy • Exposures to peer interactions in safe environments

CONSIDERATIONS FOR ACADEMIC PLACEMENTS	
Hospital-based school	*Does not qualify based on medical need*
Online school	*Not good option due to age/academic demands of child/grade level*
Homebound services	*Good option to consider until seizures are medically controlled* — Start with 4 weeks of homebound instruction for 1 hour five times a week — Academic support that includes 504 accommodations for extra time and decreased workload, concentrating on mastery of skills — Use of technology to allow peer-to-peer interactions at times he feels comfortable — Flexibility to attend medical/psychological follow-up appointments
Flexible instruction	*Good option to consider once seizures are medically controlled* — Allow time to build up tolerance — Academic support that includes 504 accommodations — Plan for when Knox misses school for medical appointments or when he has increased drowsiness from breakthrough seizures or medication

CONCLUSION

When deciding which academic placement best serves a child, there are several important factors to consider. The first step is to understand the child's chronic illness (onset, severity, duration, treatment, and prognosis) and how the illness affects learning. It is important to consider not only the immediate effects of compromised access to learning, but also the cumulative effect over time. For example, compromised mastery of single-digit multiplication in third grade could make fifth-grade multiple-digit multiplication more challenging. Next, it is important to delineate the most vital academic and social objectives for the child's given age and grade, and to use that list to guide alternative placements. For instance, socialization to peers and routine is a key objective of kindergarten education. Thus, the alternative educational setting should attempt to meet this objective to the extent possible within the constraints of its setting. Finally, it is important to be flexible and to adjust to the changing circumstances of the student's chronic illness. For instance, an adolescent with epilepsy that was previously well-managed with medication but who is experiencing breakthrough seizures may need his educational placement adjusted until seizures are better controlled again. Timely collaboration is critical to adjust academic requirements in a manner that does not embarrass the student or prohibit academic progression.

Ongoing collaboration among the medical team, teachers, the student, and the family is another key ingredient for a successful transition across alternative academic settings (Sexson & Madan-Swain, 1993). Once a team of individuals have been designated to assist the student in achieving academic success, the next step is identifying potential barriers to access for instruction, such as ongoing medical appointments or upcoming medical procedures. Incorporating necessary accommodations into a 504 or IEP plan is crucial. Additionally, school staff are encouraged to be creative in allowing for school engagement. The use of technology can bridge the gap between the classroom and alternative academic settings, with the ultimate goal being reintegration into the classroom. Research has shown a large part of social and emotional development is fostered within the school setting (Weitzman, 1984). For a child with chronic illness, school may serve as the only environment where he or she can be viewed as a typical child who is more than just an existing medical condition. Thus, it is important to delineate school interventions and supports that will ultimately maximize school attendance and foster the child's educational and social growth and success.

REFERENCES

A'Bear, D. (2014). Supporting the learning of children with chronic illness. *Canadian Journal of Action Research, 15*, 22–39.

American Academy of Pediatrics, Committee on School Health. (1993). In P. R. Nader (Ed.), *School Health: Policy and Practice,* 5th ed. Elk Grove Village, Ill.: American Academy of Pediatrics.

American Academy of Pediatrics, Committee on School Health. (2000). Home, hospital, nd other non-school-based instruction for children and adolescents who are medically unable to attend school. *Pediatrics, 106*, 1154–1155.

Bessell, A. G. (2001). Children surviving cancer: Psychosocial adjustment, quality of life, and school experiences. *Exceptional Children, 67*, 345–359.

Boonen, H., & Petry, K. (2011). How do children with a chronic or long-term illness perceive their school re-entry after a period of homebound instruction? *Child: Care, Health and Development, 38*, 490–496. doi:10.1111/j.1365-2214.2011.01279.x

Broderick, A., Mehta-Parekh, H., & Reid, D. K. (2005). Differentiating instruction for disabled students in inclusive classrooms. *Theory Into Practice, 44*(3), 194–202. doi:10.1207/s15430421tip4403_3

Champaloux, S. W., & Young, D. R. (2015). Childhood chronic health conditions and educational attainment: A social ecological approach. *Journal of Adolescent Health, 56*, 98–105. doi:10.1016/j.jadohealth.2014.07.016

Clay, D. L., Cortina, S., Harper, D. C., Cocco, K. M., & Drotar, D. (2004). Schoolteachers' experiences with childhood chronic illness. *Children's Health Care, 33*, 227–239. doi:10.1207/s15326888chc3303_5

Condie, R., & Munro, R. (2007). The impact of ICT in schools-a landscape review; Coventry, Becta. Retrieved September 2018 from http://webarchieve.nationalarchivs. gov.uk/2010110210364/publications.becta.org.uk.//display.cfm?resID=28221.

Forrest, C. B., Bevans, K. B., Riley, A. W., Crespo, R., & Louis, T. A. (2011). School outcomes of children with special health care needs. *Pediatrics, 128*, 303–312. doi:10.1542/peds.2010-3347

Frieman, B. B., & Settel, J. (1994). What the classroom teacher needs to know about children with chronic medical problems. *Childhood Education, 70*, 196–201. doi:10.1080/00094056.1994.10521807

Gadanidis, G., Graham, L., McDougall, D., & Roulet, G. (2002). *On-line mathematics: Visions and opportunities, issues and challenges, and recommendations.* Toronto, Canada: The Fields Institute for Research in Mathematical Sciences.

Gerhardt, C. A., Dixon, M., Miller, K., Vannatta, K., Valerius, K. S., Correll, J., & Noll, R. B. (2007). Educational and occupational outcomes among survivors of childhood cancer during the transition to emerging adulthood. *Journal of Developmental and Behavioral Pediatrics, 28*(6), 448–455.

Hay, G. H., Nabors, M. L., Sullivan, A., & Zygmund, A. (2015). Students with pediatric cancer: A prescription for school success. *Physical Disabilities: Education and Related Services, 34*(2), 1–13. doi:10.14434/pders.v34i2.19643

Hokkanen, H., Eriksson, E., Ahonen, O., & Salantera, S. (2004). Adolescents with cancer: Experience of life and how it could be made easier. *Cancer Nursing, 27*, 325–335. doi:10.1097/00002820-200407000-00010

Lancashire, E., Frobisher, C., Reulen, R., Winter, D., Glaser, A., & Hawkins, M. (2010). Educational attainment among adult survivors of childhood cancer in Great Britain: A population-based cohort study. *Journal of the National Cancer Institute, 102*, 254–270.

Madan-Swain, A., Katz, E. R., & LaGory, J. (2004). School and social reintegration after a serious illness or injury. In R. T. Brown (Ed.), *Handbook of pediatric psychology in school settings* (pp. 637–655). Mahwah, NJ: Lawrence Erlbaum Associates.

Martinez, W., Carter, J. S., & Legato, L. J. (2011). Social competence in children with chronic illness: A meta-analytic review. *Journal of Pediatric Psychology, 36*, 878–890.

Maslow, G., Haydon, A. A., McRee, A., & Halpern, C. T. (2012). Protective connections and educational attainment among young adults with childhood-onset chronic illness. *Journal of School Health, 82,* 364–370. doi:10.1111/j.1746-1561.2012.00710.x

Means, B., Toyama, Y., Murphy, R., Bakia, M., & Jones, K. (2010). *Evaluation of evidence-based practices in online learning: A meta-analysis and review of online learning studies.* Retrieved from https://www2.ed.gov/rschstat/eval/tech/evidence-based-practices/finalreport.pdf

Moody, G., Eaden, J. A., & Mayberry, J. F. (1999). Social implications of childhood Crohn's disease. *Journal of Pediatric Gastroenterology and Nutrition, 28,* S43–S45.

Mukherjee, S., Lightfoot, J., & Sloper, P. (2000). The inclusion of pupils with a chronic health condition in mainstream school: What does it mean for teachers? *Educational Research, 42,* 59–72. doi:10.1080/001318800363917

National Education Association. (2002). *Guide to online high school courses.* Retrieved from http://www.nea.org/assets/docs/onlinecourses.pdf

Nevile, M., & Roberts, J. (1999). School children with chronic illness. *Exceptionality Education Canada, 9*(3), 41–47.

O'Connor, M., Howell-Meurs, S., Kvalsvig, A., & Goldfeld, S. (2015). Understanding the impact of special health care needs on early school functioning: A conceptual model. *Child Care, Health and Development, 41,* 15–22.

Rowland, J. (2014). *Number of instructional days/hours in the school year.* Report prepared by Education Commission of the States. Denver, CO: ECS Distribution Center.

Searle, N. S., Askins, M., & Bleyer, W. A. (2003). Homebound schooling is the least favorite option for continued education of adolescent cancer patients: A preliminary report. *Pediatric Blood & Cancer, 40,* 380–384. doi:10.1002/mpo.10270

Sentenac, M., Gavin, A., Gabhainn, S. N., Molcho, M., Due, P., Ravens-Sieberer, U., . . . Godeau, E. (2013). Peer victimization and subjective health among students reporting disability or chronic illness in 11 Western countries. *The European Journal of Public Health, 23,* 421–426.

Sexson, S. B., & Madan-Swain, A. (1993). School reentry for the child with chronic illness. *Journal of Leaning Disabilities, 26,* 115–125. doi:10.1177/002221949302600204

Shaw, S. R., & Brown, M. B. (2011). Advances in collaboration with medical professionals: Theory and applications. *Journal of Educational and Psychological Consultation, 21,* 79–87. doi:10.1080/10474412.2011.571549

Shaw, S. R., & McCabe, P. C. (2008). Hospital-to-school transition for children with chronic illness: Meeting the new challenges of an evolving health care system. *Psychology in the Schools, 45,* 74–87. doi:10.1002/pits.20280

Stein, R. E., Bauman, L. J., Westbrook, L. E., Coupey, S. M., & Irey, H. T. (1993). Framework for identifying children who have chronic conditions: The case for a new definition. *The Journal of Pediatrics, 122,* 342–347. doi:10.1016/S0022-3476(05)83414-6

Stein, R. E., & Silver, E. J. (1999). Operationalizing a conceptually based noncategorical definition: A first look at US children with chronic conditions. *Archives of Pediatric Adolescent Medicine, 153,* 68–74. doi:10.1001/archpedi.153.1.68

Tate, J. O. (2000). Court decisions and IDEA 1997 compliance issues that affect special education programs in rural schools. *Rural Special Education Quarterly, 19,* 3–9.

Van Cleave, J., Gortmaker, S. L., & Perrin, J. M. (2010). Dynamics of obesity and chronic health conditions among children and youth. *JAMA, 303,* 623–630. doi:10.1001/jama.2010.104

Van der Lee, J. H., Mokkink, L. B., Grootenhuis, M. A., Heymans, H. S. A., & Offringa, M. (2007). Definitions and measurement of chronic health conditions in childhood. *JAMA, 297*, 2741–2751. doi:10.1001/jama.297.24.2741

Vila, G., Hayder, R., Bertrand, C., Falissard, B., De Blic, J., Mouren-Simeoni, M.-C., & Scheinmann, P. (2003). Psychopathology and quality of life for adolescents with asthma and their parents. *Psychosomatics, 44*, 319–328.

Weiss, P., Whiteley, C. P., Treviranus, J., & Fels, D. I. (2001). PEBBLES: A personal technology for meeting educational, social and emotional needs of hospitalised children. *Personal and Ubiquitous Computing, 5*(3), 157–168.

Weitzman, M. (1984). School and peer relations. *Pediatric Clinics of North America, 31*, 59–69. doi:10.1016/S0031-3955(16)34536-9

Weller, W. E., Minkwovitz, C. S., & Anderson, G. F. (2003). Utilization of medical and health-related services among school age children and adolescents with special health care needs (1994 National Health Interview Survey on Disability [NHIS-D] baseline data). *Pediatrics, 112*, 593–603.

Wenger, E. (1998). Communities of practice: Learning as a social system. *Systems Thinker, 9*(5), 1–5. doi:10.1017/cbo9780511803932

Wilkie, K. J. (2011). Academic continuity through online collaboration: Mathematics teachers support the learning of pupils with chronic illness during school absence. *Interactive Learning Environments, 19*(5), 519–535. doi:10.1080/10494820903545542

Assessment and Intervention Strategies

ection II focuses on prevention, assessment, intervention, and consultation strategies for individual students and entire school systems. Chapters in this section discuss specific models for initial assessment and monitoring progress over time at the individual level and for a population of students. Chapters focused on intervention detail intervention approaches for working with students with pediatric health conditions, reintegrating them into the school setting after a change in medical status or prolonged absence, and helping students experiencing loss and/or grief.

7

Assessment of Needs and Intervention Effectiveness

LISA HAYUTIN, CAITLIN E. WALSH,
AND ELIZABETH BENNETT ■

Children and adolescents with chronic medical conditions demonstrate lower levels of academic, physical, and social functioning than their healthy peers, and over the past decade there has been increasing recognition that addressing students' physical health and behavior is a necessary part of successful education (Lewallen, Hunt, Potts-Datema, Zaza, & Giles, 2015; Basch, 2011; Pinquart & Teubert, 2012). Because students with medical conditions are at higher risk for underperforming, they may need ongoing monitoring and assessment to help determine the need for school-based interventions and supports (Litt & McCormick, 2016). This chapter discusses considerations unique to students with medical conditions in the school-based assessment and monitoring process.

School-based assessments are typically a snapshot view of a student's functioning and are aimed at understanding the student's abilities and current performance, as well as identifying the interventions, supports, and accommodations or modifications that must be put in place to enable the student to perform to his or her academic potential. For children with medical conditions, information gathered during an assessment must be understood in the context of the medical condition. The examiner must consider the impact of symptoms, disease course, and illness-related absences. In addition to the primary effects of the medical condition, the related factors that should be considered include side effects of treatment, the child's adjustment to new treatments and what that looks like, related stress or anxiety for the child and family, and the effects of possible changes in peer and family relationships (Immelt, 2006; Vermaes, van Susante, & van Bakel, 2013).

APPROACHES TO ASSESSMENT

In conducting any evaluation, combining information from multiple domains and perspectives is critical (Sattler, 2018). Although there will be variability in what "multiple domains" means based on setting and individual circumstances, a good assessment should include a balance of objective data (e.g., norm-referenced tests and rating scales, behavioral observations, academic records) and background information and current perspectives from those who know the student well (e.g., parent and teacher interviews and questionnaires, as well as consultation with medical providers, such as the school nurse or the child's treating physician). The information gathered does not need to align perfectly, and patterns and discrepancies in the information obtained often convey important information.

For a child with medical complexity, collaboration must often be a larger and more intentional part of the assessment process, and it may involve adding medical providers to the team. Although many parents truly become experts on their child's diagnosis, they must not bear the sole responsibility for educating the team about their child's medical diagnoses. The school team is encouraged to self-educate and to check their understanding with a medical provider to avoid attributing all symptoms to the diagnosis, which could result in missing additional important concerns, or underestimating the reach of the diagnosis and failing to provide adequate accommodations. A child with chronic pain, for example, may have a variety of factors contributing to functional impairment, such as severity of the condition, pain-related anxiety, avoidance, and parents' desire to protect their child (Claar, Simons, & Logan, 2008; Peterson & Palermo, 2004). Well-rounded insight into these factors can assist with accurate conceptualization and intervention planning that will most effectively promote a student's progress.

Common assessment procedures include 1) screening instruments that are brief and help guide the need for more in-depth assessment; 2) individually administered, standardized assessments; 3) questionnaires and rating scales; 4) interviews; 5) behavioral observations; and 6) record reviews. These approaches may be used in varying proportions depending on the setting and the individual child and family. Having some flexibility in approach is often useful, especially for students whose attendance or performance may be variable. For example, in a setting that provides limited time for interviewing and direct assessment, reliance on questionnaires may allow access to more information with less face-to-face time. In the case of a family with questionable literacy skills, questionnaires and rating scales may need to be replaced with more interviewing and observation. The challenge for the examiner is to integrate all of the pieces of the evaluation into a helpful and coherent narrative about the child.

Some children with medical conditions have undergone clinical evaluations from providers in the community. It is often helpful to request and review their reports, as they may have information pertinent for understanding the child and meeting educational needs. They may also help reduce redundancies in assessment. For example, if a child was given a valid cognitive assessment in a medical setting 6 months ago, the school team may opt to adopt those results in lieu of conducting a repeat evaluation of cognitive abilities. On the other hand, clinical and school-based evaluations are not one and the same, particularly when it comes to intervention recommendations. This distinction can often be confusing for families, and upfront and clear discussion about this may go a long way in reducing frustrations and aligning shared goals and objectives. Here is an example of how the team might explain this distinction:

> When a child has a clinical evaluation, the goals are usually to find a unifying diagnosis or conceptualization to explain areas of difficulty or concern. This often comes along with recommendations aimed at maximizing functioning across a broad range of areas (e.g., learning, social, emotional, daily living). Our focus in the schools is really on the child's ability to learn and appropriately access education. For example, if a 10-year-old child has delays in speech articulation (e.g., saying |w| instead of |r|), a clinic-based speech therapist might recommend speech therapy to target proper articulation. Our school-based speech therapist might conduct the same evaluation and obtain the same results; however, school-based speech therapy will only be recommended if that articulation delay is interfering with education (e.g., others cannot understand what the student says; the student is being teased by classmates or is not participating in class due to embarrassment). This does not mean that we don't think the student should receive speech therapy. It simply means that the speech delay is not interfering with education and therefore the student won't receive school-based speech services.

Considering this school-based perspective on assessment, an evaluation serves the role of better understanding current strengths and weaknesses, areas in which intervention is needed, accommodations and modifications needed for the student to access education, and appropriate goals and expectations. Sometimes, determining what a student needs is simple and straightforward and requires only gathering basic information (i.e., talking to parents, teachers, and medical providers) and providing a rather circumscribed level of support (e.g., allowing an elevator pass for a student who cannot safely and independently take the stairs). At the other end of the spectrum, sometimes a comprehensive assessment is needed. It is up to the team to ascertain the impact of the medical condition on day-to-day school performance and to determine what type of assessment is needed. This tiered approach aligns well with the tiered intervention framework used in most schools.

DOMAINS OF ASSESSMENT

To develop an appropriate assessment plan, it is helpful to review an outline of factors to consider with each child. In this section, we review areas of consideration and various approaches to assessment that may fit. When evaluating a child with a medical condition, there are three main junctures at which an examiner should pause and consider the impact of the students' medical condition: during battery selection, when considering modifications to assessment administration, and when interpreting results. It is wise to remain aware that the assessment plan is a starting point, and that adjusting the plan in response to new information is also a critical component of conducting an appropriate assessment.

Medical Background and History

It is critical to obtain background information from those who know the child best. This may include a parent or caregiver, a teacher, and, in the case of a child with a medical condition, a clinician who best understands how the child's condition affects daily functioning. Please note that exchanging information with anyone other than the child's parent or guardian requires a signed consent for release of information, and that the parent has the right to refuse. When obtaining consent, it is important that the examiners and family have a clear shared understanding of what information will be exchanged. It is also important that school representatives consider the relevance of their questions to the child's school functioning.

BACKGROUND QUESTIONNAIRE
A background questionnaire is often a quick and efficient way to gather a range of detailed information. Although it is valuable to try to minimize paperwork for families, parents often need time to think and perhaps review their own records to answer questions about medical history and development. Sending questionnaires in advance of an in-person meeting allows for this. The examiner can then review this information prior to interviewing the family and use it to shape the focal points for the parent interview. The team is encouraged to share information gathered with one another to prevent duplication of work, which can feel disorganized and redundant to a parent.

INTERVIEWS
A brief (i.e., 20–30 minute) consultation/interview can paint a richer picture than a questionnaire and is often time well spent. Table 7.1 reflects some areas of inquiry along with sample questions that are generally transferrable across a range of potential informants.

RECORD REVIEW
Other sources for background information may include medical records and reports from previous evaluations.

Table 7.1. SAMPLE PARENT INTERVIEW QUESTIONS

Area	Sample Questions
Strengths	What are the child's strengths? What comes easily and is effortlessly engaging? In what situations does the child seem most joyful?
Challenges/Concerns	What are the child's greatest challenges? What are your greatest areas of concern? If we could magically change one or two things for this child, what would produce the greatest change/relief?
Medical Considerations (more relevant for caregiver/clinician interviews)	Tell me about the diagnosis. What is involved in the care/treatment? Who is responsible for care-management tasks? How might the diagnosis or treatment(s) affect pain? Sleep? Describe (the child's) attitude toward/understanding of the medical condition. What does the school need to know about this condition? What do the teachers need to look for? *Note that other aspects of a child's medical diagnosis may not be as relevant (How did he get this condition? How long will he live? Do his siblings have this condition?) and these questions should be avoided, because their personal nature may make some families uncomfortable.* Also, are there any hearing or vision impairments?
Nonacademic Functional Impairment	In what ways does the child's medical condition affect nonacademic factors at school? Consider attendance, tardiness, alertness, attention, memory, mental organization, energy level, and participation in field trips and other special activities. Also, how can the school best support (the child) at school in areas of need?
Academic Application	How do you think these factors affect the child's academic experience? Consider attention, emotion regulation, fine motor skills, sensory processing, alertness, memory, stamina, and attendance.
Social/Emotional Factors	How has the medical condition affected anxiety? Social relationships? Self-esteem (including body image)? What are the child's coping and support resources? How can the school team best support the child socially/emotionally?

(*continued*)

Table 7.1. CONTINUED

Area	Sample Questions
Other	What am I forgetting to ask you? What else do you think I need to know to understand (the child) well?
Reflection	Before concluding an interview, it is always good to summarize the conversation in a few sentences to ensure that the informant's insights and observations were properly captured.

Cognitive/Developmental Assessments

Cognitive assessments measure aspects of thinking that predict academic success, and they are typically administered and interpreted by a psychologist. Unlike academic skills that are learned in a classroom, cognitive abilities are those aspects of thinking that are not taught explicitly, such as the ability to make associations between concepts or to understand patterns and sequencing (Ellingsen, 2016). Cognitive assessments usually include some measure of verbal abilities, nonverbal abilities, or spatial reasoning abilities, and they may also include measures of thinking efficiency (i.e., how quickly and accurately one can perform a task, how one can store and process information while doing a task). Examples of cognitive tests include the Wechsler Intelligence Scales for Children-Fifth Edition (WISC-V; Wechsler, 2014), the Differential Abilities Scales-Second Edition (DAS-II; Elliott, 2007), and the Stanford Binet Intelligence Scales-Fifth Edition (SB:V; Roid, 2003).

For very young children (less than 3 years old) and/or older children with more significant developmental delays, the demands of a cognitive assessment may be too sophisticated. Cognitive assessments require the ability to tolerate an adult-led task, focus for the duration of a task, and manage frustration associated with answering challenging items. An assessment that measures early development can be used when a cognitive assessment is not appropriate for a student due to age or ability. Although these instruments do not have norm-referenced standard scores when administered out of age range (i.e., for older children with more significant developmental delays), they produce age equivalents that may serve as a helpful reference point for understanding a child's current abilities. Examples of assessment instruments that capture early developmental skills include the Mullen Scales of Early Learning (MSEL; Mullen, 1995) and the Bayley Scales of Infant and Toddler Development-Third Edition (Bayley-III; Bayley, 2006). In schools, when these instruments are needed, it can be helpful to enlist the help of a colleague who assesses younger children and has access to and familiarity with the instruments.

Cognitive and developmental assessments provide a useful reference point for understanding a child's abilities, for comparing other aspects of functioning to conceptualize the child's needs, and for informing appropriate intervention plans. For example, a child with average cognitive abilities should typically have age-appropriate self-help skills. A discrepancy would suggest that a barrier exists. Examples of barriers may include (but are not limited to) impaired physical motor skills, anxiety, executive function deficits, pain, sleep disturbance, or sensory impairments.

Adaptive Skills Assessment

An adaptive skills assessment provides information about an individual's independence across areas of everyday functioning, ranging from navigating social interactions to maintaining adequate hygiene. Having a medical condition can complicate the usual course of acquiring independence. Sometimes the problem may be a direct result of the medical condition or its treatment (e.g., a child with a severe tremor might not have independence with safely using the stove or cutting with knives). Secondary factors may also be contributing (e.g., the child and family may view the child as vulnerable and may limit independence and access to situations perceived as risky). Again, having insight into the nature of the medical condition will help with accurate interpretation of scores on these measures. Examples of adaptive skills instruments include the Vineland Adaptive Behavior Scales-Third Edition (VABS-III; Sparrow, Cicchetti, & Saulnier, 2016), the Adaptive Behavior Assessment System-Third Edition (ABAS-3; Harrison & Oakland, 2015), and the Scales of Independent Behavior (SIB-R; Bruininks, Woodcock, Weatherman, & Hill, 1996).

Language and Motor Assessment

Speech and language skills are often assessed by the speech-language provider. This professional can be a valuable support when there are important differences between language and other skills, and modification of curriculum, visual supports, or preteaching of vocabulary are needed. Motor skills are typically assessed by an occupational or physical therapist, and the assessment will focus on the motor skills needed for school achievement. Handwriting is often an area of focus, and the professional can be an asset in making motor modifications and providing adaptive equipment or strategies to compensate when motor skills are an area of concern.

Academic Assessment

For our purposes, academic assessment refers to individually administered tests of academic proficiency, and most often it focuses on core aspects of reading, writing, and math. In the school setting, the assessments are often administered by a special education teacher or learning specialist. Often, the tests tap various aspects of each subject area, such as basic skills (e.g., word reading), applied skills (e.g., reading comprehension), and efficiency (e.g., reading fluency). Assessment can range from a broad review of all areas, to a more in-depth review in an area of specific concern. Examples of broad academic assessment instruments include the Wechsler Individual Achievement Test-Third Edition (WIAT-III; Psychological Corporation, 2009) and the Woodcock Johnson Tests of Achievement-Fourth Edition (WJ IV ACH; Schrank, Mather, McGrew, 2014). Examples of more in-depth assessment in a particular area include the Comprehensive Test of Phonological Processing-Second Edition (CTOPP-2; Wagner, Torgesen, Rashotte, & Pearson, 2013) and the Test of Mathematical Abilities-Third Edition (TOMA-3; Brown, Cronin, & Bryant, 2013). A common pitfall in educational testing is to use these scores alone to determine whether a student qualifies for supports. It is important to remember that testing is done under ideal circumstances, such as a quiet environment, and that the examiner provides one-on-one support to regulate attention and task engagement. Along with the individually administered tests, examiners should consider measures of everyday performance, such as report cards, school-administered standardized tests, and parent and teacher interviews.

Social, Emotional, and Behavioral Assessment

Having a chronic medical condition can be a severe stressor, and children and adolescents with medical conditions are at higher risk for social and emotional difficulties (Shin & Cho, 2012). Learning and behavioral difficulties may follow. It will be important to understand the social, emotional, and behavioral difficulties and to integrate them into the conceptualization and intervention planning for the child. Much can be gleaned from parent and teacher interviews and behavioral observations of the child. The usefulness of a child interview is variable depending on the child's skills; however, this should also be considered when planning the assessment. Behavior rating scales are often one of the most efficient ways to gather this information, and they have the benefit of providing a score as a reference of severity or concern. They also can be re-administered at multiple time points so that progress can be tracked. Rating scales often provide a springboard for additional interviewing. Examples of broad behavior rating scales include The Behavior Assessment System for Children-Third Edition (BASC-3; Reynolds & Kamphaus, 2015) and the Child Behavior Checklist (CBCL; Achenbach & Rescorla, 2001). Examples of more in-depth rating scales include the Screen for Child Anxiety Related Disorders (SCARED; Birmaher, Khetarpal, Cully, Brent, & Mackenzie, 1997) and the Conners Third Edition (Conners 3; Conners, 2008), a rating scale for ADHD symptoms. Note that self-, parent, and teacher report measures also invariably measure subjective aspects, such as distress, opinion about the reason for the behavior, and social desirability.

Observations

Observations of behavior by a trained, experienced, and a "fresh set of eyes" is a valuable component of assessment. This may include a description of behavior during assessment procedures (e.g., social skills at the time of greeting, language use, attention, and activity level). In the school setting, this often includes some observation of behavior during structured and unstructured times of the school day. On occasion, parents may bring in video recordings of behavior that occurs at home, which can be a helpful glimpse into behaviors that might not be revealed in the school setting.

Functional behavior analysis (FBA) is another useful approach to understanding the factors underlying a child's behavior (Sugai, Lewis-Palmer, & Hagan-Burke, 2000). In FBA, a behavioral specialist gathers information about concerning behaviors (e.g., destroying notebooks, breaking pencils, throwing objects), and then examines the surrounding factors. This might include: where the behavior occurs (e.g., language arts class), what tasks or events seem to precede the behavior (e.g., writing workshop), what the early warning signs might be (e.g., increased restlessness), and what happens afterward (e.g., the child is sent to the school counselor to cool down). The specialist then analyzes and interprets the information to provide the team with a better understanding of what is contributing to and maintaining the concerning behavior. For example, a student may be struggling with writing and has low frustration tolerance or advocacy skills. Disruptive behavior has been reinforced by going to the counselor's office and avoiding the writing assignment. The team can then work to change this sequence toward a better outcome. This could include skills intervention (e.g., writing help), modifications to demands (e.g., adjusting the task to be at a more manageable level), intervening early (e.g., assisting the student when he starts to fidget), and crafting responses that reinforce desired behavior (e.g., rewarding good effort, praise for "keeping your cool" and task completion; if a behavioral disturbance occurs, requiring the student to return to complete his work). For children with medical concerns, there may be specific symptoms related to their illness, that are not readily apparent to teachers or other adults, but that are affecting their behavior (e.g., stomach aches, nausea, migraines). These are often "setting events" or precipitating factors for challenging behaviors in children.

CONSIDERATIONS FOR BATTERY SELECTION, TESTING MODIFICATIONS, AND INTERPRETATION

Battery Selection

After becoming familiar with the student's history and current concerns, the examiner's next step is test selection. Many good test instruments exist, and examiners must make predictions regarding the goodness of fit between a child and the format and content of the test.

One of the challenges in choosing evaluation procedures is balancing assessment aimed at extracting the best of specific, isolated abilities versus gaining an understanding of functional ability. In most situations, tailoring the assessment to be more comprehensive and to capture more functional ability is advised. For example, when choosing a cognitive test for a child with a language disorder, it may be tempting to administer a test of nonverbal ability—such as the Wechsler Nonverbal Scale of Ability (WNV; Wechsler, & Naglieri, 2006) or the Leiter International Performance Scale-Third Edition (Roid, Miller, Pomplun, & Koch, 2013)—so that the student does not get penalized for limited language. There are times when this might be appropriate; however, the examiner must be cautious when presenting data, so as not to allow the team to confuse a score that reflects only nonverbal abilities with a more general indicator of intelligence. The effects of the student's language limitations must be captured elsewhere in the evaluation and considered when setting expectations and identifying appropriate supports. Another approach would be to administer a more comprehensive test of cognitive abilities, such as the WISC-V, which would say less about the child's "pure" nonverbal thinking abilities, but would offer insight into how the child might function and what supports might be needed within a classroom, where most of the instruction and performance is mediated by language (i.e., teachers explain concepts and students provide answers orally). Each of these approaches provides valuable information, and test selection may be determined by the specific questions that need to be answered.

Children thought to be developmentally close to age level can often be served well by a language-intensive measure, such as a WISC-V. Children for whom there are more broad developmental concerns may be better served by a test that has fewer language demands, such as the DAS-II. By reducing the language demands, the examiner will have to make fewer nonstandardized modifications to administration and is also less likely to mistakenly identify a language deficit as an overall cognitive deficit. It is also important to remember that many assessments are not validated for children with various developmental or medical conditions (e.g., children who are vision or hearing impaired, language impaired, or bilingual). In these cases, it may be important to work with a specialist (if available) who is familiar with best practices for assessment of children for whom the measures are not standardized.

In addition to choosing the best instrument to fit with the assessment questions, battery selection is also determined by logistic constraints. In the school setting, these may include parents' ability to participate in a clinical interview, time available to the examiners, student attendance, and access to materials and consultants that would facilitate the most appropriate assessment. Maintaining a flexible approach and shifting procedures to meet these logistic constraints is important. For example, with non-English-speaking parents, conducting a more robust clinical interview (with interpreter services) may be necessary in lieu of behavioral rating scales that may not be available in their language. If clinical providers are unavailable for consultation, it may be possible to send a list of questions and request that the provider leave a detailed confidential voice message with their thoughts.

Modifications

Since many testing instruments are developed and normed with a typical population, the standard procedures may be a poor fit for a student with a medical condition. There are times when the student's condition renders an assessment instrument utterly inappropriate (e.g., administering a visual reasoning task to a student who is blind). There are many more scenarios, however, in which useful information may be gained by making modifications to the standardized assessment procedures. These changes must always be explained in the report, and there must always be an accompanying note of caution regarding interpretation. Some modifications and examples are outlined below:

PHYSICAL STRUCTURE

Sometimes children who are very young or restless need the physical testing set-up to be different from standard procedures. It might be helpful to sit adjacent to, rather than across from, a student who gets up frequently, and perhaps position the furniture in a way that helps corral him or her. A student with low muscle tone might require carefully adjusted seating in order to remain engaged and to reduce fatigue. A student who is highly distractible may need objects removed from the room or furniture positioned in a way that simplifies the visual field. Some children may work best while standing, and many can benefit from the careful use of fidget toys.

ORGANIZATIONAL STRUCTURE

Sometimes, children who are reluctant, anxious, or have a hard time with task persistence need forecasting about what is happening. A simple visual schedule (empty boxes or circles, one for each task) can provide reassurance about progress, as subtests are "marked off" and steps to the next break are clearly laid out.

REINFORCEMENT

Often, students who struggle with attention, engagement, fatigue, or negativity will respond well to reinforcers, adjusted to the child's needs (e.g., a sticker after each subtest, an M&M after each item). This is also useful information when informing a starting point for interventions. A child who can delay gratification to receive a prize at the end of testing has different self-regulation skills from a child who needs an M&M after each item. While food reinforcers can be problematic when used daily, evaluation is a rare enough event that it can often be justified.

BEHAVIORAL REGULATION

With appropriate test selection and modifications, very few children are "untestable" due to behavior. Sometimes the test being administered is a poor fit for the child's skills, and behavioral dysregulation is a sign of frustration or confusion. Sometimes a student is slow to warm up but acts out instead of presenting as shy. In such cases, spending more time at the front-end building trust and rapport is needed. Sometimes students have primary problems with behavioral regulation, and the examiner must take steps to structure the assessment to allow an appropriate outlet for physical activity and self-directed behavior. For students with challenging behaviors, the examiner should readily consider basic accommodations, such as taking frequent physical breaks with the child (e.g., take a walk, do sprints in the hallway, run up and down a flight of stairs) and allowing alternative seating (e.g., allowing a child to stand up or lie on the floor during a subtest that does not require table work). Sometimes children require a higher level of modification, such as taking a stimulus book into the hall and answering one item after each sprint down the hallway. For an older child who is impulsive, gently placing your hands over the student's hands for several seconds may encourage him to consider all possible options before pointing to his answer. Examiners may be concerned that these modifications invalidate the assessment. While it is certainly important to document what was needed to support the student in completing the task, having a glimpse into the student's potential (with supports) is of greater value than a failed score and no good insight into whether the failure was due to lack of skills versus behavioral dysregulation. Additionally, students who take medications to improve behavioral regulation should take the medications as regularly prescribed, and efforts should be made to schedule the assessment at a time when the medication is active in their system.

TASK INSTRUCTIONS

Instructions should always be given in the standardized way first; however, the examiner must use judgment to determine the child's comprehension of instruction, and the examiner should make and document modifications if the child appears to not understand the standardized instructions. For example, if a child has a language impairment, it might be appropriate to use nonverbal gesture to "show" terms like *next to* or *on top of* when explaining a visual reasoning task. Similarly, if a child is showing evidence of slow processing, then giving an extra "teaching" or "sample" item at the beginning of a verbal reasoning task is an appropriate modification.

When making these changes, it is important to consider whether the modification is affecting the skill that is being assessed. For example, during a working memory task, a child might struggle to keep the rules in mind. In this situation, keeping rules in one's head is part of working memory. Therefore, making the modification of repeating the rules throughout the test would be inappropriate. In contrast, giving reminders about rules for tasks measuring visuospatial reasoning may be appropriate. Later, when interpreting, it is critical to describe the baseline response before modifications, the modifications made, and whatever change seemed to follow from those modifications.

INTERPRETATION AND RECOMMENDATIONS

Once the child's medical condition has been considered with regard to assessment procedures and modifications, the third area that requires consideration is interpretation of information gathered. This includes numeric scores as well as qualitative information, such as interview information, behavioral observations, and any modifications that were needed during the assessment. It may be helpful to keep a list of symptoms, medication side effects, and other medically related comments gathered from interviews that are helpful to have in mind. Referencing this list may be helpful when interpreting results.

Parents and teachers are often eager to understand whether a student's difficulties are attributable to a particular cause. Unfortunately, an assessment at one point in time usually cannot provide the answers. What it can do, however, is offer guidance regarding recommended next steps.

School-based evaluations are uniquely suited to provide useful recommendations, as the examiner is intimately familiar with the setting and the practical realities of implementation. The school team is encouraged to consider the options for interventions, accommodations, and modifications that are commonly offered in school, but also to consider new suggestions unique to the child. It may be helpful to draw from the modifications and supports trialed during the evaluation to promote successful participation.

The team must also consider the consistency with which supports must be provided. Some needs require that supports be provided consistently (e.g., a student with low muscle tone might need specialized seating throughout the day to reduce fatigue). Other needs may only require occasional support (e.g., a student with migraines receiving a teacher's class notes only during episodes of migraine).

MONITORING PROGRESS

Monitoring progress is a critical component of determining if a student is benefiting from intervention strategies. The monitoring occurs after the original assessment is complete and intervention approaches have been put into place for a period of time. When making a plan to monitor progress, goals should be "appropriate and measurable," meaning they should relate to the child's present level of performance and there should be a way to quantify them and to communicate results to parents and other team members. Teachers are active collectors and reporters in this process and, as such, it is important to make data collection tools "user friendly." Case managers must consider practical factors when designing a plan for monitoring progress. An example of this is a communication notebook that goes back and forth from home to school and highlights major areas of difficulty or improvements. Teachers and families can make weekly entries to promote communication and consistency in approaches. The book does not have to involve free-form writing. It can use personalized checklists to track certain behaviors and interventions. Handout 7.1 contains a sample checklist that can be individualized for students with a variety of health issues and minimizes the time needed for teachers or case managers to complete it each week.

It is important to keep in mind that there may be many goals or intervention strategies for a child, and monitoring all of the strategies at once may not be feasible. Therefore, the school team can choose one or two strategies to focus on and monitor, then, once specific goals have been met, the team can move on to implementing and monitoring others. The case manager can make this accessible to the busy teacher by creating a system that requires only the checking of boxes (similar to the format in the example above), perhaps weekly.

When determining a time frame to assess progress, a general starting point is to collect information monthly. For a student with an individualized education plan (IEP), progress will be monitored based on the IEP goals, which should also be specific, attainable, and measurable. For students without an IEP, their progress will be monitored along with their peers' progress. The monitoring frequency (e.g., weekly, daily, every 6 weeks) can also be guided by the likely rate of change for the particular intervention. For example, scheduling physical breaks to promote alertness and task completion may yield more immediate results, and the team may have an impression about progress made after a week or two. In contrast, teaching and implementing self-advocacy skills needed to effectively catch up on learning and assignments after an absence will need a longer monitoring interval.

There may also be different types of progress monitoring, ranging from less structured weekly check-ins with the student's teacher to highly structured, data-based approaches. Creating a checklist of all of the components of an intervention that must be in place could be helpful in tracking the success of interventions. School teams may have their own measures that are routinely used. At other times, it might be most useful to develop an individualized data collection measure to track a child's progress over time. When selecting a tool for monitoring progress, the instrument should be closely tied to the specific intervention strategies and able to pick up improvements or changes made through intervention, have a format that is usable for teachers, and not interfere with the teacher's other classroom responsibilities.

For students with medical conditions, it is important to frame progress within the context of the condition, particularly if progress is slowed. The school team will likely need to track related areas of concern for children with medical complexities like absences, exacerbations of their condition, or medication changes. The team may find it helpful to track these factors on a calendar to monitor changes over time. Parents and caregivers will also be helpful in monitoring changes outside of school. As part of this process, it is important that the school team have ongoing communication with families and other providers involved in the child's care (e.g., doctors, outside therapists). Furthermore, new issues may arise after the assessment phase that may need to be addressed with specific interventions (e.g., school refusal, behavioral challenges, new learning concerns), and consistent monitoring will allow the school team to pick up on these changes.

If a child is making less progress, is it because the medical condition is producing more symptoms, or because there is an inherent challenge with the intervention strategies being used? For example, a child with poorly controlled type 1 diabetes may continue to exhibit academic challenges despite certain intervention strategies. The challenges may be due to behavioral issues or underlying learning issues, for example. Behavior challenges that are secondary to a medical condition may actually affect learning more than the medical condition alone (McCarthy, Lindgren, Mengeling, Tsalikian, & Engvall, 2002). For a child with type 1 diabetes and concurrent behavior challenges, glucose management may be difficult due to resistant behaviors, resulting in increased episodes of hyperglycemia, which affect cognitive skills, attention, working memory, and sleep (Kucera & Sullivan, 2011).

Case Example of Monitoring Progress

Haley is a 9-year-old girl with inflammatory bowel disease. Her school team determined that she would benefit from unlimited bathroom passes, access to the clinic throughout the day, and a behavioral strategy. Below is the monitoring form the team developed to track her progress:

Date	Tardy or absent	Number of times leaving the classroom	Difficulty participating in class activity (yes/no)

Hayley's teacher was asked to fill out this brief form each day, collecting information from the classroom's restroom sign-out sheet, and her case manager was responsible for collecting and tallying the data. Her teacher found the checklist to be very easy and quick to complete, thus increasing her ability to monitor the student over time. While school nurses develop healthcare plans that provide detailed instructions for management of health conditions within the school setting, this example addresses behavioral and learning components that are monitored by the rest of the school team.

Making Modifications to Intervention Strategies

Measuring intervention effectiveness is data-based and is driven by goals on the student's IEP or by the observations made during assessment. Measuring the outcomes of an intervention shows if the intervention is working, quantifies the changes made, and points to changes that are needed to improve effectiveness. This is meant to be a continuous process, and having a plan in place to measure progress over time will allow the team to evaluate changes throughout the school year. The student's team (i.e., case manager, teacher, school nurse, and other important providers) should meet regularly throughout the school year to share information, to discuss intervention outcomes, and to make appropriate changes. It is often helpful to chart results and track them over time to better inform future decisions.

Children with complex medical needs are likely to require a variety of interventions (e.g., medication management at school, behavioral contracts, management of absences, social and emotional support, environmental supports). Depending on the type, severity, and course of the medical condition, children may require an increase in intervention supports and changes to individualized healthcare plans (e.g., when asthma attacks increase during winter months, when transitioning back to school after a hospital stay). Consistent and frequent communication with the student's parents, caregivers, and school nurse continues to be important, particularly as the school team is evaluating whether interventions are helping. Amid complex and often overlapping factors, it is difficult but important to determine whether the interventions are indeed helping.

CONCLUSION

Serving children with medical conditions in the school setting begins with the assessment process and continues with ongoing monitoring and intervention. It is crucial to have standardized procedures for evaluation; however, there must be flexibility and room for clinical judgment when working to understand a medically complex child. This flexibility will likely lead to developing nuanced interventions that work. While this chapter provides general guidelines for school teams to follow, it is important to remember that each process should be individualized to the child. It is our hope that this information will help school teams think through some of the complexities as they work to understand their children and embark on the important task of teaching them.

REFERENCES

Achenbach, T. M., & Rescorla, L. A. (2001). *Manual for the ASEBA school-age forms & profiles.* Burlington: Research Center for Children, Youth and Families, University of Vermont.

Lewallen, T. C., Hunt, H., Potts-Datema, W., Zaza, S., & Giles, W. (2015). The whole school, whole community, whole child model: A new approach for improving educational attainment and healthy development for students. *Journal of School Health, 85*, 729–739.

Basch, C. E. (2011). Healthier students are better learners: A missing link in school reforms to close the achievement gap. *Journal of School Health, 8*, 593–598.

Bayley, N. (2006). *Bayley Scales of Infant and Toddler Development* (3rd ed.). San Antonio, TX: Harcourt Assessment.

Birmaher, B., Khetarpal, S., Cully, M., Brent, D., & Mackenzie, S. (1997). Screen for Child Anxiety Related Emotional Disorders (SCARED): Scale construction and psychometric characteristics. *Journal of the American Academy of Child & Adolescent Psychiatry, 36*, 545–553. doi:10.1097/00004583-199704000-00018

Brown, V., Cronin, M. E., & Bryant, D. (2013). *Test of Mathematical Abilities* (3rd ed.). Austin, TX: Pro-Ed.

Bruininks, R. H., Woodcock, R. W., Weatherman, R. E., & Hill, B. K. (1996). *Scales of Independent Behavior—Revised.* Itasca, IL: Riverside Publishing.

Claar, R. L., Simons, L. E., & Logan, D. E. (2008). Parental response to children's pain: The moderating impact of children's emotional distress on symptoms and disability. *Pain, 138*, 172–179.

Conners, C. K. (2008). *Conners 3rd edition manual.* Toronto, Canada: Multi-Health Systems.

Ellingsen, K. M. (2016). Standardized assessment of cognitive development. In A. Garro (Ed.), *Early childhood assessment in school and clinical child psychology.* New York, NY: Springer-Verlag.

Elliott, C. D. (2007). *Differential Ability Scales* (2nd ed). San Antonio, TX: Harcourt Assessment.

Harrison, P., & Oakland, T. (2015). *Adaptive Behavior Assessment System* (3rd ed.). Torrance, CA: Western Psychological Services.

Immelt, S. (2006). Psychological adjustment in young children with chronic medical conditions. *Journal of Pediatric Nursing, 21*, 362–377.

Kucera, M., & Sullivan, A. L. (2011). The educational implications of type 1 diabetes mellitus: A review of research and recommendations for school psychological practice. *Educational Psychology, 6*, 587–603.

Litt, J. S., & McCormick, M. C. (2016). The impact of special health care needs on academic achievement in children born prematurely. *Academic Pediatrics, 16*, 350–357.

McCarthy, A. M., Lindgren, S., Mengeling, M. A., Tsalikian, E., & Engvall, J. C. (2002). Effects of diabetes on learning in children. *Pediatrics, 109*, 1–12.

Mullen, E. M. (1995). *Mullen Scales of Early Learning* (AGS ed.). Circle Pines, MN: American Guidance Service Inc.

Peterson, C. C., & Palermo, T. M. (2004). Parental reinforcement of recurrent pain: The moderating impact of child depression and anxiety on functional disability. *Journal of Pediatric Psychology, 29*, 331–341.

Pinquart, M., & Teubert, D. (2012). Academic, physical, and social functioning of children and adolescents with chronic physical illness: A meta-analysis. *Journal of Pediatric Psychology, 37*, 376–389.

Psychological Corporation. (2009). *Wechsler Individual Achievement Test* (3rd ed.). San Antonio, TX: Pearson.

Reynolds, C. R., & Kamphaus, R. W. (2015). *Behavior Assessment System for Children* (3rd ed.; BASC-3). Bloomington, MN: Pearson.

Roid, G. H. (2003). *Stanford-Binet Intelligence Scales* (5th ed.; SB:V). Itasca, IL: Riverside Publishing.

Roid, G. H., Miller, L. J., Pomplun, M., & Koch, C. (2013). *Leiter International Performance Scale* (3rd ed.). Wood Dale, IL: Stoelting.

Sattler, J. M. (2018). *Assessment of children: Cognitive foundations and applications* (6th ed.). La Mesa, CA: Jerome M. Sattler Publisher.

Schrank, F. A., Mather, N., & McGrew, K. S. (2014). *Woodcock-Johnson IV Test of Achievement*. Rolling Meadows, IL: Riverside.

Shin, Y. M., & Cho, S. M. (2012). Emotional and behavioral problems in children with chronic physical illness. *Annals of Pediatric Endocrinology & Metabolism, 17*, 1–9.

Sparrow, S. S., Cicchetti, D. V., & Saulnier, C. A. (2016). *Vineland Adaptive Behavior Scales* (3rd ed.; VABS-III). Bloomington, MN: Pearson.

Sugai, G., Lewis-Palmer, T., & Hagan-Burke, S. (2000). Overview of the functional behavior assessment process. *Exceptionality, 8*, 149–160.

Vermaes, I. P. R, van Susante, A. M. J., & van Bakel, H. J. A. (2013). Psychological functioning of siblings in families of children with chronic health conditions: A meta-analysis. *Journal of Pediatric Psychology, 37*, 166–184.

Wagner, R., Torgesen, J., Rashotte, C., & Pearson, N. A. (2013). *Comprehensive Test of Phonological Processing* (2nd ed.). Austin, TX: Pro-Ed.

Wechsler, D. (2014). *Wechsler Intelligence Scale for Children* (5th ed.). San Antonio, TX: Psychological Corporation.

Wechsler, D., & Naglieri, J. A. (2006). *Wechsler Nonverbal Scale of Ability*. San Antonio, TX: Harcourt Assessment.

HANDOUT 7.1.

SYMPTOM TRACKER

Name:_____

Date: _____

	WORSE	SAME	BETTER
1. Migraine _____	☐	☐	☐
2. Attention in class _____	☐	☐	☐
3. Nausea _____	☐	☐	☐
4. _____	☐	☐	☐

Current Medication or Intervention

_____

_____

_____

Prescribing Physician

Name:_____

Fax: _____

Release dated: _____

8

Classroom and Schoolwide, Universal Health-Promotion Strategies

KATHY L. BRADLEY-KLUG, COURTNEY LYNN, AND KATHERINE L. WESLEY ■

It is estimated that as many as 25% of children and adolescents in the United States have a chronic health condition requiring coordination of services for them to be successful in the educational setting (Bradley-Klug & Armstrong, 2014; Miller, Coffield, Leroy, & Wallin, 2016). Furthermore, conditions like asthma, autism spectrum disorder (ASD), and attention deficit hyperactivity disorder (ADHD) are reportedly on the rise, resulting in a forecast that even greater numbers of youth in schools will be affected by a pediatric health condition (American Academy of Pediatrics, 2016). In order to address the needs of youth in our schools, school-based and health professionals must concentrate on health promotion and systems-level coordination of services.

This chapter focuses on specific classroom and schoolwide, universal health-promotion strategies that may be implemented in the educational setting. Specifically, the topics of healthy eating and exercise are covered, followed by a discussion of sleep hygiene and the integration of mindfulness training into the educational curriculum. The chapter concludes with a focus on school-based consultation and the role of mental health professionals in providing services to students with chronic health conditions.

HEALTHY EATING

The National Health and Nutrition Examination Survey (NHANES) reported that the prevalence of obesity among children and adolescents 2 to 19 years old is

17% (Ogden et al., 2016). Healthy eating is essential to growth, development, and wellness across the lifespan. It is also linked to a variety of positive outcomes, including reduced risk of health problems like cardiovascular disease, type 2 diabetes, obesity, and some cancers (U.S. Department of Health and Human Services [DHHS] and U.S. Department of Agriculture [USDA], 2015). Healthy eating patterns may be particularly relevant for children and adolescents with health conditions involving the metabolic, cardiovascular, pulmonary, or gastrointestinal systems, which can be negatively affected by obesity (Centers for Disease Control and Prevention [CDC], 2016; Daniels, 2006).

Student and Family Education

The *Dietary Guidelines for Americans 2015–2020* (DHHS & USDA, 2015) defined a healthy diet as one that includes a variety of vegetables, fruits, grains (especially whole grains), fat-free or low-fat dairy, oils, and a variety of proteins. Additionally, a nutritious diet limits added fats, sugars, and sodium (DHHS & USDA, 2015). Schools can play a foundational role in helping children learn healthy eating patterns and to make good choices when eating. Universal interventions for healthy eating should focus on promoting awareness and education about healthy eating patterns in the classroom and implementing policies or practices that can improve consumption of nutritious foods throughout the educational system.

The USDA has provided several tools and resources for teachers and schools to use in the classroom to provide education about healthy eating and to increase awareness of healthy eating patterns among children and adolescents. In 2010, the USDA introduced the MyPlate symbol, along with the 2010 *Dietary Guidelines for Americans,* as a visual tool to increase awareness and to provide education about making healthy eating choices (USDA, 2011). The MyPlate symbol outlines the five food groups and shows recommended amounts of each food group to include on your plate. Further information about each of the food groups, how to choose healthy foods, ways to change eating habits, and ways to create a healthy eating pattern, as well as classroom resources, can be found on the MyPlate website (see Table 8.1). For high school teachers, nutrition lesson plans are available using SuperTracker, a food and physical activity tracking tool (USDA, 2016). Each lesson plan is composed of preparation steps, learning objectives, teaching instructions, and a handout for students.

The CDC (2011) recommends that health-education programs address student knowledge, attitudes, skills, and experiences in order to promote healthy eating. Health-education nutrition programs should focus on targeting specific behaviors, should have multiple components (e.g., food service, classroom nutrition education, physical activity, parent or peer involvement), should include family involvement, should be age, culturally, and developmentally appropriate, should offer interactive learning approaches, and should provide professional development to teachers and staff (Briggs, Fleischhacker, & Mueller, 2010; CDC, 2011; Roseman, Riddell, & Haynes, 2011). The CDC Health Education Curriculum Analysis Tool

Table 8.1. Universal Health-Promotion Resources

Topic	Resource	Description
Healthy Eating	MyPlate (USDA, 2015) www.ChooseMyPlate.gov	Information about each of the food groups, how to choose healthy foods, and ways to change eating habits and create a healthy eating pattern. Provides games, activities, and recipes for children that can be used during nutrition lessons in the classroom.
Healthy Eating	SuperTracker (USDA, 2016) www.SuperTracker.usda.gov	Six lesson plans on healthy snacks, the five food groups, daily recommended calorie intake, tracking and analyzing nutrition intake, how to plan and create a healthy menu, the importance of physical activity, and information on personal calorie needs.
Healthy Eating	Health Education Curriculum Analysis Tool (HECAT; CDC, 2012) www.cdc.gov/healthyyouth/ HECAT/	A tool for educators to analyze health education curricula.
Physical Education	Physical Education Curriculum Analysis Tool (PECAT; CDC, 2006) https://www.cdc.gov/ healthyschools/pecat/ index.htm	A tool for educators to compare physical education curricula to the national physical education standards. It also can assist educators in choosing, modifying, or creating a quality physical education curriculum.
Sleep	Sleep Disturbance Scale for Children (SDSC; Bruni et al., 1996)	A 27-item scale that is completed by parents of children and adolescents and consists of six factors: initiating and maintaining sleep, sleep breathing disorders, disorders of arousal, sleep–wake transition disorders, disorders of excessive somnolence, and sleep hyperhidrosis.
Sleep	Pediatric Daytime Sleepiness Scale (PDSS; Drake et al., 2003) http://corporate.psionline. com/support/talent- assessment-test-support/ tos/develop-local-norms/	An 8-item, self-report measure that can be used in schools to assess for sleepiness in children 11–15 years old. Clinicians can create local norms by identifying students at or above the 95th percentile for their individual school on the PDSS website.

(continued)

Table 8.1. CONTINUED

Topic	Resource	Description
Sleep	Sleep Disorders Inventory for Students (SDIS; Luginbuehl et al., 2008) http://sleepdisorderhelp.com/	A screening measure for sleep disorders with two forms, the SDIS-Children's Form (for children 2–10 years old) and SDIS-Adolescent Form (for those 11–18 years old). Contains 25–30 items assessing a variety of sleep disorders along with an additional 10 general health questions.
Sleep	American Academy of Sleep Medicine (n.d.) http://school.sleepeducation.com/	Lesson plans for teachers on sleep hygiene, sleep disorders, animals and biomes and sleep, and sleep careers.
Mindfulness	Mindful Moment Program (Holistic Life Foundation, 2016) http://hlfinc.org/programs-services/mindful-moment-program/	Consists of a 15-minute breath work and meditation recording that plays over the school intercom every morning. Includes training for educators and parents.
Mindfulness	MindUp (The Hawn Foundation, n.d.) https://mindup.org	A mindfulness-based social and emotional learning program that includes 15 lesson plans for grades K–8, divided into four units. The units focus on 1) learning about the brain and an introduction to mindfulness, 2) broadening mindfulness to the senses, 3) developing a positive mindset through social and emotional skills, and 4) putting mindfulness into action by engaging in activities like random acts of kindness. Offers in-service training for educators.

(HECAT; CDC, 2012) is a resource for school and district personnel to help them analyze health-education curricula and make decisions regarding selecting, developing, or improving health-education curricula.

Environmental Supports

In addition to health and nutrition education, the school environment is an important component of helping students make healthy eating choices.

Recommendations to encourage a healthy eating environment include providing ample time to gather and eat meals, scheduling recess before lunch, reducing wait times in food lines, providing opportunities to wash or sanitize hands before meals, offering safe and sufficient space and facilities for eating, providing students access to drinking fountains, allowing students to carry water bottles in class, and ensuring water fountains are clean and functioning properly (CDC, 2011; Cook-Cottone, Tribole, & Tylaka, 2013).

School Gardens

Another environmental intervention with promise is school gardens. School gardens are designed to be a hands-on instructional environment to increase exposure to, access to, and consumption of fruits and vegetables in children and adolescents by improving their knowledge of, and attitudes toward, healthy foods. A review of school garden programs suggests they can improve fruit and vegetable consumption by students, provide opportunities for hands-on learning, and increase knowledge of agriculture (Berezowitz, Bontrager Yoder, & Schoeller, 2015).

Food Offerings

A number of strategies focusing on choice and marketing also have been shown to be effective in increasing selection and consumption of fruits and vegetables and improving healthy eating behaviors in school cafeterias. Offering students a selection of more than one fruit or vegetable increases fruit and vegetable consumption. Schools can implement this strategy by allowing students to choose one fruit or vegetable from a selection of three (Hakim & Meissen, 2013) or by providing a salad bar (Slusser, Cumberland, Browdy, Lange, & Neumann, 2007). Another strategy utilizing choice is to have students choose their lunch entrée in the morning. Elementary students who preordered their lunch entrée chose a healthier option more frequently than students who chose their entrée in the lunch line (Hanks, Just, & Wansink, 2013). Preordering can be implemented using paper-and-pencil or computer-based systems. Marketing also can be an effective tool in increasing healthy eating behaviors. Labeling healthy foods with creative names (e.g., "X-ray Vision Carrots", "Silly Dilly Green Beans") can both increase selection and consumption of vegetables in elementary schools (Wansink, Just, Payne, & Klinger, 2012) and serve as a cost- and labor-effective intervention.

Nutritious eating practices are essential to the health and development of all children and adolescents. Establishing positive eating patterns in childhood improves healthy eating across the lifespan and can improve outcomes and decrease risk for certain health conditions. Schools are an optimal environment for providing education and knowledge about, and improving attitudes toward, healthy eating. In addition, a variety of cost-effective interventions can be implemented in the school environment to increase exposure and access and to improve consumption of fruits and vegetables.

PHYSICAL ACTIVITY AND EXERCISE

In addition to nutritious eating, a healthy lifestyle also includes regular physical activity and exercise. Children 6 years old and older should engage in 60 minutes of exercise a day (DHHS, 2008). For children, the best form of exercise is active play that is moderate to vigorous in intensity, such as playing tag, walking, riding a bike to school, or playing soccer. Although a variety of aerobic, muscle-strengthening, and bone-strengthening activities should be included in daily physical activity, the amount of time spent in physical activity is most important for a healthy lifestyle (DHHS, 2008). Schools provide an excellent opportunity for children to engage in a variety of physical activities during recess, physical education (PE) class, physical activity breaks, before-school and after-school programs, and walk- and bicycle-to-school programs (CDC, 2011). Educators are able to promote physical activity by providing opportunities for both structured and unstructured play, encouraging staff to be active role models for students, teaching skills needed to safely engage in physical activities, encouraging activities that promote engagement in physical activity throughout students' lives, and providing a comprehensive school-based physical activity program (CDC, 2009; DHHS, 2008).

Physical Activity Programs

A comprehensive physical activity program begins with quality PE and includes recess, physical activity breaks, intramural sports, interscholastic sports, and walk- and bike-to-school programs (CDC, 2009). Quality PE is age and skill appropriate, meets all skill levels and needs, teaches skills, promotes knowledge for a lifetime of physical activity, requires students to be active more than 50% of class, and is fun for students (CDC, 2009). Educators should choose an evidence-based PE curriculum as the foundation of interventions and strategies to improve physical activity at school. The Physical Education Curriculum Analysis Tool (PECAT) can be used by educators to help select an appropriate curriculum (see Table 8.1).

Physical Activity Breaks

One strategy to increase physical activity throughout the school day is incorporating physical activity into the classroom. Teacher implementation of activity breaks is related to increased physical activity (Whitt-Glover, Ham, & Yancey, 2011). This can be accomplished by incorporating physical activity into academic lessons and instruction time or by building in physical activity breaks in the classroom.

Programs like TAKE 10! (Stewart, Dennison, Kohl, & Doyle, 2004) and Instant Recess (Whitt-Glover et al., 2011) are evidence-based programs that incorporate 10-minute activity breaks and physical movement into academic lessons and are shown to increase student physical activity. Activity breaks use physical activity to reinforce academic skills being taught and are implemented during regular class time in place of a seated or sedentary activity. Multiple activity breaks throughout the day can play a key role in helping children achieve the recommended 60 minutes of physical activity per day. Students who engaged in more than one physical activity break had a small, but significant, increase in moderate to vigorous physical activity per day at school compared to students who did not engage in physical activity breaks or only engaged in one activity break (Carlson et al., 2015).

Recess

Another opportunity for schools to promote physical activity is during recess. Recess allows children opportunities to engage in games and to use skills they learned in PE class (CDC, 2009). Ready for Recess (Huberty et al., 2011) is an intervention designed to make the playground/recess environment more conducive to physical activity by using activity zones. For this intervention, the playground is divided into activity zones, with each zone containing a different activity along with the appropriate equipment and space to engage in the activity. Each zone should allow for multiple games and repetitions of the same activity. Zones are labeled with the activity and students help set up each zone prior to recess. Recess monitors are trained on the rules and games in each zone, PE teachers and recess monitors develop and plan for the zones, and activities are changed when a zone shows less participation over time. A pilot study of Ready for Recess indicates that this program can increase both moderate and vigorous physical activity in children during recess (Huberty et al., 2011).

A significant concern in the literature is the decrease in PE and recess in the schools. Currently, only Oregon and the District of Columbia meet the weekly recommendations for PE at the elementary and middle school levels (SHAPE America, 2016). In addition, most states allow students to waive, receive an exemption, or use a substitute for PE. A comprehensive physical activity program addresses policy, curriculum, instruction, and assessment of student PE and provides equal opportunities for all students to learn and establish healthy habits at school. Educators should be active in not only implementing strategies to improve physical activity in the classroom, but also advocating for policy decisions that support comprehensive physical activity programs.

SLEEP

The American Academy of Sleep Medicine recommends that children 3 to 5 years old sleep 10 to 13 hours per 24 hours, including naps (Paruthi et al., 2016).

School-age children 6 to 12 years old should sleep 9 to 12 hours per 24 hours and adolescents 13 to 18 years old should sleep 8 to 10 hours per 24 hours in order to promote optimal health (Paruthi et al., 2016). However, in a national poll conducted by the National Sleep Foundation (2014), parents estimated that their children 6 to 10 years old receive 8.9 hours of sleep per night on average, children 11 to 12 years old sleep 8.2 hours, children 13 to 14 years old sleep 7.7 hours, and children 15 to 17 years old sleep 7.1 hours. Clearly, there is a discrepancy between the recommended hours of sleep per night and the estimated hours of sleep per night.

The detriments of obtaining insufficient sleep are numerous and include increased conduct problems (Chervin, Dillon, Archbold, & Ruzicka, 2003), poor working memory performance (Steenari et al., 2003), and anxiety and depression (Alfano, Zakem, Costa, Taylor, & Weems, 2009). Insufficient sleep is also associated with self-harm, obesity, inattentiveness, and hyperactivity (Paruthi et al., 2016). In a prospective study of 1,046 children, sleep duration and executive function, behavior, and social-emotional functioning were assessed at 1, 2, 4, 5, and 6 years after birth (Taveras, Rifas-Shiman, Bub, Gillman, & Oken, 2017). Children who received insufficient sleep from ages 3 to 4 years and 5 to 7 years had worse maternal and teacher-reported scores on measures of executive functioning, behavior, and social-emotional functioning than children who received sufficient sleep (Taveras et al., 2017). It is clear that sleep plays a primary role in children's success in school. Therefore, a universal program for sleep hygiene should be implemented in schools to promote better academic and behavioral performance.

Sleep Education Programs

A high-quality sleep education program includes various topics, such as sleep knowledge, weekend and weekday sleep behavior, and sleep hygiene (Chung, Chan, Lam, Lai, & Yeung, 2017). Several programs have been implemented in schools (see Beijamini & Louzada, 2012; Rigney et al., 2015; Wing et al., 2015) and a systematic review showed benefits in total weekend and weekday sleep and mood immediately after the intervention, but the effects were not sustained long term (Chung et al., 2017). Several do's and don'ts regarding sleep education program implementation were identified by Blunden and Rigney (2015) that could help to create more lasting positive changes.

Parental Involvement

One way to increase the chances of success for sleep education programs is to involve parents, because they are often part of the sleep routines established at home (Blunden & Rigney, 2015). A simple strategy to increase parental involvement is to send home handouts of information discussed in the program. The handouts can include information about the suggested amount of sleep per night, tips for sleep hygiene (e.g., removing the television from the bedroom, limiting electronic use after a certain time), as well as how to complete a sleep diary. Another way to involve families is to invite them to an information evening and have students present different information they have learned about sleep.

Class Curriculum

To reinforce sleep education, the information should be included in other curriculum areas besides PE and health classes (Blunden & Rigney, 2015). When possible, examples of the benefits of sleep, as well as the detriments of too little sleep, should be used in science, math, and reading lessons, among others. For example, in math, students could keep a sleep diary and graph the number of hours of sleep per night. The class could then compile their data and the teacher could guide the class in drawing conclusions about the data. The teacher can also use the data to illustrate concepts like mean, median, and mode. In science, teachers could discuss the similarities and differences in sleep patterns among various species and have students complete a Venn diagram.

Universal Screening

Universal screening for sleep insufficiency and sleep hygiene using validated instruments is recommended to identify individuals at risk for sleep problems, as well as to assess the overall effectiveness of a school's sleep intervention program. Universal screening procedures are intended to be administered to all students to identify those at risk for future difficulties (Albers & Kettler, 2014), in this instance difficulties with sleep hygiene or sleep insufficiency. Screening for sleep insufficiency and sleep hygiene can be incorporated into existing structures for universal screening (e.g., screening for reading difficulties, mental health screening) already established at schools. The screening data are then easily integrated into a multitiered system of supports (MTSS) delivery framework.

Screening procedures for social, emotional, behavioral, and academic difficulties have been implemented in primary care settings with children as young as 6 months old (Briggs et al., 2012). In a school setting, screening for sleep difficulties should begin as early as pre-kindergarten, with parents as informants. Parents can remain the primary informants until children are around 11 years old, at which age both parents and children can provide reports. Depending on the exact sleep measure selected by the school, there will be different responses to a positive or negative screen. Various measures, such as the Sleep Disorders Inventory for Students (SDIS; Luginbuehl, Bradley-Klug, Ferron, Anderson, & Benbadis, 2008), have clinical cut-off scores for having normal sleep, caution range of sleep, or high risk of a sleep disorder. The ranges can correspond to Tier 1, 2, and 3, respectively, in the MTSS framework. For measures without predetermined cut-off scores, schools can create their own local norms to identify the top 2% to 7% of students who are high risk, the 15% of students at medium risk, and the bottom 80% of students at low risk of sleep difficulties. Schools also can use a predetermined criterion for identifying students at risk of sleep difficulties. For example, in screening for the number of hours of sleep per night, students can screen positive if they fall below the American Academy of Sleep Medicine's sleep recommendations for their age group.

MINDFULNESS

Originally derived from Buddhist tradition, mindfulness is described as being fully present in the moment without judgment (Kabat-Zinn, 1994). Mindfulness has gained attention in the scientific literature and has been used in many interventions to help treat several disorders in adults, including depression, anxiety, and chronic pain (Baer, 2003).

Mindfulness Education

School-based mindfulness programs are gaining popularity. Zenner, Herrnleben-Kurz, and Walach (2014) conducted a meta-analysis of mindfulness-based interventions in schools. Results indicated that these interventions were able to increase cognitive performance for attention and learning as well as to increase resilience and decrease stress, especially when interventions were delivered frequently and students practiced at home. These results are considered preliminary given the small number of studies included in the analyses. Components of school-based mindfulness programs include breath awareness, body-scan, yoga, and psychoeducation (Zenner et al., 2014). Various individuals can deliver mindfulness activities. Zenner and colleagues (2014) found that most programs were delivered by an outside (non-school-related) trainer (63%), followed by a classroom teacher (29%) and a combination of teacher and outside trainer (8%). Mindfulness programs can be implemented at a targeted level for students at high risk of mental health difficulties; however, all students may benefit from universal mindfulness practices. In addition, when teachers take part in personal mindfulness practices, they can indirectly benefit students by increasing teachers' self-efficacy (Poulin, Mackenzie, Soloway, & Karayolas, 2008) as well as by increasing teachers' overall well-being and their effectiveness in delivering emotional and academic support to students (Jennings & Greenberg, 2009).

Teacher Practices

Several comprehensive mindfulness programs exist for teachers that focus on active listening, emotional awareness, empathy, and compassion (Meiklejohn et al.,

2012). Teachers can utilize loving-kindness practices in which they imagine different individuals being healthy, happy, and at peace; first they imagine themselves, then a loved one, then a neutral person, and last someone they find challenging (Jennings, Snowberg, Coccia, & Greenberg, 2011). Teachers also can develop a meditation practice of their own, either by using an application on their phone or by finding materials online. In addition, schools can offer teachers mindfulness practices, such as yoga, before or after school.

Classwide Practices

Many structured mindfulness programs occur at a classroom level. Practices incorporated in these programs include present-moment awareness as well as kindness and compassion. Random acts of kindness or creating a gratitude journal are two interventions that have been shown to increase well-being (Bono, Froh, & Forrett, 2014; Layous, Nelson, Oberle, Schonert-Reichl, & Lyubomirsky, 2012) and these practices can be used as a way to cultivate kindness and compassion. Another activity is a guided imagery practice, in which students imagine another person in a place that makes them happy and where they are safe (Flook et al., 2010). In order to cultivate present-moment awareness, teachers can lead students in a mindfulness-of-sound activity in which students each raise a hand, the teacher rings a bell, and the students put their hands down when they can no longer hear the bell's tone. The teacher can then ring the bell again when everyone's hand is down. Students will likely put their hands down at different times and the teacher can lead a class discussion about what the experience was like, prompting and modeling such things as the mind's wandering and thinking about other topics or students' comparing themselves to other students in the class (Turrell, Bell, & Wilson, 2016). Another mindfulness activity that promotes nonjudgmental awareness is observation of objects. For this activity, each student can look at their palm for a specified period of time and practice objectively observing what they see (e.g., the color of the skin) without making assumptions (e.g., "My palm is red, so I must be hot" ; Turrell et al., 2016).

Schoolwide Practices

In addition to comprehensive mindfulness curricula, there are several practices that schools can implement to create an environment that promotes mindfulness (see Table 8.1). For example, schools can dedicate a certain time of day for a moment of mindfulness and breath work. Mindfulness recordings and breathing exercises can be played over the school's intercom system or in individual classrooms. In addition, schools can send home psychoeducational materials about mindfulness to parents, including tips for ways to practice mindfulness at home.

SCHOOL-BASED CONSULTATION AND IMPLEMENTATION OF UNIVERSAL HEALTH-PROMOTION PROGRAMS

School-based teams, including school psychologists, nurses, guidance counselors, social workers, and administrators, are trained professionals who can provide support within the school system for youth and their families, particularly those with chronic healthcare concerns (Bradley-Klug & Armstrong, 2014; Miller et al., 2016). When collaborative efforts across disciplines are increased within a problem-solving framework, the efficiency and effectiveness of prevention and intervention strategies will increase. A comprehensive, integrated student service model that engages students, teachers, school staff, parents, and community stakeholders (such as medical providers) will be most practical, particularly for implementing universal health-promotion and prevention strategies.

For the interdisciplinary partnership to exist, all parties must communicate and collaborate. In this case, *communication* is defined as a one-way sharing of information related to a particular student, whereas *collaboration* is defined as bidirectional, ongoing sharing of information to promote positive outcomes (Bradley-Klug et al., 2013). Studies to date have shown that, although professionals may see the benefits of communication and collaboration across disciplines, a number of obstacles prevent interdisciplinary partnership from occurring on a regular basis, such as limited resources, different perceptions of child development and needs, and lack of a structured framework to promote service integration (Bradley-Klug et al., 2013; Hernández Finch, Finch, Mcintosh, Thomas, & Maughan, 2015; Villarreal, 2017). A model for interdisciplinary partnership is the Team-Based Pediatric Care Model (Katkin et al., 2017). According to the model, "Team-based care for children aims to address the unique aspects of childhood, such as preventive care, health promotion, and health maintenance to promote long-term health, as well as child development and its influence on disease presentation and management" (Katkin et al., 2017, p. 2). In applying the model to the educational setting, the school psychologist could serve as the facilitator and the liaison between the educational team and the community-based medical providers. Given school psychologists' training, the interdisciplinary model would place the school psychologist in the position of promoting data-based decision-making, ensuring implementation integrity, and progress monitoring of outcomes.

CONCLUSION

Prevention at the universal level is designed for all children and typically includes components of health promotion and risk reduction. This chapter focuses on healthy eating, physical activity and exercise, and integration of sleep education and mindfulness programming into the curriculum. The successful implementation of universal health-promotion programs in the classroom and schoolwide requires the collaboration of individuals both within and outside of the educational system. Although mental health professionals in the educational setting have the knowledge and skills to spearhead these efforts when provided with a framework for interdisciplinary partnerships, school psychologists are uniquely trained to serve as facilitators for team-based efforts to promote wellness and to reduce risk for all students.

REFERENCES

Albers, C. A., & Kettler, R. J. (2014). Best practices in universal screening. In P. Harrison & A. Thomas (Eds.), *Best practices in school psychology: Data-based and collaborative decision making* (pp. 121–131). Bethesda, MD: National Association of School Psychologists Publications.

Alfano, C. A., Zakem, A. H., Costa, N. M., Taylor, L. K., & Weems, C. F. (2009). Sleep problems and their relation to cognitive factors, anxiety, and depressive symptoms in children and adolescents. *Depression and Anxiety, 26*, 503–512. doi:10.1002/da.20443

American Academy of Pediatrics. (2016, April 30). Percentage of US children who have chronic health conditions on the rise: Diseases such as asthma and attention deficit hyperactivity disorder have increased at a disproportionate rate among children living in poverty, according to new research being presented at the Pediatric Academic Societies 2016 Meeting. *ScienceDaily*. Retrieved from www.sciencedaily.com/releases/2016/04/160430100357.htm

American Academy of Sleep Medicine. (n.d.). *Sleep education for school*. Retrieved from http://school.sleepeducation.com/default.aspx

Baer, R. A. (2003). Mindfulness training as a clinical intervention: A conceptual and empirical review. *Clinical Psychological Sciences Practice, 10*, 125–143. doi:10.1093/clipsy/bpg015

Beijamini, F., & Louzada, F. M. (2012). Are educational interventions able to prevent excessive daytime sleepiness in adolescents? *Biological Rhythm Research, 43*(6), 603–613. doi:10.1080/09291016.2011.630183

Berezowitz, C. K., Bontrager Yoder, A. B., & Schoeller, D. A. (2015). School gardens enhance academic performance and dietary outcomes in children. *Journal of School Health, 85*(8), 508–518.

Blunden, S., & Rigney, G. (2015). Lessons learned from sleep education in schools: A review of dos and don'ts. *Journal of Clinical Sleep Medicine, 11*(6), 671–680. doi:10.5664/jcsm.4782

Bono, G., Froh, J. J., & Forrett, R. (2014). Gratitude in school: Benefits to students and schools. In M. Furlong, R. Gilman, & E. S. Heubner (Eds.), *Handbook of positive psychology in the schools* (2nd ed., pp. 67–81). New York, NY: Wiley.

Bradley-Klug, K. L., & Armstrong, K. (2014). Preparing school psychologists as partners in integrated health care delivery. *Trainers Forum: Journal of the Trainers of School Psychologists, 32*, 67–83.

Bradley-Klug, K. L., Jeffries-DeLoatche, K. L., Walsh, A. S. J., Bateman, L. P., Nadeau, J., Powers, D. J., & Cunningham, J. (2013). School psychologists' perceptions of primary care partnerships: Implications for building the collaborative bridge. *Advances in School Mental Health Promotion, 6*(1), 51–67.

Briggs, M., Fleischhacker, S., & Mueller, C. G. (2010). Position of the American Dietetic Association, School Nutrition Association, and Society for Nutrition Education: Comprehensive school nutrition services. *Journal of Nutrition Education and Behavior, 42*(6), 360–371. doi:10.1016/j.jneb.2010.08.007

Briggs, R. D., Stettler, E. M., Silver, E. J., Schrag, R. D. A., Nayak, M., Chinitz, S., & Racine, A. D. (2012). Social-emotional screening for infants and toddlers in primary care. *Pediatrics, 129*(2), e377–e384. doi:10.1542/peds.2010-2211

Bruni, O., Ottaviano, S., Guidetti, V., Romoli, M., Innocenzi M., Cortesi, F., & Giannotti, F. (1996). The Sleep Disturbance Scale for Children (SDSC): Construction and validation of an instrument to evaluate sleep disturbances in childhood and adolescence. *Journal of Sleep Research, 5*, 251–261.

Carlson, J. A., Engelberg, J. K., Cain, K. L., Conway, T. L., Mignano, A. M., Bonilla, E. A., . . . Sallis, J. F. (2015). Implementing classroom physical activity breaks: Associations with student physical activity and classroom behavior. *Preventive Medicine, 81*, 67–72. doi:10.1016/j.ypmed.2015.08.006

Centers for Disease Control and Prevention. (2006). *Physical education curriculum analysis tool*. Retrieved from https://www.cdc.gov/healthyschools/pecat/pdf/pecat.pdf

Centers for Disease Control and Prevention. (2009). *Youth physical activity: The role of schools*. Retrieved from https://www.cdc.gov/healthyschools/physicalactivity/toolkit/factsheet_pa_guidelines_schools.pdf

Centers for Disease Control and Prevention. (2011). School health guidelines to promote healthy eating and physical activity. *Morbidity and Mortality Weekly Report (MMWR), 60*(5), 1–74.

Centers for Disease Control and Prevention. (2012). *Health education curriculum analysis tool*. Retrieved from https://www.cdc.gov/healthyyouth/HECAT/

Centers for Disease Control and Prevention. (2016). *Childhood obesity causes & consequences*. Retrieved from https://www.cdc.gov/obesity/childhood/causes.html

Chervin, R. D., Dillon, J. E., Archbold, K. H., & Ruzicka, D. L. (2003). Conduct problems and symptoms of sleep disorders in children. *Journal of the American Academy of Child & Adolescent Psychiatry, 42*(2), 201–208. doi:10.1097/00004583-200302000-00014

Chung, K., Chan, M., Lam, Y., Lai, C. S., & Yeung, W. (2017). School-based sleep education programs for short sleep duration in adolescents: A systematic review and meta-analysis. *Journal of School Health, 87*(6), 401–408. doi:10.1111/josh.12509

Cook-Cottone, C. P., Tribole, E., & Tylka, T. L. (2013). *Healthy eating in schools: Evidence-based interventions to help kids thrive*. Washington, DC: American Psychological Association.

Daniels, S. R. (2006). The consequences of childhood overweight and obesity. *The Future of Children, 16*(1), 47–67.

Drake, C., Nickel, C., Burduvali, E., Roth, T., Jefferson, C., & Badia, P. (2003). The Pediatric Daytime Sleepiness Scale (PDSS): Sleep habits and outcomes in middle-school children. *Sleep, 26*(4), 455–458.

Flook, L., Smalley, S. L., Kitil, J., Galla, B. M., Kaiser-Greenland, S., Locke, J., . . . Kasari, C. (2010). Effects of mindful awareness practices on executive functions in elementary school children. *Journal of Applied School Psychology, 26*(1), 70–95. doi:10.1080/15377900903379125

Hakim, S. M., & Meissen, G. (2013). Increasing consumption of fruits and vegetables in the school cafeteria: The influence of active choice. *Journal of Health Care for the Poor and Underserved*, *24*(2), 145–157.

Hanks, A. S., Just, D. R., & Wansink, B. (2013). Preordering school lunch encourages better food choices by children. *JAMA Pediatrics*, *167*(7), 673–674.

Hernández Finch, M. E., Finch, W., Mcintosh, C. E., Thomas, C., & Maughan, E. (2015). Enhancing collaboration between school nurses and school psychologists when providing a continuum of care for children with medical needs. *Psychology in the Schools*, *57*, 635–647.

Holistic Life Foundation. (2016). *Mindful moment program*. Retrieved from http://hlfinc.org/programs-services/mindful-moment-program/

Huberty, J. L., Siahpush, M., Beighle, A., Fuhrmeister, E., Silva, P., & Welk, G. (2011). Ready for Recess: A pilot study to increase physical activity in elementary school. *Journal of School Health*, *81*(5), 251–257.

Jennings, P. A., & Greenberg, M. T. (2009). The prosocial classroom: Teacher social and emotional competence in relation to student and classroom outcomes. *Review of Educational Research*, *79*(1), 491–525. doi:10.3102/0034654308325693

Jennings, P. A., Snowberg, K. E., Coccia, M. A., & Greenberg, M. T. (2011). Improving classroom learning environments by Cultivating Awareness and Resilience in Education (CARE): Results of two pilot studies. *The Journal of Classroom Interaction*, *46*(1), 37–48.

Kabat-Zinn, J. (1994). *Wherever you go, there you are: Mindfulness meditation in everyday life*. New York, NY: Hyperion.

Katkin, J. P., Kressly, S. J., Edwards, A. R., Perrin, J. M., Kraft, C. A., Richerson, J. E., . . . Wall, L. (2017). Guiding principles for team-based pediatric care. *Pediatrics*, *140*(2), 1–7. doi:10.1542/peds.2017-1489.

Layous, K., Nelson, S. K., Oberle, E., Schonert-Reichl, K. A., & Lyubomirsky, S. (2012). Kindness counts: Prompting prosocial behavior in preadolescents boosts peer acceptance and well-being. *PLoS One 7*, e51380. doi:10.1371/journal.pone.00513

Luginbuehl, M., Bradley-Klug, K. L., Ferron, J., Anderson, W. M., & Benbadis, S. R. (2008). Pediatric sleep disorders: Validation of the Sleep Disorders Inventory for Students. *School Psychology Review*, *37*(3), 409–431.

Meiklejohn, J., Phillips, C., Freedman, M. L., Griffin, M. L., Biegel, G., Roach, A., . . . Saltzman, A. (2012). Integrating mindfulness training into K-12 education: Fostering the resilience of teachers and students. *Mindfulness*, *3*(4), 291–307. doi:10.1007/s12671-012-0094-5

Miller, G. F., Coffield, E., Leroy, Z., & Wallin, R. (2016). Prevalence and costs of five chronic conditions in children. *The Journal of School Nursing*, *32*, 357–364. doi:10.1177/1059840516641190.

National Sleep Foundation. (2014). *National Sleep Foundation 2014 Sleep in America poll finds children sleep better when parents establish rules, limit technology and set a good example*. Retrieved from https://sleepfoundation.org/media-center/press-release/national-sleep-foundation-2014-sleep-america-poll-finds-children-sleep

Ogden, C. L., Carroll, M. D., Lawman, H. G., Fryar, C. D., Kruszon-Moran, D., Brian, K., & Flegal, K. M. (2016). Trends in obesity prevalence among children and adolescents in the United States, 1988–1994 through 2013–2014. *JAMA*, *315*(21), 2292–2299. doi:10.1001/jama.2016.6361

Paruthi, S., Brooks, L. J., D'Ambrosio, C., Hall, W. A., Kotagal, S., . . . Wise, M. S. (2016). Recommended amount of sleep for pediatric populations: A consensus statement of the American Academy of Sleep Medicine. *Journal of Clinical Sleep Medicine, 12*(6), 785–786. doi:10.5664/jcsm.5866

Poulin, P. A., Mackenzie, C. S., Soloway, G., & Karayolas, E. (2008). Mindfulness training as an evidenced-based approach to reducing stress and promoting well-being among human services professionals. *International Journal of Health Promotion and Education, 46*(2), 72–80. doi:10.1080/14635240.2008.10708132

Rigney, G., Blunden, S., Maher, C., Dollman, J., Parvazian, S., Matricciani, L., & Olds, T. (2015). Can a school-based sleep education programme improve sleep knowledge, hygiene and behaviours using a randomised controlled trial. *Sleep Medicine, 16*(6), 736–745. doi:10.1016/j.sleep.2015.02.534

Roseman, M. G., Riddell, M. C., & Haynes, J. N. (2011). A content analysis of kindergarten-12th grade school-based nutrition interventions: Taking advantage of past learning. *Journal of Nutrition Education and Behavior, 43*(1), 2–18. doi:10.1016/j.jneb.2010.07.009

SHAPE America. (2016). Shape of the nation: Status of physical education in the USA. Retrieved from http://www.shapeamerica.org/advocacy/son/2016/upload/Shape-of-the-Nation-2016_web.pdf

Slusser, W. M., Cumberland, W. G., Browdy, B. L., Lange, L., & Neumann, C. (2007). A school salad bar increases frequency of fruit and vegetable consumption among children living in low-income households. *Public Health Nutrition, 10*(12), 1490–1496. doi:10.1017/S1368980007000444

Steenari, M. R., Vuontela, V., Paavonen, J., Carlson, S., Fjallberg, M., & Aronen, E. T. (2003). Working memory and sleep in 6- to 13-year-old schoolchildren. *Journal of the American Academy of Child & Adolescent Psychiatry, 42*(1), 85–92. doi:10.1097/00004583-200301000-00014

Stewart, J. A., Dennison, D. A., Kohl, H. W., & Doyle, A. (2004). Exercise level and energy expenditure in the TAKE 10!® in-class physical activity program. *Journal of School Health, 74*(10), 397–400.

Taveras, E. M., Rifas-Shiman, S. L., Bub, K. L., Gillman, M. W., & Oken, E. (2017). Prospective study of insufficient sleep and neurobehavioral functioning among school-age children. *Academic Pediatrics.* doi:10.1016/j.acap.2017.02.001

The Hawn Foundation. (n.d). *MindUp.* Retrieved from https://mindup.org

Turrell, S. L., Bell, M., & Wilson, K. G. (2016). ACT for adolescents: Treating teens and adolescents in individual and group therapy. Oakland, CA: New Harbinger Publications.

U.S. Department of Agriculture. (2015). *MyPlate kids' place.* Retrieved from https://www.choosemyplate.gov/kids

U.S. Department of Agriculture, Center for Nutrition Policy and Promotion. (2011). *A brief history of USDA food guides.* Retrieved from https://choosemyplate-prod.azureedge.net/sites/default/files/printablematerials/ABriefHistoryOfUSDAFoodGuides.pdf

U.S. Department of Agriculture, Center for Nutrition Policy and Promotion. (2016). *SuperTracker nutrition lesson plans for high school students.* Retrieved from https://choosemyplateprod.azureedge.net/sites/default/files/printablematerials/SuperTrackerHighSchoolLessonPlans2016Updates-FINAL.pdf

U.S. Department of Health and Human Services. (2008). *2008 Physical activity guidelines for Americans* (ODPHP Publication No. U0036). Retrieved from https://health.gov/paguidelines/pdf/paguide.pdf

U.S. Department of Health and Human Services & U.S. Department of Agriculture. (2015). *Dietary guidelines for Americans 2015–2020* (HHS Publication No. HHS-ODPHP-2015-2020-01-DGA-A). Retrieved from https://health.gov/dietaryguidelines/2015/guidelines/

Villarreal, V. (2017). Mental health collaboration: A survey of practicing school psychologists. *Journal of Applied School Psychology.* doi:10.1080/15377903.2017.1328626

Wansink, B., Just, D. R., Payne, C. R., & Klinger, M. Z. (2012). Attractive names sustain increased vegetable intake in schools. *Preventive Medicine, 55*, 330–332.

Whitt-Glover, M. C., Ham, S. A., & Yancey, A. K. (2011). Instant Recess®: A practical tool for increasing physical activity during the school day. *Progress in Community Health Partnerships: Research, Education, and Action, 5*(3), 289–297.

Wing, Y., Chan, N., Yu, M., Lam, S., Zhang, J., . . . Li, A. (2015). A school-based sleep education program for adolescents: A cluster randomized trial. *Pediatrics*, e1–e9.

Zenner, C., Herrnleben-Kurz, S., & Walach, H. (2014). Mindfulness-based interventions in schools: A systematic review and meta-analysis. *Frontiers in Psychology, 5*, 603.

9

Cognitive-Behavioral Interventions for Pediatric Health Concerns in Schools

MICHAEL L. SULKOWSKI, GRAI BLUEZ, ARIEL MCKINNEY, AND JACLYN WOLF ■

Thanks to advances in medicine that allow for the successful treatment and management of previously debilitating or fatal childhood illnesses, the mental health and educational needs of many children with chronic medical conditions— about 20%–30% of this population—can be prioritized (van der Lee, Mokkink, Grootenhuis, Heymans, & Offringa, 2007). However, despite the advancements, an alarming number of youth with co-occurring physical and mental health concerns do not receive adequate treatment. In general, children with chronic medical conditions need, yet often do not receive, more mental health supports than their peers without health problems. Overall, about 25% of individuals with chronic medical conditions have clinically significant mental health symptoms that impede their social, academic, or occupational functioning, yet only a fraction of these individuals receive effective mental health interventions (Hippisley-Cox, Fielding, & Pringle, 1998; Newacheck et al., 1998). Additionally, it is important to note that children with chronic medical conditions often face high levels of stress related to the uncertainty of their health, frequent absences from school, and other demands associated with the treatment or management of their illness that collectively exert a deleterious effect on their psychosocial functioning (White, 2001).

Current laws do, however, provide some solace and support for youth with co-occurring health and mental health concerns. Children with chronic medical conditions are mandated a free and appropriate public education (FAPE) under the category of other health impairment (OHI) in the Individuals with Disabilities Education Improvement Act (IDEIA; 2004). Therefore, public schools are mandated to address both physical health problems and mental health problems that can limit students' ability to learn, engage the curriculum, and succeed in school. Additionally, as required by current federal education law, school-based practitioners (e.g., school psychologists, social workers, counselors) must address the varied needs of students with pediatric health concerns. Of course, addressing these needs involves the use of evidence-based interventions.

Currently, compared to other mental health interventions, the most empirical support exists for using cognitive-behavioral therapy (CBT) to treat most mood and anxiety concerns in pediatric populations (Chambless & Hollon, 1998; Kashikar-Zuck et al., 2012; Safren et al., 2009; Salloum, Sulkowski, Sirrine, & Storch, 2009). Research supports the efficacy of using CBT in school settings with a range of student populations as well as in medical settings with students displaying varied chronic medical conditions (Albano & Kendall, 2002; Joyce-Beaulieu & Sulkowski, 2015; Kashikar-Zuck et al., 2012; Robins, Smith, Glutting, & Bishop, 2005; Safren et al., 2009; Salloum et al., 2009; Sulkowski, McGuire, & Tesoro, 2015; White, 2001). Additionally, an emerging body of research suggests that CBT is effective in reducing mental health problems co-occurring or associated with chronic health problems in pediatric populations. To bolster the CBT intervention approach, this chapter reviews research, scholarship, and clinically relevant information on the use of CBT for pediatric health concerns in school-age youth. In particular, the following evidence-based CBT components are discussed: psychoeducation, cognitive restructuring, relaxation training and stress management, and behavioral exposure.

THE CBT MODEL

Undergirding the CBT model is the interconnection of thoughts, feelings, and behaviors (the CBT triad; Kendall, 2012; Kendall & Hedtke, 2006). Consistent with this model, thoughts (i.e., cognitions) can be either adaptive if they foster healthy emotions and behavior, or maladaptive if they contribute to emotional distress or unhealthy behavior. For example, children with type 1 diabetes face daily challenges related to diet and medication management and must be mindful of their blood sugar levels. An example of an adaptive thought a child with diabetes might have is: "My friends understand that I need to check my blood sugar because it is important to my health." This thought is adaptive because it appropriately appraises the situation and is likely to promote healthy behaviors related to disease management. Conversely, the thought, "My friends don't have to test their blood sugar so I shouldn't either," is maladaptive and potentially could contribute to emotional distress.

Unlike nondirective or unstructured psychotherapies, CBT is typically conceptualized as a structured, skill-based, and time-limed intervention (Kendall, 2012). The skill-based nature of CBT makes it well suited for school settings in which learning, instruction, and orderly conduct are parts of the culture and are expected. Additionally, time-limited therapeutic approaches are also most suited for practitioners working in school settings with children who transition between educational and medical settings each quarter, semester, or year. However, it is worth noting that, despite the inherently structured nature of CBT, this approach can also be individualized for children based on their needs. For example, a child presenting with mild anxiety symptoms after an asthma attack during class would likely require and receive a different intervention than would a child who develops panic attacks and school phobia after an asthma attack (Joyce-Beaulieu & Sulkowski, 2015).

CORE COMPONENTS OF CBT

Core components of CBT include psychoeducation (particularly as it relates to normalizing health problems for youth experiencing pediatric illness and promoting awareness of the mind–body connection), cognitive restructuring, relaxation training and stress management, and behavioral exposure (Joyce-Beaulieu & Sulkowski, 2015; Kendall, 2012; Kendall & Hedtke, 2006). However, based on the combined presentation of physical and mental health concerns, children will display unique needs that require different CBT options. Therefore, consistent with current literature, it is important for clinicians to tailor CBT protocols to meet the specific needs of youth and to flexibly implement various CBT components (Kendall, 2012). Doing so involves addressing and implementing core CBT components, yet it also involves the artful selection of the components. Handout 9.1 provides a sample overview of a CBT protocol for working with a child with a chronic illness. Of course, this is a general guide and therapists have latitude to structure and pace CBT based on the child's individual needs.

Psychoeducation

In the CBT literature, psychoeducation is used to address a cognitive deficiency or a lack of information in a client, patient, or student. Often, psychoeducation involves describing a range of symptoms an individual is experiencing, the nature of treatment, expected treatment outcomes, and the stigma associated with physical and mental health problems, as well as addressing any questions the person may have. Additionally, motivation for, and barriers to, treatment may be explored, as well as the role of key caregivers, family members, and educational professionals who may be involved in the treatment process. Children and families affected by co-occurring physical and mental health conditions may feel like the challenges they face are overwhelming and insurmountable, which then warrants that the provider suggest otherwise. Overall, the psychoeducational part of the CBT process involves disabusing children and families of feelings of hopelessness by providing accurate information related to the treatment process. (For example, the provider can tell the child and parents, "Many people with similar concerns have benefitted from CBT and have experienced a higher quality of life.")

The impact of a client's emotional state on his or her health outcomes, including pain, recovery, and the ability to combat disease (as well as manage related sequelae), has been empirically investigated (Tagge et al., 2013). In general, research suggests that children who have been provided more information about their physical and mental health conditions develop more positive attitudes than do children who are unaware of the adversities they might experience (Nussey, Pistrang, & Murphy, 2013). Moreover, providing clients with information about their injury or illness in early stages of pathology and treatment has been linked to the overall recovery process, and it also has been found to buffer against experiencing anxiety and distress (Kenardy, Thompson, Le Brocque, & Olsson, 2008). Therefore, the nexus between physical and psychological concerns is real and established. However, more research and scholarship is needed to delineate how the psychoeducational CBT process pertains most directly to youth who are experiencing chronic illness and related concerns. For example, in contrast to CBT for mood and anxiety concerns without co-occurring health problems, the process of normalizing illness appears to be particularly important for successful outcomes in youth with health concerns.

NORMALIZATION

Normalization has been identified as a key part of the psychoeducational process for children and families coping with childhood chronic illness (Burns, Erickson, & Brenner, 2014; Knafl, Darney, Gallo, & Angst, 2010). Normalization of chronic pediatric illness includes both the process by which families create a normal family life as well as the meaning and value associated with overcoming suffering associated with illness. In this regard, normalization of pediatric health concerns often involves working within the constraints of the established religious and philosophical belief systems of children and families. Therefore, considerable care and compassion are needed to help affected individuals find meaning in illness and recovery, as well as cope with adversity. As a clinical focus, kernels of wisdom or meaning associated with (and embraced through the recovery and coping process) can be identified and reinforced as part of the overall treatment process (Knafl et al., 2010).

PROMOTING AWARENESS OF THE MIND–BODY CONNECTION

Awareness of the mind–body connection allows individuals to feel more empowered to cope with distressing thoughts, feelings, and sensations associated with illness. Thus, a student who can make the link between excessive worrying and symptoms associated with a chronic health condition can be taught cognitive interventions, relaxation strategies, or stress-management skills to reduce his or her suffering. (These skills are all covered in this chapter.)

Although the connection between the mind and body has been discussed for centuries, recent research has more firmly established an indelible link between the two. For example, some findings from the field of neuroendocrinology suggests that there is considerable plasticity in the mind–body connection and that the relationship between the mind and body is dynamic, amenable to modification, and a potential point of intervention (Fosha, Siegel, & Solomon, 2009; Pally, 1998). Therefore, by providing psychoeducation about the mind–body connection, clinicians can persuade youth to be more receptive to a range of CBT interventions that can help them with co-occurring physical and mental health problems (Astin, Shapiro, Eisenberg, & Forys, 2003).

Several therapeutic strategies exist to promote awareness of the mind–body connection. As a salient example, mindfulness-based interventions have gained increasing attention in recent years. This is primarily because of evidence supporting the utility of the mindfulness-based approach in helping patients to accept their thoughts, feelings, sensations, and symptoms as well as to embrace the present moment (Baer, 2003). Mindfulness-based stress reduction (MBSR) is a structured mindfulness intervention that has been used to help reduce pain sensations in youth by improving their physical and emotional well-being. Specific components of MBSR include sitting meditation, body scan, and mindful yoga, and research supports the efficacy of the MBSR approach. A review of research on MBSR found that the approach improved the mental health of participants in 11 studies where MBSR was compared to wait-list control treatments or treatment-as-usual conditions (Fjorback, Arendt, Ørnbøl, & Walach, 2011). Additionally, in the same review, MBSR was found to be superior to active and alternative control treatment conditions in three studies. In further support of MBSR, Sauer-Zavala, Walsh, Eisenlohr-Mòul, and Lykins (2013) found that participants in a 3-week intervention program who were treated with MBSR displayed increased psychological well-being, less rumination, and increased willingness to describe their emotional experiences.

Cognitive Restructuring

Cognitive restructuring is a core component of CBT that is used to address cognitive distortions, thinking errors, or maladaptive thinking patterns. Although different texts use different names to describe these distortions, common terms include *all-or-nothing thinking, discounting the positive, magnifying, minimizing, catastrophizing, labeling, overgeneralizing, emotional reasoning, jumping to conclusions, fortune telling, filtering, control and fairness fallacy,* and *personalizing.* As an example of how cognitive distortions might influence a child with a chronic health condition, the child might think: "Because of my diabetes, I am doomed and I will always be sick and unhappy, and do poorly in school." In this brief example, several cognitive distortions are present: catastrophizing ("I'm doomed"), all-or-nothing thinking, and fortune telling ("I will always be sick and unhappy, and do poorly in school"). Collectively, if the distortions go unchallenged, they could result in feelings of helplessness, hopelessness, or even despair.

Cognitive restructuring to challenge cognitive distortions first involves helping a student understand and recognize the thinking errors that he or she is taking for granted and may not identify as distortions. Because school-age children's linguistic and metacognitive abilities are variable, clinicians need to individualize cognitive restructuring interventions to fit students' developmental levels. In general, adolescents who have at least average intellectual abilities or cognitive functioning, as well as insight into their own thinking patterns, tend to benefit the most from cognitive restructuring. In contrast, young children, children with cognitive impairments or limitations, and children with neurodevelopmental or communication disorders likely will derive limited benefit from this intervention approach (Joyce-Beaulieu & Sulkowski, 2015).

To help a student identify cognitive distortions, the therapist needs to use a variety of strategies that can slow down, make more transparent, and demystify maladaptive thinking patterns. In this regard, thought journals and logs often are used by clinicians to help youth identify their maladaptive cognitions. Essentially, the therapist can have the youth focus on identifying when his or her emotions are changing markedly or when he or she experiences strong feelings. Then, using a thought log or journal, the child can document the feeling, what was happening right before the change in affect, the thoughts at the time, and what he or she did afterward. After the youth can identify the emotions successfully, the therapist can then work with him or her to identify possible cognitive distortions and antecedents to the distortions, as well as how maladaptive thoughts tend to influence feelings and behaviors.

Furthermore, once youth understand that thinking errors exist, therapists can help restructure negative thought patterns through specific cognitive interventions. However, this process should be subtle so that the child does not feel coerced and instead independently comes up with different ways to think about a situation or context. Essentially, the therapist should help the child evaluate his or her own thoughts and choose more adaptive ones, which can be guided by simple paraphrasing followed by prompts like "What is another way to think of that?" or "What might someone else think?" Additionally, Socratic questioning, or asking questions that encourage self-reflection and evaluating one's own thoughts, also can help youth restructure their thoughts. One Socratic questioning strategy involves having youth engage in "for/against guessing" associated with maintaining certain thoughts or positions. For example, a child who is experiencing maladies associated with pediatric obesity might be encouraged to evaluate arguments for and against adopting and implementing a new, healthy lifestyle intervention. For more information on the application of cognitive restructuring to help school-age youth, see Joyce-Beaulieu and Sulkowski (2015).

Relaxation Training

Several relaxation techniques can be used to reduce the stress, distress, and anxiety associated with experiencing a chronic medical condition. Most saliently, the techniques include diaphragmatic breathing, guided imagery (also called creative visualization), and progressive muscle relaxation (PMR). Diaphragmatic breathing (also called belly or deep breathing) involves having a child sit or lie down with good spinal alignment. Then, the child is instructed to breathe slowly and deeply through his or her nose, hold his or her breath, and finally slowly exhale. As a rule of thumb, each part of the process should take at least 3 seconds, which causes a slowing down of breathing and greater relaxation. The purpose of diaphragmatic breathing is to counteract the shallow and fast breathing that individuals who are prone to negative emotions tend to display and that can cause hyperventilation, dizziness, or even fainting in children with chronic medical conditions (Katon, Richardson, Lozano, & McCauley, 2004).

Guided imagery involves replacing intrusive thoughts with a calming mental image or picture that can temporarily alleviate emotional distress. This relaxation approach often involves having the child identify a favorite place to imagine, mentally visit, and inhabit psychologically (van Tilburg et al., 2009). Essentially, guided imagery involves distancing oneself from difficult and overwhelming emotional experiences by refocusing on images that produce feelings of calmness, balance, and control. For additional information on guided imagery, the Children's Hospital of Orange County (CHOC) provides complimentary guided imagery recordings on their website (www.choc.org).

Last, PMR involves tensing muscle groups and then relaxing them to reduce stress, tension, and anxiety. PMR is done systematically under the direction of a therapist, who guides the child through the process; individuals are taught to identify areas in which they hold tension and then to mitigate the tension through systematic relaxation strategies. Often, PMR involves having a therapist read or use a script with instructions for releasing tension in sequential muscle groups. However, depending on the presentation of the child's chronic medical condition and potential physical limitations, PMR can be modified to address specific needs or particular clients (Emery, France, Harris, Norman, & VanArsdalen, 2008). For example, scripts can be modified for youth with physical or mobility limitations. Handout 9.2 provides information on using PMR with children.

Stress-Management Training

The effects of chronic stress and illness often are interrelated; individuals who are stressed are prone to illness, and being ill can be stressful. Considering this, children experiencing chronic health conditions are more likely to experience stress than are their healthy peers (Christian, 2016; Johnston-Brooks, Lewis, Evans, & Whalen, 1998). Moreover, stress associated with experiencing chronic illness and intensive treatment has been linked to the development of mental health problems that can negatively affect treatment outcomes (Compas, Jaser, Dunn, & Rodriguez, 2012). Chronic health conditions and related sequelae often are exacerbated by other life stressors, such as co-occurring mental health problems, financial stress, familial conflict, and interpersonal stress (Compas et al., 2012; Currie & Lin, 2007; El-Sheikh, Harger, & Whitson, 2001; Garasky, Stewart, Gundersen, Lohman, & Eisenmann, 2009). In general, chronic illnesses present a unique source of stress because they are unanticipated and often are uncontrollable (Compas et al., 2012).

IDENTIFYING STRESSORS

Children with chronic health conditions usually experience two types of stressors: stressors associated with illness and stressors associated with daily life/regular functioning. The distinction is important, yet it is worth noting that the two types of stressors are not necessarily mutually exclusive. A study by Rodriguez et al. (2012) examined stressors in children with cancer and found that daily-life stressors included falling behind at school, not being able to participate in activities that the children previously engaged in, and concerns about the well-being of family and friends. In contrast, stressors associated with chronic illness included feeling sick after treatments and pain and soreness associated with medical procedures. General uncertainty, such as confusion about what cancer is and what causes it, was also identified as an illness-specific stressor. Importantly, results indicated that the children rated stressors associated with their daily functioning as more pervasive than their illness-specific stressors. Thus, this finding highlights the importance of adopting a flexible and holistic approach to addressing stress when working with children affected by chronic illness or health concerns.

COPING WITH STRESS

Dellenmark-Blom et al. (2016) conducted a focus group study to assess coping strategies used by children with a chronic illness. Results of the investigation identified nine strategies that were used regularly. The most popular strategies were problem-solving (i.e., finding alternative solutions to health-related problems), avoidance (e.g., behaviors to avoid situations, concealed emotions), recognition of responsibility (e.g., taking the initiative to learn more about their health or treatment, taking care of health-related problems), and seeking social support from parents, peers, teachers, and medical professionals to help cope with chronic illness.

In addition to the previously mentioned general strategies, there are specific interventions that can help youth with chronic illness to cope with stress. In this vein, a review by Ndetan, Willard Evans, Williams, Woolsey, and Swartz (2014) of movement therapies (e.g., yoga and Pilates, Tai Chi) and relaxation techniques (e.g., meditation, deep breathing) found that both approaches were useful in managing anxiety and stress associated with chronic pediatric illness. Essentially, both approaches empowered youth to reduce their stress proactively as opposed to feeling incapable of doing so. Additionally, a strategy that seems to be particularly useful for reducing stress in youth experiencing chronic illness is imaginal coping, which appears to have distinct clinical utility (Rindstedt, 2014). Imaginal coping involves the use of imagination to transform and reframe the challenges associated with chronic illness, and it appears to be useful for young children and adolescents (Clark, 2003). Imaginal coping often involves using and focusing on specific objects to reduce stress. For example, after being diagnosed with diabetes, a child might decide that a teddy bear shares the same diagnosis and treatment regimen, and then the child can be taught to imagine the bear undergoing and responding to treatment (e.g., receiving pretend insulin injections, avoiding certain foods, adopting other healthy lifestyle choices, etc.; Clark, 2003). Overall, imaginal coping strategies can help increase a sense of control and stability in the lives of youth faced with a lot of uncertainty related to their chronic health concerns.

Behavioral Exposure

Although the existing literature is relatively devoid of content related to the use of behavioral exposure for treating stress and anxiety related to chronic pediatric health concerns, significant empirical support exists for this intervention in a range of mental health conditions that commonly co-occur with chronic illness (for a review, see Jordan, Reid, Mariaskin, Augusto, and Sulkowski, 2012). Behavioral exposure can help reduce stress and anxiety by breaking associations that maintain fear or anxiety-based beliefs and that result in avoidant or compulsive behavior.

Behavioral exposure may be particularly crucial to the application of CBT for youth with anxiety related to actual or perceived threats to their health or safety. Additionally, after overcoming or recuperating from a chronic health condition, some youth are prone to developing illness anxiety disorder (formally health anxiety disorder), which involves being preoccupied with having, or getting, a serious disease or health condition and worrying that minor symptoms or body sensations mean you have a serious illness (American Psychiatric Association, 2013). For example, a child who recovers from leukemia may interpret typical fatigue, joint pain, bruising, or a fever as being indicative of a resurgence of the disease. Additionally, after being out of school for a significant time period to receive treatment, a child may struggle to transition back to school and may experience anxiety about this process (Bussing, Burket, & Kelleher, 1996).

Behavioral exposure involves facing fear and stressors in a gradual and systematic manner that follows a hierarchy. Thus, a child with worries about illness or getting sick can gradually be exposed to feared places (e.g., hospitals, a physician's office), stimuli (e.g., contaminated objects), and sensations (e.g., rapid heart rate, dizziness). It is important for a therapist to monitor the subjective units of distress that the child is experiencing to ensure that the child is experiencing anxiety but is not feeling flooded (Sulkowski, Jacob, & Storch, 2013). Ultimately, the goal of behavioral exposure is for the child to face his or her fears in a therapeutically safe environment and to habituate to anxiety-producing settings, stimuli, sensations, and thoughts (Pence, Sulkowski, Jordan, & Storch, 2010). Therefore, through the process of habituation, behavioral exposure breaks two key anxiety-maintaining associations: (1) that a legitimate threat is present and worth worrying about, and (2) that the child needs to perform some form of compulsive, avoidant, or otherwise anxiety-reducing behavior (Jordan, Reid, Guzick, Simmons, & Sulkowski, 2017).

CONCLUSION

Although chronic medical conditions often cause youth to experience considerable stress, anxiety, and depression, CBT interventions can be employed to help this at-risk population. Over the past few decades, considerable advancements have been made in the development of, access to, and delivery of such interventions, and an increasing body of research supports the efficacy of CBT (Chambless et al., 1998; Joyce-Beaulieu & Sulkowski, 2015). Specifically, the following CBT components have been found to alleviate different forms of distress in youth populations: psychoeducation, cognitive restructuring, relaxation training, stress management, and behavioral exposure. Although it is still an emerging area for research and applied clinical practice, the use of CBT for maladies associated with pediatric health problems displays considerable promise. Coping with a chronic health condition is never easy; however, learning ways to think and act more adaptively can have a profound impact on the emotional burden associated with childhood illness.

REFERENCES

Albano, A. M., & Kendall, P. C. (2002). Cognitive behavioural therapy for children and adolescents with anxiety disorders: Clinical research advances. *International Review of Psychiatry, 14*, 129–134. doi:10.1080/09540260220132644

American Psychiatric Association. (2013). *Diagnostic and statistical manual of mental disorders* (5th ed.; DSM-5®). Washington, DC: American Psychiatric Association.

Astin, J. A., Shapiro, S. L., Eisenberg, D. M., & Forys, K. L. (2003). Mind-body medicine: State of the science, implications for practice. *Journal of the American Board of Family Practice, 16*, 131–147. doi:10.3122/jabfm.16.2.131

Baer, R. A. (2003). Mindfulness training as a clinical intervention: A conceptual and empirical review. *Clinical Psychology: Science and Practice, 10*, 125–143. doi:10.1093/clipsy.bpg015

Burns, A. M., Erickson, D. H., & Brenner, C. A. (2014). Cognitive-behavioral therapy for medication-resistant psychosis: A meta-analytic review. *Psychiatric Services, 65*, 874–880. doi:10.1176/appi.ps.201300213

Bussing, R., Burket, R. C., & Kelleher, E. T. (1996). Prevalence of anxiety disorders in a clinic-based sample of pediatric asthma patients. *Psychosomatics, 37*, 108–115. doi:10.1016/S0033-3182(96)71576-1

Chambless, D. L., & Hollon, S. D. (1998). Defining empirically supported therapies. *Journal of Consulting and Clinical Psychology, 66*, 7–18. doi:10.1037/0022-006X.66.1.7

Children's Hospital of Orange County. (n.d.). *Guided imagery for kids.* Retrieved from http://www.choc.org/programs-services/integrative-health/guided-imagery/

Christian, B. J. (2016). Translational research—Adapting to the stress and challenges of chronic conditions in children and adolescents. *Journal of Pediatric Nursing, 31*, 736–739. doi:10.1016/j.pedn.2016.09.006

Clark, C. D. (2003). *In sickness and in play: Children coping with chronic illness.* New Brunswick, NJ: Rutgers University Press.

Compas, B. E., Jaser, S. S., Dunn, M. J., & Rodriguez, E. M. (2012). Coping with chronic illness in childhood and adolescence. *Annual Review of Clinical Psychology, 8,* 455–480. doi:10.1146/annurev-clinpsy-032511-143108

Currie, J., & Lin, W. (2007). Chipping away at health: More on the relationship between income and child health. *Health Affairs, 26,* 331–344. doi:10.1377/hlthaff.26.2.331

Dellenmark-Blom, M., Chaplin, J. E., Jönsson, L., Gatzinsky, V., Quitmann, J. H., & Abrahamsson, K. (2016). Coping strategies used by children and adolescents born with esophageal atresia—A focus group study obtaining the child and parent perspective. *Child Care, Health and Development, 42,* 759–767. doi:10.1111/cch.12372

El-Sheikh, M., Harger, J., & Whitson, S. M. (2001). Exposure to interparental conflict and children's adjustment and physical health: The moderating role of vagal tone. *Child Development, 72,* 1617–1636. doi:10.1111/1467-8624.00369

Emery, C. F., France, C. R., Harris, J., Norman, G., & VanArsdalen, C. (2008). Effects of progressive muscle relaxation training on nociceptive flexion reflex threshold in healthy young adults: A randomized trial. *Pain, 138,* 375–379. doi:10.1016/j.pain.2008.01.015

Fjorback, L. O., Arendt, M., Ørnbøl, E., Fink, P., & Walach, H. (2011). Mindfulness-based stress reduction and mindfulness-based cognitive therapy—A systematic review of randomized controlled trials. *Acta Psychiatrica Scandinavica, 124,* 102–119. doi:10.1111/j.1600-0447.2011.01704.x

Fosha, D., Siegel, D. J., & Solomon, M. (2009). *The healing power of emotion: Affective neuroscience, development & clinical practice.* New York, NY: WW Norton.

Friedberg, R. D., & McClure, J. M. (2015). *Clinical practice of cognitive therapy with children and adolescents: The nuts and bolts.* New York, NY: Guilford Press.

Garasky, S., Stewart, S. D., Gundersen, C., Lohman, B. J., & Eisenmann, J. C. (2009). Family stressors and child obesity. *Social Science Research, 38,* 755–766. doi:10.1016/j.ssresearch.2009.06.002

Goldfried, M. R., & Davidson, G. C. (1976). *The therapeutic relationship. Clinical behavior therapy.* New York, NY: Holt, Rinehart & Winston.

Hippisley-Cox, J., Fielding, K., & Pringle, M. (1998). Depression as a risk factor for ischaemic heart disease in men: Population based case-control study. *British Medical Journal, 316,* 1714–1719. doi:10.1136/bmj.316.7146.1714

Individuals with Disabilities Education Improvement Act of 2004, 20 U.S.C. § 1400 *et seq.*

Johnston-Brooks, C. H., Lewis, M. A., Evans, G. W., & Whalen, C. K. (1998). Chronic stress and illness in children: The role of allostatic load. *Psychosomatic Medicine, 60,* 597–603.

Jordan, C., Reid, A. M., Guzick, A. G., Simmons, J., & Sulkowski, M. L. (2017). When exposures go right: Effective exposure-based treatment for obsessive-compulsive disorder. *Journal of Contemporary Psychotherapy, 47,* 31–39. doi:10.1007/s10879-016-9339-2

Jordan, C., Reid, A., Mariaskin, A., Augusto, B., & Sulkowski, M. L. (2012). First-line treatments for pediatric obsessive-compulsive disorder. *Journal of Contemporary Psychotherapy, 42,* 243–248. doi:10.1007/s10879-012-9210-z

Joyce-Beaulieu, D. J., & Sulkowski, M. L. (2015). *Cognitive behavioral therapy in K-12 school settings: A practitioner's toolkit.* New York, NY: Springer.

Kashikar-Zuck, S., Ting, T. V., Arnold, L. M., Bean, J., Powers, S. W., Graham, T. B., . . . Lynch-Jordan, A. M. (2012). Cognitive behavioral therapy for the treatment of juvenile fibromyalgia: A multisite, single-blind, randomized, controlled clinical trial. *Arthritis & Rheumatology, 64*, 297–305. doi:10.1002/art.30644

Katon, W. J., Richardson, L., Lozano, P., & McCauley, E. (2004). The relationship of asthma and anxiety disorders. *Psychosomatic Medicine, 66*, 349–355.

Kenardy, J., Thompson, K., Le Brocque, R., & Olsson, K. (2008). Information–provision intervention for children and their parents following pediatric accidental injury. *European Child & Adolescent Psychiatry, 17*, 316–325. doi:10.1007/s00787-007-0673-5

Kendall, P. C. (2012). *Child and adolescent therapy: Cognitive-behavioral procedures* (4th ed.). New York, NY: Guilford Press.

Kendall, P. C., & Hedtke, K. (2006). *Coping Cat workbook* (2nd ed). Ardmore, PA: Workbook Publishing.

Knafl, K. A., Darney, B. G., Gallo, A. M., & Angst, D. B. (2010). Parental perceptions of the outcome and meaning of normalization. *Research in Nursing & Health, 33*, 87–98. doi:10.1002/nur.20367

Ndetan, H., Willard Evans, M., Williams, R. D., Woolsey, C., & Swartz, J. H. (2014). Use of movement therapies and relaxation techniques and management of health conditions among children. *Alternative Therapies, 20*, 44–50. doi:1078-6791

Newacheck, P., Strickland, B., Shonkoff, J., Perrin, J., McPherson, M., McManus, M., . . . Arango, P. (1998). An epidemiologic profile of children with special health care needs, *Pediatrics, 102*, 117–123.

Nussey, C., Pistrang, N., & Murphy, T. (2013). How does psychoeducation help? A review of the effects of providing information about Tourette syndrome and attention-deficit/hyperactivity disorder. *Child Care, Health and Development, 39*, 617–627. doi:10.1111/cch.12039

Pally, R. (1998). Emotional processing: The mind-body connection. *International Journal of Psycho-analysis 79*, 349.

Pence, S. L., Jr., Sulkowski, M. L., Jordan, C., & Storch, E. A. (2010). When exposures go wrong: Trouble-shooting guidelines for managing difficult scenarios that arise in exposure-based treatment for obsessive-compulsive disorder. *American Journal of Psychotherapy, 64*, 39–53.

Rindstedt, C. (2014). Children's strategies to handle cancer: A video ethnography of imaginal coping. *Child Care, Health and Development, 40*, 580–586. doi:10.1111/cch.12064

Robins, P. M., Smith, S. M., Glutting, J. J., & Bishop, C. T. (2005). A randomized controlled trial of a cognitive-behavioral family intervention for pediatric recurrent abdominal pain. *Journal of Pediatric Psychology, 30*, 397–408. doi:10.1093/jpepsy/jsi063

Rodriguez, E. M., Dunn, M. J., Zuckerman, T., Vannatta, K., Gerhardt, C. A., & Compas, B. E. (2012). Cancer-related sources of stress for children with cancer and their parents. *Journal of Pediatric Psychology, 37*, 185–197. doi:10.1093/jpepsy/jsr054

Safren, S. A., O'cleirigh, C., Tan, J. Y., Raminani, S. R., Reilly, L. C., Otto, M. W., & Mayer, K. H. (2009). A randomized controlled trial of cognitive behavioral therapy for adherence and depression (CBT-AD) in HIV-infected individuals. *Health Psychology, 28*, 1–10. doi:10.1037/a0012715

Salloum, A., Sulkowski, M. L., Sirrine, E., & Storch, E. A. (2009). Overcoming barriers to using empirically supported therapies to treat childhood anxiety disorders in social work practice. *Child and Adolescent Social Work Journal, 26,* 259–273. doi:10.1007/s10560-009-0173-1

Sauer-Zavala, S. E., Walsh, E. C., Eisenlohr-Moul, T. A., & Lykins, E. L. (2013). Comparing mindfulness-based intervention strategies: Differential effects of sitting meditation, body scan, and mindful yoga. *Mindfulness, 4,* 383–388. doi:10.1007/s12671-012-0139-9

Sulkowski, M. L., Jacob, M. L., & Storch, E. A. (2013). Exposure and response prevention and habit reversal training: Commonalities, differential use, and combined applications. *Journal of Contemporary Psychotherapy, 43,* 179–185. doi:10.1007/s10879-013-9234-z

Sulkowski, M. L., McGuire, J. F., & Tesoro, A. (2015). Treating tics and Tourette's disorder in school settings. *Canadian Journal of School Psychology, 31,* 47–62. doi:10.1177/0829573515601820

Tagge, E. P., Natali, E. L., Lima, E., Leek, D., Neece, C. L., & Randall, K. F. (2013). Psychoneuroimmunology and the pediatric surgeon. *Seminars in Pediatric Surgery, 22,* 144–148. doi:10.1053/j.sempedsurg.2013.05.002

van der Lee, J. H., Mokkink, L. B., Grootenhuis, M. A., Heymans, H. S., & Offringa, M. (2007). Definitions and measurement of chronic health conditions in childhood: A systematic review. *Journal of the American Medical Association, 297,* 2741–2751. doi:10.1001/jama.297.24.2741

Van Tilburg, M. A., Chitkara, D. K., Palsson, O. S., Turner, M., Blois-Martin, N., Ulshen, M., & Whitehead, W. E. (2009). Audio-recorded guided imagery treatment reduces functional abdominal pain in children: A pilot study. *Pediatrics, 124,* e890–e897.

White, C. A. (2001). Cognitive behavioral principles in managing chronic disease. *Western Journal of Medicine, 175,* 338–342.

HANDOUT 9.1.

A BRIEF CBT SESSION OVERVIEW

Session 1
- Get consent and assent for treatment and establish the limits of confidentiality
- Develop rapport with the child
- Collect needed background information to help with treatment planning and goal setting (e.g., mental health history, medical history, developmental history, family history and supports, academic or school performance, previous experience with therapy)
- Begin the psychoeducation process and answer any questions the child and family might have about treatment

Session 2
- Continue the psychoeducation process:
  - Normalize the child's experience
  - Provide hope for improvement and reduce feelings of hopelessness
  - Promote awareness of the mind–body connection
  - Cover the CBT model (if it has not already been covered)
- Establish measurable treatment goals (if they have not already been established)

Session 3
Based on a child's presenting issues, consider:

- Relaxation training and stress management (e.g., progressive muscle relaxation, diaphragmatic breathing, guided imagery)
  - Utilize or create relaxation scripts
  - Practice relaxation and stress-management strategies
- Cognitive restructuring
  - Teach about cognitive distortions and maladaptive thinking
- Behavioral exposure
  - Develop an exposure hierarchy and teach about subjective units of distress
- Assign practice or session-related homework

Sessions 4–7
- Assess practice/homework completion from the previous session
- Continue to implement active CBT components
- Consider switching to different components based on the child's treatment response

Session 8+
- Assess treatment response and progress toward goals
- Evaluate whether to terminate therapy or continue
- Discuss managing potential setbacks and regressions
- Discuss booster sessions
- Process termination with the child

Handout 9.2.

Progressive Muscle Relaxation

Progressive muscle relaxation (PMR) involves deep muscle relaxation. It is easy to do, and it can help youth experiencing stress related to chronic medical issues. Therapeutically, PMR is based on the premise that muscle tension is the body's response to anxiety-provoking thoughts and feelings and that relaxing our muscles can help reducing our overall tension, stress, and anxiety. PMR is easy to learn and to use with children to induce a sense of relaxation.

Using PMR involves learning to identify and to monitor tension in specific muscle groups. Common areas where muscle tension tends to accumulate include the shoulders, neck, chest, arms, and back. However, tension can easily be reduced in these areas using PMR. Implementing PMR involves systematically tightening and loosening muscles to produce a sensation of relaxation in the previously mentioned muscle groups. Essentially, through tightening and relaxation of muscle groups, PMR helps to promote relaxation through complex physiological and psychological interactions. Furthermore, PMR can be modified for a child who has a physical disability by avoiding focusing on muscle groups that cause excessive pain or that are impaired.

Sample PMR Script

Sit back, close your eyes, and get comfortable—try to allow your worries and stressors to melt away as you become relaxed.

Take some very deep breaths. Try to imagine your chest inflating like a large balloon—fill up your balloon as much as you possibly can.

Now release your breath slowly—very slowly—and imagine exhaling your tension, all of your tension. Then, completely empty your tension so you're ready to breathe deeply again.
[*Repeat several times until the client starts feeling more relaxed*]

Now turn your attention to your feet. Begin to tense your feet by curling your toes and the arch of your foot. Notice and witness the tension.
[*Have the client stay tense for about 5–10 seconds, followed by about 20 seconds of relaxation*]

Now release the tension in your feet. Notice the new feeling of relaxation. Notice how you feel different than you did when you were tense.

Now begin to focus on your lower legs. Tense the muscles in the back of your legs. Get your muscles really hard and pay attention to the tension.
[*Have the client stay tense for about 5–10 seconds, followed by about 20 seconds of relaxation*]

Now release the tension in your legs and pay attention to the feeling of relaxation again. Remember to keep taking deep breaths.

Now tense the muscles of your upper leg and in the middle of your body. You can do this by tightly squeezing your thighs together. Make sure you feel the tension. [*Have the client stay tense for about 5–10 seconds, followed by about 20 seconds of relaxation*]

And now release. Feel the tension leaving your muscles.

The previous process can be continued to target tension through the rest of the body. For example, the next muscle group could be stomach or torso. Moreover, this approach is easy to teach to students of a range of different ages and backgrounds (Joyce-Beaulieu & Sulkowski, 2015).

Factors to Consider When Using PMR

How long PMR sessions should be can vary, although it usually takes at least 15 to 20 minutes to induce sufficient relaxation. In general, shorter PMR scripts should be used with younger individuals, and such scripts usually focus on fewer or less nuanced muscle groups than are the focus of scripts used with adolescents and adults. Instead of using long scripts, shorter scripts can be repeated multiple times in a session to ensure learning and correct application. Regarding specific delivery guidelines, Goldfried and Davidson (1976) recommend that approximately 20 seconds of relaxation follow each 5 to 10 seconds of muscle tension. Additionally, to prevent injury or serious discomfort, especially with children with medical problems or chronic illness, they recommend that the trainer advise the child to tense 75% of the way to full tension during muscle tensing. Furthermore, a wealth of literature recommends that the trainer speak slowly, melodically, and in a calm and warm voice while delivering PMR (Friedberg & McClure, 2015).

Recommendations for Using the Intervention

Structure
1. Develop rapport with the child and provide psychoeducation or information about the PMR process. This generally involves discussing the treatment, assessing symptoms and current functioning, normalizing treatment, coming up with treatment goals, addressing questions from the child or parents, and playing a brief game.
2. Determine an appropriate script or create one. Factors to consider are: The presenting problems (e.g., anxiety, anger), the developmental level of the child, the amount of time available to do the intervention, availability of resources (e.g., reliable Internet connection, tape recorder, etc.), and cultural and linguistic factors that can influence treatment.
3. Implement the script. Allow for adequate cycles of tension and relaxation, speak in a soft yet warm voice, assess the child's response to the intervention, and use metaphors to illustrate therapeutic concepts, as well as consider imagery, cue-controlled relaxation, or biofeedback.

4. Make adjustments to the script (if needed) and record it. Address any parts of the script that the child finds confusing, assess for any difficulties with understanding the therapeutic process, record the script, and provide the child access to the script for practice.
5. Assign practice. Encourage the child to practice using the script, problem-solve, resolve any barriers to practice, and schedule follow-up meetings with the child to ensure success with PMR.
6. Evaluate the child's response to the intervention. Assess and determine the efficacy of treatment, if additional training is needed, or if another intervention approach might be more appropriate or effective.

Finally, it important to note that PMR should not be used to address compulsive or anxiety-related disorders, such as obsessive-compulsive disorder (Joyce-Beaulieu & Sulkowski, 2015), because of the risk that PMR strategies might be misapplied and become new compulsive behaviors, which can lead to further complications and treatment setbacks. Additionally, although not much is known about why it happens, a small number of individuals experience heightened anxiety when engaging in PMR or relaxation strategies more generally. Therefore, if a child appears to be becoming increasingly anxious, as opposed to experiencing relaxation, during PMR, the intervention should be discontinued.

Recommended Resources

Print Resources
Friednerg, R. D., & McClure, J. M. (2016). *Clinical practice with cognitive therapy with children and adolescents: The nuts and bolts.* New York, NY: Guilford Press.
Joyce-Beaulieu, D. J., & Sulkowski, M. L. (2015). *Cognitive behavioral therapy in K-12 schools: A practitioner's workbook.* New York, NY: Springer.
Kendall, P. C. (2012). *Child and adolescent therapy: Cognitive-behavioral procedures* (4th ed.). New York, NY: Guilford Press.

Web Resources
The Association of Behavioral and Cognitive Therapies (ABCT) provides resources on evidence-based treatments for a range of disorders and mental health problems. Also, ABCT maintains an active database of expert providers: http://www.abct.org/Home/
In an initiative encouraging professionals from a range of disciplines to learn, teach, and implement evidence-based behavioral practice (EBBP), the EBBP.org project provides training resources to help therapists learn and apply EBBP: http://www.ebbp.org/

10

Acceptance and Commitment Therapy

GLENN M. SLOMAN AND MICHAEL C. SELBST ■

Acceptance and commitment therapy, or ACT (pronounced as the entire word), helps individuals manage their chronic pain through changing their relationship with unpleasant thoughts, feelings, sensations, urges, and memories in the service of engaging in values-based actions. ACT utilizes an experiential approach to help people connect with what they have struggled, how they address the issue, and an alternative approach to living. As an example, imagine a student and therapist are standing and each is holding one end of the same rope. This student has experienced secondary headaches caused by chronic sinus infections that often contribute to her missing class. In the therapist's room, there is a line of paper on the floor separating the therapist and the student.

> THERAPIST: *"Imagine that you are in a tug-of-war match with an enormous headache monster. You are holding one end of the rope and I am the monster that has the other end. Between the two of us lies a deep ravine. As you pull backward as hard as you can, the monster pulls harder, moving you ever closer to the edge. What do you do?"*
> STUDENT: *"I'll pull even harder."* [Student pulls on the rope.]
> THERAPIST: *"Makes sense, so the monster in turn pulls harder. You pull harder, and the monster pulls harder.* [Therapist tugs on the rope.] *I'm sure that you could keep this up for a while. How long do you think you could do this before becoming tired?"*
> STUDENT: *"Probably a couple of minutes."*
> THERAPIST: *"How would you feel in a couple of hours?"*
> STUDENT: *"I would be exhausted."*

THERAPIST: "*So, you're stuck in this tug-of-war match, trying very hard to win, but as the monster, I can do this forever.*" [Therapist and student are each pulling on the rope.] "*What could you do instead?*"

STUDENT: "*I guess I could let go of the rope.*" [Student drops the rope to the floor.]

THERAPIST: [Therapist, still playing the monster, tells the student to pick up the rope, telling her that the only way to get rid of the monster is to join the tug-of-war match again.] "*When you drop the rope, the monster does not go away. On the other hand, you have stopped struggling with the monster and can instead do something more useful.*"

STUDENT: "*So, what else can I do?*"

THERAPIST: "*Well, that is a great question and something that we will explore together.*"

OVERVIEW OF THE ACT PROCESS

In the brief exchange above, the therapist uses a metaphor and an experiential exercise, adapted from Hayes, Strosahl, and Wilson (1999), to help the student notice how emotional and thought-control strategies limit life and induce additional anguish, as she struggles with challenging private/covert experiences (i.e., thoughts, feelings, sensations, urges, and memories). An alternative to the continued struggle is offered by ACT. Developed by Hayes and colleagues in the early 1980s, ACT is a treatment approach that focuses on workability (i.e., doing what works) to promote psychological flexibility. Psychological flexibility is the "ability to contact the present more fully as a conscious human being, and to either change or persist when doing so serves valued ends" (Hayes, Strosahl, Bunting, Twohig, & Wilson, 2005, p. 5). A shorter definition of psychological flexibility is offered by Harris (2009) as the ability "to be present, open up, and do what matters" (p. 12).

In the metaphor, one must acknowledge first the unworkable action that has been historically and currently used to end suffering through attempts to control private experiences. For example, the student in the "tug-of-war" match avoids class in response to the headache, yet the headache does not improve. The cost of avoidance is life-restricting, as the student's social supports in school are not contacted as frequently and the absences from class become lost learning opportunities. The avoidance/escape strategies can be healthy, or harmful to the student if used in excess, and they may include distracting oneself with television/social media, withdrawing from friends and family, disengaging from things that are important (e.g., school and community life), or self-harm, all of which function to gain relief from what one does not want to have (e.g., unwanted private experiences, such as sadness, nervousness, thoughts of "I can't stand/do this," anger, etc.) by temporarily escaping or avoiding them.

ACT uses metaphors, such as the metaphor of the monster in the example, to help change one's relationship to thoughts, feelings, sensations, urges, and memories and to help loosen the struggle with them and engage in behaviors that are value-oriented. The approach assumes that suffering is part of the human experience and, at times, may be inescapable even when engaging in actions predicated on what is meaningful. The individual learns through experience that avoiding or escaping suffering is impossible and that attempting to do so costs him/her the opportunity to live a life of vitality. For children with a health condition, ACT may help them to re-engage with actions directed toward educational and social aspects of school, over which they have more control, instead of focusing on attempting to modify how they feel and think.

Empirical Support for ACT

Currently, there are over 170 randomized controlled trials (RCTs) as well as a number of meta-analytic and systematic reviews of the research (e.g., Halliburton & Cooper, 2015; Swain, Hancock, Dixon, & Bowman, 2015) that support the effectiveness of ACT for individuals with a variety of conditions. For children and adolescents, ACT has been applied to many socially significant concerns, including obsessive-compulsive disorder, emotional dysregulation, anxiety, high-functioning autism spectrum disorder, pain, anorexia nervosa, depression, tic disorders, trichotillomania, stress, post-traumatic stress disorder, attention deficit hyperactivity disorder, sickle cell disease, and sexualized behavior (Swain et al., 2015). At the time of this writing, ACT has shown promising outcomes by increasing school attendance and quality of life and decreasing stress, anxiety, rumination, depressive symptoms, and reports of pain intensity and discomfort (Swain et al., 2015).

THE MIND: NOT YOUR FRIEND, NOT YOUR ENEMY

From an ACT perspective, the mind consists of thoughts and language. Humans utilize their minds for survival purposes in managing the external world to solve a wide range of problems effectively. The downside of language, and its virtue in solving problems, is that humans use their mind to target problems residing inside the skin (e.g., difficult thoughts, unpleasant feelings) because it works well for outside-the-skin issues (such as fixing a flat tire, inventing new technologies, and navigating social and environmental contexts).

When humans attempt to solve internal problems by using a generalized approach to problem-solving, the solutions sometimes become the problem. Our minds engage the problem (as if it were a physical problem) and encourage us to pull the rope harder or to pick it up again to escape from or to avoid difficult private experiences. In the short term, behaviors based on attempts to reduce or eliminate private experiences bring short-term relief. In the long term, if the struggle with private events becomes the focus, it is at the expense of living a values-guided life. In ACT, the two major issues that can contribute to being stuck in the short-term relief cycle are experiential avoidance and cognitive fusion, both of which are described more fully later in this section.

The ACT model posits that psychological difficulties arise from psychological inflexibility or "the inability to change or persist in behavior in the service of long term valued ends" (Hayes, Luoma, Bond, Masuda, & Lillis, 2006, p. 6). As meantioned, the major culprits that prevent individuals from behaving in a fashion that is meaningful to them are experiential avoidance and cognitive fusion. The two culprits are often experienced in tandem and are a helpful illustration of how many people become stuck in unworkable patterns of behavior.

Experiential Avoidance

Experiential avoidance is the attempt to control or alter the form, frequency, or situational sensitivity of internal experiences, even when doing so causes harm (Hayes, Wilson, Gifford, Follette, & Strosahl, 1996). In other words, experiential avoidance occurs when one is unwilling to experience internal discomfort that cannot be avoided, but from which one may temporarily escape. For example, a child diagnosed with cancer may struggle to manage and accept the physical pain, fatigue, fear, and uncertainty he experiences during the long car ride to access necessary treatment and while meeting with the pediatric oncologist. Instead of noticing and accepting the discomfort, he may display extreme anxiety, throw a tantrum, or elope from the office as an attempt to avoid the uncomfortable experiences.

Cognitive Fusion

Cognitive fusion occurs when one's behavior is largely dominated by rules, reasons, judgments, and evaluations rather than contact with direct environmental contingencies. When people are fused with thoughts, thoughts greatly influence our behavior. For example, a child who self-administers insulin for diabetes management may be faced with both emotional discomfort and thoughts that interfere with behavioral adherence to blood glucose testing and daily injections. A difficult thought, such as "I can't do this today [daily injection]," if taken literally and resulting in nonadherence to the self-care regimen, may have serious health consequences.

Cognitive Behavioral Therapy and ACT: A Short Comparison

Cognitive behavioral therapy (CBT) aims to modify distorted thoughts and beliefs directly through cognitive restructuring, disputation, evaluating the rationality of thoughts, and thought stopping. Alternatively, ACT helps individuals begin to relate to thoughts and feelings in new ways, rather than change them, in the service of doing what is workable. A CBT practitioner may have a client test if a belief is true by examining the evidence for the belief through looking at its content. For example, the thought, "I can't go to school when I am in pain" may be disputed by examining a history of times when the student went to school while in pain. An evidentiary approach may then convince the client he/she has gone to school, and can go to school, based on previous experiences. In contrast, an ACT practitioner may have the individual become aware of, and then label, the sensations of pain and approach them with curiosity; thereafter, the practitioner may ask the client both to notice the sensations and to go to school to see what happens. Additionally, the ACT practitioner may then connect going to school to values that the young person has, such as interacting with friends and a love of learning new ideas.

Both CBT and ACT use experiential exercises, but for different purposes. CBT may have a student test the validity of a belief outside the therapy session. For example, the aforementioned student who self-administers insulin and believes that peers will tease him about his diabetes may be asked to arrange a play date and later to record what the peer said and did to determine whether the teasing really occurred. On the other hand, ACT examines the workability of avoiding fear stimuli in meeting valued life ends by participating fully during the play date while having the student notice the thoughts and feelings that show up for him. While the topography of the exercise and the outcome (child attends play date) may look the same, the underlying purpose or function of the exercise is different. One aims to challenge the belief directly and to reduce the symptoms of anxiety or fear (CBT), whereas the other (ACT) attempts to foster flexibility through the experience of accepting discomfort and distancing from thoughts (not disputing them) to connect with what is meaningful to the individual. In this example, CBT targets symptom reduction specifically, while ACT does not. The ACT approach incorporates successful action and workability, while avoiding a focus on symptom elimination (although many times this does occur as a byproduct).

DANCING AROUND THE HEXA-FLEX

Because the ACT practitioner is constantly seeking to foster psychological flexibility in the client, the practitioner embodies the core processes of psychological flexibility during treatment sessions. There are six interdependent processes that contribute to psychological flexibility as an outcome; three are mindfulness and acceptance-based processes and three are behavior-change processes. These processes are typically presented in the model called the Hexa-Flex (see Figure 10.1). The three mindfulness and acceptance-based processes are defusion, acceptance, and contact with the present moment, and the three behavior-change processes are self-as-context, values, and committed action. For example, the skill of contacting the present moment may be compared with the skill of noticing without evaluation or judgment one's bodily sensations while they are occurring

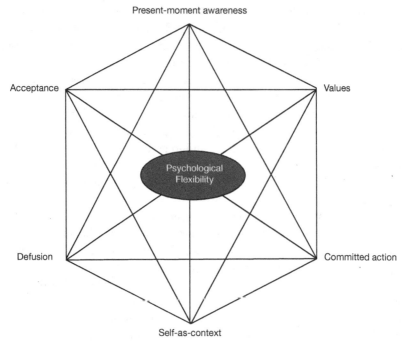

Figure 10.1. ACT Hexa-Flex representing the interconnected processes of psychological flexibility.

in real time. The student with diabetes, therefore, would notice the physical sensations associated with administering insulin, as well as where he experiences pain in his body throughout the day. Each of the core processes of psychological flexibility can be thought of as a skill, and they are described below.

Due to ACT's nonlinear model, practitioners often refer to attempts to engender psychological flexibility in session as "dancing around the Hexa-Flex." As the ACT practitioner attempts to move a person to psychological flexibility, the person may become stuck in a process/skill. ACT practitioners can demonstrate psychological flexibility by switching to a different process within the Hexa-Flex to help foster the client's meaningful engagement in his life through performing committed actions aligned with values.

Defusion

Defusion is the skill that allows people to notice that thoughts simply are pictures and words that float through the mind, rather than being the truth and representing the literal meaning of the words. The skill of defusion may be introduced by describing the protective nature of language and how, at times, it can lead to life-constricting behavioral repertories. Alternatively, the power of words may be reduced by having the student sing a thought aloud, thereby helping him or her to relate to the thought differently. To illustrate defusion, often saying the word *lice*, especially in the school setting, will evoke private images associated with lice (i.e., little crawly bugs in hair) and potentially some behavioral correlates, such as scratching or itching. One method to disarm the word *lice* is to highlight its acoustic properties by repeating it aloud for 45 seconds. The exercise transforms the word from its aversive function to a repeated sound with little to no impact. In a sense, the process reduces the "minding" of the word and increases the sensory properties of the word.

For example, a student with cystic fibrosis may say, "I can't complete the math problems or participate in class because I'm too tired and weak." If taken literally (fused with the thought), the student will have to wait until she is awake, alert, and breathing better to more fully participate in math class. However, if the student is defused from the thought, then she notices that her mind is telling her that she is too tired and weak, but that she can make the choice to work and participate. The defusion skill allows her to increase awareness of her thoughts as they happen, rather than seeing through them and buying into them. Defusion allows students to respond to thoughts in terms of workability and not the literal truth (Luoma, Hayes, & Walser, 2007, p. 58).

Another example is when a student has a strong belief that she is not good enough. Picture attempting to help a student apply to college, but the student says, "What's the use in even applying? Who would possibly accept someone with cystic fibrosis who coughs and has trouble breathing? They would see me as too disruptive." The ACT practitioner can compassionately empathize with the student while helping her defuse from the thought by saying, "It sounds like your mind is really trying to beat you up right now. What would happen if we listened to your mind?" If the student replies, "I'd leave your office and not submit an application," the ACT practitioner can say, "Yeah, you're right. See if you can thank your mind for those thoughts and let's open the application for the first college you listed."

Acceptance

Acceptance is a critical skill that means the individual learns how to actively become aware of, and accept, his/her private events without trying to change the form or frequency. Thus, the individual does not try to reduce or eliminate the discomfort they are experiencing. Instead, the individual learns how to feel worry, fear, sadness, and any other feeling completely. The therapist provides the individual with approaches that will help him or her turn off the "struggle switch" so that he or she is no longer struggling with the debilitating emotions. This allows the student with cystic fibrosis, for example, to notice her chest pain and uncomfortable breathing while continuing with her treatment, attending class, and participating in valued social interactions. Fundamentally, this contrasts with EA, since she makes no attempt to control her private events, which would effectively move her away from that what she values (Luoma et al., 2007).

The ACT practitioner teaches the student that suffering is a normal part of existing and being human, while demonstrating compassion throughout the sessions. The student learns that it is important to be willing to be fully and actively open to the entirety of experiences. Often, it is helpful to use the terms *acceptance* and *willingness* interchangeably, since many individuals have preconceived notions of acceptance, thinking that they need to "just be okay" with their circumstances, ignore their feelings, and "move on." Instead, the therapist helps the student to choose to move in the direction of who and what he or she identifies as important, while accepting (or being willing to experience) the thoughts and feelings that show up.

For example, choosing to attend school and to participate fully may require the student with cystic fibrosis to accept that she may have the thought that she is exhausted and to recognize that it would be a lot easier to just stay in bed; however, if she focuses on eliminating her negative thoughts and feelings, she may continue to miss school, to avoid valued peer interactions, and not move toward what she has identified as most important in her life. The ACT therapist helps the student create valuable opportunities to actively practice and to foster willingness skills in situations where the student previously avoided negative, unwanted internal experiences.

Contact with the Present Moment/Mindfulness

Mindfulness practice is a skill that helps an individual come in contact with experiences as they are, rather than as what he or she expects or evaluates them to be. If one enhances one's noticing skills by discriminating or labeling a thought or feeling as a thought or feeling as it happens, one begins to understand that one can either struggle with the experience or simply have it as it is. Experiences are both physiological and psychological (language-based), which facilitates allowing the "experience to be [the] guide" (Hayes et al., 1999).

It is important for both the ACT practitioner and the student to be nonjudgmental throughout the experiences. This promotes "present moment awareness." Luoma et al. (2007) stated, "When in contact with the present moment, humans are flexible, responsive, and aware of the possibilities and learning opportunities afforded by the current situation" (p. 19). Alternatively, if the individual does not successfully contact the present moment, he or she is likely to continue to engage in the same behaviors, which historically relieve symptoms only for the short term at best and which are inconsistent with the individual's values. The therapist helps the student focus on the "here and now," that his or her life is happening now, in the moment, and that the relationship with the present moment is paramount. The goal is to help the student understand and appreciate that he or she does not need to eliminate or change past, present, or future thinking or feeling. Rather, he or she benefits by being mindful of the present experiences, observing and describing such experiences without judgment. This yields greater psychological flexibility. Structured therapeutic activities may include mindfulness/meditation exercises to focus on present-moment awareness. For example, a student may be asked to practice mindful awareness of everyday activities, such as brushing teeth, eating, walking to school, opening a locker, waiting in the cafeteria line, etc. Other activities may involve keeping a journal of thoughts and feelings related to daily events, various meditations (while sitting or walking), and metaphors, such as imagining clouds moving through the sky, leaves falling from a tree, or leaves floating down a stream. The student is guided to imagine placing his or her thoughts on the clouds or leaves as they gradually move along, allowing the thoughts to "go."

Self-as-Context

A goal of ACT is for individuals to develop a sense of themselves as observers, noticers, and experiencers, unrelated to the specific private event they are experiencing in the present moment. While individuals are aware of their experiences, they are taught to be careful not to become attached to such experiences. Over time, they learn to observe and accept all their experiences without equating themselves to the experience. For example, the student who fails a test may privately think, "I am stupid," "I am a failure," or "I am never good at studying." The adolescent who struggles with sports due to low muscle tone, poor speed and agility, and poor hand–eye coordination may say "I am a terrible athlete" and avoid any group activities that involve gross-motor movement. Both students in these examples have come to believe their stories about themselves, stories that they wrote and perpetuated. The "I am" statement becomes a belief statement about oneself that the student is certain is true, complete, and undeniable. This is powerful and debilitating, resulting in the individual's digging a greater proverbial hole for themselves rather than putting aside the shovel and simply becoming aware of the present moment while observing his or her thoughts.

In ACT, the practitioner helps the individual to learn to attend to a continuous sense of self. The ongoing private events (thoughts, feelings) are observed with a greater awareness of the context in which they are occurring, instead of as facts that define who the person "is" or "is not." Students may be taught to notice thoughts or feelings, so that noticing their stories and developing self-as-context allow them to become unstuck and no longer struggle (Luoma et al., 2007).
For example, a student with chronic pain may learn to say, "I'm noticing I'm having the thought that this game is really difficult," "I'm observing that my legs feel sore and my body is sweating profusely," or "I'm aware that my eyes are closing and paying attention is hard to do when I haven't had a good night's sleep." An ACT exercise may include having the student recall a memory of something he did at school recently, noticing what he was doing, where he was, who else was present, and recalling the smells, sounds, sights, etc. As he is remembering the event, noticing all the details, he is encouraged to notice who is noticing all of this.

This helps the student better observe his thoughts and feelings without experiential avoidance or cognitive fusion. Thus, he is better able to choose and to commit to actions consistent with his values.

Values

When taking steps in a value-driven direction, the student moves toward who and what is important to him or her. In ACT, a commonly used metaphor is to think of values as a compass. Values are the cardinal directions (north, south, etc.) of our lives, and goals are the places we find when heading in one direction or another (Harris, 2009). A compass includes directions and keeps you on track when you are traveling. If you decide that traveling west is important to you, then you take committed steps moving in that direction. If you begin in New York and get to California, then you have been traveling west and your journey has not ended. Instead, you can continue to travel further and further west, experiencing, noticing, and accepting the discomfort that may come along (rough waters, bad weather, roadblocks, and fatigue) while persisting in your values-based action.

Our chosen values that provide us with direction in life commonly include family relations, intimate relations, parenting, friendships, career, educational growth, recreation/leisure, health, spirituality, and community life (Harris, 2009). After considering and choosing which values are important (which could include some or all of those listed), each person can choose which goals he or she wants to achieve on his or her journey.

The student with cystic fibrosis, who values learning and helping others, moves in this direction by showing up in class, paying attention, working diligently, asking questions, and seeking assistance when needed. When she achieves her high school diploma, undergraduate degree, graduate degree, and her first job opportunity, she has achieved many goals, but she can continue her journey consistent with her values by learning from others (e.g., attending seminars, speaking with colleagues, reading) and helping others in many ways (e.g., volunteering at a soup kitchen, providing a free workshop, coaching a youth sports team). Meanwhile, she also notices her private events, which may include financial hardships, fatigue, illness, time away from loved ones, etc.

It is also important to differentiate between having a value-driven life and happiness. The same student described above may have straight A's, serve as president of her high school class, be captain of a sports team, have many friends, and be considered highly attractive. Yet, she may be mindful of frequent negative thoughts and feelings with which she is struggling. This occurs because accumulating "things," having titles and awards, and doing "things" do not necessarily equate to happiness. Instead, the ACT practitioner helps the student strive to have a life that is meaningful, with committed actions toward what she values, while being willing to experience discomfort that shows up along the way.

Committed Action

Committed action, an integral component of ACT, helps the individual change his or her behavior in order to move forward consistent with his or her chosen values, while noticing and accepting his or her private experiences (thoughts, feelings, and other "stuff" that shows up along the way). Yet, committed action is often challenging for the student who has been experiencing significant health conditions. The student may have avoided going to school many days, skipped school events (dances, sports events), stopped studying, and procrastinated about returning phone calls, text messages, or social media communications. The ACT therapist outlines specific steps of the journey for the individual, employing empirically based behavioral methods. A detailed description of the approaches is beyond the scope of this book; however, it is common to include exposure, skills training, behavioral activation, and other empirically supported interventions for problems related to school avoidance, fear of public speaking or class participation, difficulty working in groups, executive functioning deficits, obsessive-compulsive disorder, anxiety related to participation in a sport, teasing or bullying, depression, generalized anxiety disorder, substance abuse, etc. (see Weisz & Kazdin, 2017, for a comprehensive assessment and treatment guide to many psychological difficulties experienced by children, adolescents, and their families).

A METHOD FOR PRESENTING ACT

There have been many useful approaches to conceptualizing ACT processes while communicating the processes to the client. One is the ACT Matrix described by Polk and Schoendorff (2014). Other variations include the DNA-V Model developed by Hayes and Ciarrochi (2015) and the Choice Point 2.0 originally created by Bailey, Ciarrochi, and Harris (2013) and then modified by Harris (2017). These approaches utilize the skills identified in the Hexa-Flex while presenting the skills to the client in different ways. Please note that no ACT variation is superior to the others, and determining which variation to select depends on what the clinician judges would be most helpful to the client in fostering psychological flexibility. The ACT Matrix is discussed below with an embedded case illustration.

ACT Matrix

The ACT Matrix (see Figure 10.2) is a tool created by Kevin Polk to teach others how to sort inside and outside experiences and behavior toward values or away from difficult inside experiences, while bringing awareness to the impact of short-term "away moves." Sorting involves becoming aware of experiences, discriminating

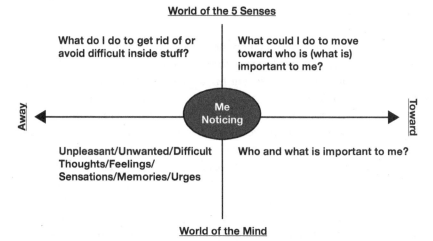

Figure 10.2. The ACT Matrix with accompanying questions by Polk and Schoendorff (2014).

the experiences, and performing some action based on the experiences. The 13 steps in using the ACT Matrix are illustrated in the case study below.

Alice, an 11-year-old girl in the sixth grade, was diagnosed with Type 1 diabetes when she was 10 years old, following her admission to a hospital for diabetic ketoacidosis (DKA). After being stabilized and receiving psychoeducation on diabetes and diabetes management, Alice was informed that to help monitor her blood glucose levels, a small drop of blood must be extracted via a tiny needlestick in the side of her finger. Although she was not phobic about needles, over time Alice began skipping days of her self-monitoring during the next summer, due to the aversiveness of self-testing, and she started lying to her mother about testing her glucose levels. This resulted in another hospital admittance during September to stabilize her glucose control. After Alice received clearance to return to school, she participates in a meeting with her mother, the school nurse, and the school psychologist (SP), who was familiar with ACT and the ACT Matrix. The goal of the meeting is to discuss Alice's issues and to help Alice adhere to blood glucose monitoring. SP starts by inviting Alice to use the ACT Matrix in 13 steps.

Step 1: *The SP stands up and draws a vertical line on a large white board. At the top of the line is the label "World of the 5 Senses." The SP asks Alice to hold a pencil and notice how the pencil feels/smells/looks/sounds, pausing for 5 seconds between each sense (taste is not included because it may be unhygienic).*

Step 2: *The SP labels the bottom part of the vertical line "World of the Mind." This time, the exercise is for Alice to close her eyes, place the pencil aside, and imagine the pencil, including the pencil's taste. The SP asks, "Did you notice any differences?" and "Who notices the differences?" These two questions help to promote present-moment awareness and self-as-context* *(that is, Alice steps back from her experience while not being defined by her experience).*

Step 3: *The SP writes "Me noticing," in the middle of the vertical line and circles the words.*

Step 4: *The SP draws a horizontal line through the vertical line and labels the right side "Toward." The SP asks, "Have you ever had the experience of picking up a loved one at the airport or seeing a good friend whom you haven't seen in a while, such as on the first day of school?" and "How do you feel recalling moving toward them?" The questions asked are to generate a sense of what it feels like to engage in "toward" moves (i.e., values-based actions).*

Step 5: *Then the SP writes "Away," on the left side of the horizontal line. The SP asks, "Have you ever seen a scary movie where there is a really scary part with a lot of suspense?" Alice indicates that she has, and she sometimes leaves the room because the tension she feels makes her uncomfortable. Alice reports that, after she leaves the room, she feels a sense of relief from being scared.*

Step 6: *The SP notes that Alice's feeling sounds like "relief from grief" and asks Alice to notice the difference between toward and away moves, as well as, again, who notices the difference.*

Step 7: *The SP writes in the lower right-hand quadrant "Who/what is important to you?" and then writes down Alice's answers (such as her parents, friends, music, artwork, an art class she takes at school, and her health).*

Step 8: *The SP then asks, "What kind of unwanted or painful stuff shows up inside of you and gets in the way?" and records what Alice says in the lower left-hand quadrant. Alice describes her daily blood check as painful and worries that she may have to go to the hospital again. The SP reflects that many painful thoughts, feelings, and memories show up.*

Step 9: *The SP inquires what Alice does when the painful stuff shows up and records Alice's reported actions in the upper left-hand quadrant, such as not following through with her diabetes management plan and eating food that she is supposed to avoid. The SP validates these actions as understandable, because people attempt to get rid of, or move away from, painful inside stuff by engaging in many different actions.*

Step 10: *The SP then asks Alice if responding to her painful inside experiences eliminates them forever. Alice reports that it does not, while the SP draws arrows first from the lower left to the upper left and then an arrow from the upper left back down to the lower left, indicating that painful inside experiences return even when people desperately attempt to avoid them through various actions. This process demonstrates how people "get stuck" and struggle endlessly in the attempt to control the way they think and feel. It also creates awareness of the futility of these actions and, as step 11 exemplifies, the need to do something radically different in managing unwanted internal experiences.*

Step 11: *The SP encourages Alice to be on the lookout for hooks in step 10. Hooks occur when our attention focuses on dealing with unwanted inside stuff directly, which may lead to unhelpful, values-inconsistent actions. Step 11 involves completing the upper right quadrant by answering the question, "What could you do instead to move toward who or what is important to you?" The SP initiates this process by asking the question and by pointing from the lower right to the upper right quadrant. This type of active problem-solving concentrates on values-based actions rather than directing problem-solving efforts toward alleviating internal experiences. Alice comments that she can schedule a time to check her blood glucose and and she can conduct the checks in front of her mother because her health is important to her. Alice also states that she will follow her dietary plan and reward herself for sticking to it by doing something fun, like texting a friend pictures using a new filter on her phone's camera. She connects these behaviors to being able to attend an art class at school while not having to go to the hospital to be monitored.*

Step 12: *The SP asks Alice to estimate the time she spends engaging in away moves as compared to toward moves and to write down her estimates on the corresponding sides of the Matrix (i.e., on the toward side or the away side). Alice notes that, including sleep, she spends approximately 16 hours engaging in away moves and 8 hours engaging in toward moves. This step allows students to become aware of how much time they use to control internal experiences and hints that the moves they make can be predicated on choice, not history.*

Step 13: *The Matrix activity session ends with a homework assignment. The SP asks Alice to notice what she does when unwanted thoughts and feelings show up as she goes about her day. The homework assignment is designed to be unobtrusive and relatively easy, and it is used as a bridge to conducting another Matrix exercise at the next meeting.*

CONCLUSION

Overall, ACT is a case conceptualization tool and treatment approach that offers a practical method for school-based professionals to help children and adolescents who experience chronic health conditions reduce suffering and engage in life-affirming, values-based actions. This chapter aims to help professionals understand how they may incorporate ACT in their practices with the populations they dedicatedly serve.

ADDITIONAL RESOURCES

To learn more about ACT and to access resources on ACT, visit the Association for Contextual Behavioral Science at https://contextualscience.org.

REFERENCES

Bailey, A., Ciarrochi, J., & Harris, R. (2013). *The weight escape: How to stop dieting and start living.* Boulder, CO: Shambhala.

Halliburton, A. E., & Cooper, L. D. (2015). Applications and adaptations of acceptance and commitment therapy (ACT) for adolescents. *Journal of Contextual Behavioral Science, 4,* 1–11.

Harris, R. (2009). *ACT made simple.* Oakland, CA: New Harbinger.

Harris, R. (2017). *Choice Point 2.0.* Retrieved from https://www.actmindfully.com.au

Hayes, L., & Ciarrochi, J. (2015). *The thriving adolescent: Using acceptance and commitment therapy and positive psychology to help teens manage emotions, achieve goals, and build connection.* Oakland, CA: New Harbinger.

Hayes, S. C., Luoma, J. B., Bond, F. W., Masuda, A., & Lillis, J. (2006). Acceptance and commitment therapy: Model, processes, and outcomes. *Behaviour Research and Therapy, 44,* 1–25.

Hayes, S. C., Strosahl, K. D., Bunting, K., Twohig, M., & Wilson, K. G. (2005). What is acceptance and commitment therapy? In S.C. Hayes & K. D. Strosahl (Eds.), *A practical guide to acceptance and commitment therapy* (pp. 3–31). New York, NY: Springer-Verlag.

Hayes, S. C., Strosahl, K. D., & Wilson, K. G. (1999). *Acceptance and commitment therapy: An experiential approach to behavior change.* New York, NY: Guilford Press.

Hayes, S. C., Wilson, K. G., Gifford, E. V., Follette, V. M., & Strosahl, K. (1996). Experiential avoidance and behavioral disorders: A functional dimensional approach to diagnosis and treatment. *Journal of Consulting and Clinical Psychology, 64*(6), 1152–1168.

Luoma, J. B., Hayes, S. C., & Walser, R. D. (2007). *Learning ACT: An acceptance & commitment therapy skills-training manual for therapists.* Oakland, CA: New Harbinger.

Polk, K., & Schoendorff, B. (2014). *The ACT Matrix: A new approach to building psychological flexibility across settings and populations.* Oakland, CA: Context Press/New Harbinger.

Swain, J., Hancock, K., Dixon, A., & Bowman, J. (2015). Acceptance and commitment therapy for children: A systematic review of intervention studies. *Journal of Contextual Behavioral Science, 4,* 73–85.

Weisz, J. R., & Kazdin, A. E. (Eds.). (2017). *Evidence-based psychotherapies for children and adolescents* (3rd ed.). New York, NY: Guilford Press.

Behavioral Strategies to Promote Adherence

ANGELA I. CANTO, DAVID J. CHESIRE, AND C. BAKER WRIGHT ■

Children with chronic medical conditions experience a host of symptoms that may affect their ability to be fully participatory in school and family activities. Symptoms vary greatly from one medical condition to the next, and from one child to another, but often include fatigue, pain, headache, inattentiveness, stress, anxiety, behavioral disinhibition, and low frustration tolerance. Further complicating matters, research has consistently shown that roughly 50% of all patients, including pediatric patients, are not compliant with recommended treatment (Burrell & Levy, 1985; Rapoff, 2010). This lack of adherence to medical treatment increases the likelihood of adverse outcomes and associated healthcare costs (Sokol, McGuigan, Verbrugge, & Epstein, 2005).

Thus, despite the child's having access to appropriate and needed medical treatment—a valid challenge faced by many—medical personnel, family, schools, and individuals also still face additional challenges in promoting adherence to medical treatment as prescribed. This chapter focuses on interventions to promote adherence broadly speaking and then explores behavioral interventions more specifically. A sample psychosocial interview to guide behavior intervention planning is provided for reference (Handout 11.1). Successful intervention plans incorporate condition-specific goals and targets (e.g., taking medication as prescribed, participating in physical therapy goals) in addition to broad behavioral expectations for treatment compliance and measures to increase compliance.

FACTORS AFFECTING ADHERENCE

Of course, there are a host of reasons why patients, and especially pediatric patients, may not be compliant with medical treatment. For example, negative side effects of medication may induce the very symptoms that create the daily challenges to living and learning. Other reasons include lack of understanding of the need for, and associated outcomes of, medical treatment (low motivation), forgetting to take medications, and trying to hide medical conditions from other people. McGrady and Hommel (2013) reported a direct positive relationship between medication noncompliance and increased healthcare use by children and adolescents.

Other risk factors that contribute to reduced treatment adherence relate to family and school influences (Shaw & Páez, 2002). Specific to family influences, stress (and possible grief), financial constraints, and time resources needed to care for a child with special needs can affect parents' ability to promote treatment adherence. Santer, Ring, Yardley, Geraghty, and Wyke (2014) found that caregivers' assistance with pediatric adherence to treatment was dependent on several factors, including the difficulty of treatment implementation, presence of unwanted side effects, the child's resistance to treatment, beliefs about the medical condition and benefits of treatment, and a desire to promote and maintain a "normal life" for the family.

Likewise, many school personnel may not be adequately trained and prepared to work with children who have medical needs, and they may not associate a child's scholastic problems with a medical condition. For example, Canto, Chesire, Buckley, Andrews, and Roehring (2014) highlighted several barriers in the school system that affect the management of children with traumatic brain injuries (TBI) when they return to the classroom and how these barriers may be addressed. Canto and colleagues stressed the importance of adequately educating and training school personnel for effectively reintegrating children with TBI into the classroom after injury. Certainly, providing education and support to classroom teachers is essential when it comes to promoting an effective learning environment for children with health issues. Chesire, Canto, and Buckley (2011) proposed a model to improve communication between schools and local hospitals so that schools are notified when children acquire injuries, and school personnel can then anticipate and prepare for the needs of individual children when they return. Working with school personnel using an interdisciplinary and collaborative approach with medical personnel and the family to promote adherence is key (Chesire et al., 2011).

INTERVENTIONS TO PROMOTE ADHERENCE

Kahana, Drotor, and Frazier (2008) used meta-analysis to investigate various interventions to promote treatment adherence across a variety of chronic health conditions. Their analysis included 70 studies promoting adherence-building interventions, and their results showed strongest effects for behavioral and multicomponent interventions, with smaller to negligible effect sizes associated with educational interventions. Further, the researchers found that the effects of the interventions tended to diminish over time, with less adherence to medical treatment as time passed. Similarly, in a meta-analysis by Wu and Pai (2014), results suggested that adherence improved when healthcare providers included multiple intervention modalities, including in-person or on-phone communications made by multidisciplinary team members as well as educational/behavioral strategies designed for families and patients and aimed to improve flexibility for care delivery. Clearly, the specific strategies or interventions utilized may depend on the specific condition of the pediatric patient or the specific outcome desired. That said, behavioral interventions are consistently demonstrated to have positive effects on treatment adherence across conditions.

Motivational Interviewing

As noted in condition-specific literature, many researchers have focused on the need to improve pediatric adherence to medical treatment. For example, Powell and Hilliard (2014) examined the efficacy of utilizing motivational interviewing to increase treatment adherence among children with type 1 diabetes. Motivational interviewing employs a conversational style of engagement with patients and families with the goal of increasing intrinsic motivation to develop and commit to behavior-change goals. This intervention strategy focuses on collaborative relationship-building and asking questions to encourage the patient and family to identify barriers to treatment adherence as well as possible positive outcomes associated with adhering to treatment. The patient is then encouraged to explore pathways to overcome the obstacles and to commit to treatment adherence. The authors found that motivational interviewing yielded mixed results, but outcomes were better when treatment adherence was the focus of intervention, rather than glycemic outcomes, for patients with type 1 diabetes. These results were supported in subsequent research by Hilliard, Powell, and Anderson (2016) that emphasized including family members in intervention planning that targets improved treatment adherence, with particular focus on greater sensitivity to cultural and family issues related to health. The authors also advocated for the inclusion of psychologists and behavioral scientists in the treatment regimen for pediatric patients with type 1 diabetes.

Problem-Solving Skills Training

With regard to behavioral interventions, options range from the simplistic designs of positive reinforcement for compliance—best results from which are achieved if it is used consistently and daily—to more complex interventions. For example, Greenley and colleagues (2015) utilized problem-solving skills training (PSST) to increase adherence among pediatric patients with inflammatory bowel disease (Greenley et al., 2015). PSST is a behaviorally based approach that explicitly teaches problem-solving skills, especially those that address common concerns of caregivers (e.g., increasing compliance, decreasing disruptive behaviors). Outcomes in this study suggested that PSST was both feasible and acceptable in terms of practice among patients, and there was no increased benefit from four sessions versus only two sessions. Also, older adolescents appeared to benefit more from PSST than younger patients.

Technology-Based Interventions

Wu and Hommel (2014) examined the emergence of mobile technologies that were designed to improve treatment adherence and maximize health outcomes for children with chronic illness. The authors suggested that behavioral interventions have shown efficacy in improving treatment adherence, but more work remains to be done. Although no data were presented to promote mobile technologies as more or less effective than any other intervention targeting treatment adherence, the authors provided strengths and weakness associated with text messaging, smartphone applications, electronic monitors of adherence, and illness-specific medical devices. Although each method of increasing treatment adherence had its own set of strengths and weaknesses, the common factor among the mobile technologies was that increasing mindfulness about one's health increases adherence to treatment. The effects of these technologies can also be understood behaviorally, in that the messages serve to cue the desired compliance behavior.

Behavioral Interventions

Despite the fact that roughly 50% of children and adolescents with medical needs do not adhere to recommended medical treatment, there is no single agreed-upon solution for how to intervene to improve adherence. Research has shown modest improvements when behavioral interventions are employed, such as rewards for treatment adherence and consequences for not maintaining treatment expectations, and motivational interviewing has also shown some effectiveness. Despite the challenges to reaching a consensus approach, a handout titled "Psychosocial Interview Targeting Adherence" is included at the end of this chapter and is intended to be used to facilitate understanding of the issues that may be affecting adherence. Knowledge of the issues helps to facilitate the design of appropriate behavioral interventions and supports and to identify need for multidisciplinary support (such as help from the school social worker). The interview in the handout incorporates elements from motivational interviewing.

With research supporting the effectiveness of behavioral intervention, its use in classrooms and schools to promote treatment adherence and to manage the behavioral effects of treatment is warranted. Functional behavior assessments are recommended to outline the operating antecedents and consequences that cue and foster a specified set of behaviors. In the next sections, where the overall use of behavioral interventions in schools (specifically, interventions that support educators' work with the pediatric or medically involved population) is described, emphasis is given to understanding the unique challenges faced by educators in delivering high-quality differentiated instruction to students at all levels in a high-stakes educational environment as well as the challenges presented by medically involved students.

THE BROAD ROLE OF BEHAVIORAL INTERVENTIONS IN SCHOOLS

Teachers with more than 20 years in the classroom now have students with exceptional behavioral needs for which the teachers are likely unprepared and untrained, and for whom the "standard" behavioral strategies (e.g., stickers, time out) do not work. Even with their decades of experience, teachers are challenged more than ever by their frustration with disruptive behavior, by students who are "not motivated," and by students who do not respond despite the teachers' "trying everything." The word *epidemic* has been used to describe this change over the decades (Lewis, Sugai, & Colvin, 1998), with research noting the increased prevalence of aggression and intense behavior problems in the classroom (Koop & Lundberg, 1992; Rutherford & Nelson, 1995), as well as the prevalence of other less intense but interfering problem behavior (e.g., inattention; Walker, Colvin, & Ramsey, 1995). The debate on how the problem grew over time will likely continue, and successful behavior management and intervention in the classroom will continue to play a major role in how students are educated.

In the context of discussing the role that behavioral interventions currently play in the classroom, it is important to briefly consider what was included in "behavioral interventions" in the past. Anecdotally, teachers and administrators discuss the "referral" process, detentions, suspensions, time out, being sent to the principal, and other "consequences" as the typical school-level behavior management or behavior "interventions" in the past. Classroom management strategies also seemed to reflect the approach of escalating forms of punitive strategies, within which students performed and behaved well, "or else." Of course, there have always been teachers and administrators who were exceptionally positive, had classroom procedures and routines that created environments within which appropriate behavior was most likely to occur, and for whom students responded year after year. But even these teachers have noticed the differences in students' behavioral needs and the increased time devoted to behavior management in the classroom.

With the increase in challenging behavior in mainstream classrooms, administrators and teachers have seen a rise in "new" strategies, including the flood of interest in, and implementation of, positive behavior supports (PBS) systems, general schoolwide and classroom positive behavioral strategies, and applied behavior analysis (ABA) services in schools with typically developing students as well as for students with exceptional needs. Additionally, schools have been tasked with approaching student behavior and behavior supports in a more systematic and research-based fashion through the response to intervention (RtI) process or multitiered system of supports (MTSS). Theoretically, interventions start earlier, require data and "research-based interventions," focus on positive and proactive strategies (including Tier 1 classroom and schoolwide procedures), and are much more individualized (i.e., based on the function of the behavior). Therefore, the role of behavioral interventions in schools seems to have changed in a positive way; the purpose has shifted from a system within which students either responded to the general progression of corrective "consequences" or not, to a system within which teachers more systematically assess and address the role of the environment in student behavior; enlist more proactive, positive, and individual interventions; and have a much more objective way to evaluate the effects of the interventions.

Therefore, in the interest of serving students in the least restrictive environment (LRE), and focusing on the RtI process for behavior, behavior management and intervention play a much larger role. If done correctly within the RtI/MTSS system, behavior intervention and supports begin much earlier and students are identified for further support. Focusing on the individual needs of a student, including the behavioral characteristics and effects of certain behavioral, medical, social, learning, and mental health challenges, has become a job of the mainstream or "regular education" teacher, rather than the responsibility of the special education team or school-based clinician.

Importantly, due to the unique differences in student behavior and behavioral needs, positive interventions and proactive strategies are increasingly required because, in many cases, consequences typically used in schools no longer have the intended effect. For many students with challenging behavior, going to detention, being suspended, being sent to the principal's office, or having extra work has more of a reinforcing effect (i.e., escape from aversive work or increased attention) than the intended corrective or punitive effect. It is unclear if this is the result of a shift in the way students respond to the strategies as a whole, or the fact that those who do not respond to these strategies are more prevalent in the mainstream environment. Either way, implementing behavioral change in a positive way requires an expanded repertoire of strategies from the classroom up (not necessarily administrative); hence, there has been increased focus on positive strategies from Tier 1 (classroom and schoolwide) to Tier 3 (individualized intervention prior to assessment for special education services). Thus, behavioral interventions are now at the forefront, alongside academic instruction and intervention.

BEHAVIORAL STRATEGIES FOR PROMOTING ADHERENCE AND INCREASING HEALTH BEHAVIORS

Behavioral strategies for promoting adherence and increasing health behaviors can be as varied as the conditions or specific health outcomes warranting intervention. However, all can be distilled down to the basics of quality behavioral intervention design: conducting a functional behavioral assessment, identifying specific target behaviors, identifying an appropriate (and hopefully positive) set of antecedents and consequences (used in the behavioral sense, the word *consequences* should not have a pejorative connotation), applying the intervention, measuring the effects, and facilitating maintenance and generalization over time.

Functional Behavior Assessment

Functional behavior assessment (FBA) is the systematic observation of the child in natural settings to identify specific behaviors (problem behaviors to target for intervention as well as appropriate replacement behaviors) and to identify the factors that are associated with their occurrences (both antecedents and consequences). The observational information then assists with design, implementation, and monitoring of an individualized intervention plan. Although a classroom teacher can certainly conduct the FBA independently, it is often useful to have an independent observer conduct the FBA so that instruction can continue in the typical fashion, promoting an assessment of the more authentic environment. In the FBA, the evaluator typically identifies both the problematic behaviors and the antecedents and consequences that cue and maintain them as well as noting the more desirable behaviors that may or may not be occurring in the classroom. Environmental factors to be evaluated include instructional factors (e.g., pace of delivery, complexity of curriculum), classroom factors (e.g., routines, distraction), peer factors (e.g., rate of similar behaviors, peer instigators of behaviors), individual factors (e.g., sensitivity to stimuli), and biological factors (e.g., medication side effects, pain). Typical functions of behavior include gaining access to attention, tangible reinforcers, sensory (internal) reinforcers, and escape from work demands. It is important that the FBA consider both the problematic behaviors and the desired (preferably competing) behaviors. Many FBA template forms are available online if one is desired to guide the process, and Handout 11.2 provides a simple observation form that can be used in FBA.

IDENTIFYING TARGET BEHAVIORS

Typically, educators could target a large number of behaviors for measurement and intervention. It is critical, however, to target only one to three of the highest priority behaviors for intervention at a time. In the case of children with chronic health conditions, the targets would be the behaviors that either promote increased well-being (e.g., increasing functional movements or other adherence targets) or that limit the negative effects of treatment (e.g., side effects), or escape behaviors (e.g., complaining of somatic symptoms to get out of completing a task). Preferably, target behaviors would be framed positively and would be consistent with what is realistic and appropriate given the student's medical condition and developmental level and the baseline rates of the behavior. Consultation with medical personnel may be helpful in determining what is appropriate given the student's medical condition. For example, to decrease inattention, one might frame the target behavior as increasing on-task behavior, with consideration given to the student's medical condition and developmental level. Measuring baseline rates of behavior is critical in order to identify realistic goals and rates of change. Requiring 80% on-task behavior when the student currently operates at 20% is unrealistic and, in fact, damaging, in that it can increase negativity, discouragement, and disengagement in the student and often increases the rate of observed disruptive behaviors.

Identifying Antecedents and Consequences for Behavioral Interventions

Perhaps the most underutilized and yet powerful intervention is the use of antecedent manipulations—the minor changes to the environment that decrease the likelihood of a problem behavior or increase the likelihood that a desired behavior will occur. An interventionist's "superpower," antecedent manipulations are often the easiest and most effective intervention. Typical antecedent manipulations in the behavioral literature include:

- Presenting (or removing) the discriminative stimuli that cue the desirable behaviors (or targeted problem)—for example, setting a timer on a watch that cues when a particular desired behavior should occur
- Increasing or decreasing the response effort required to engage in the problem or desirable behavior—for example, making it easier to access a needed accommodation to avoid disruptive behavior
- Manipulating the establishing operations acting on the behavior—for example, if the student is often off task due to fatigue, providing interventions that support the student's receiving adequate rest/sleep

Multiple options exist for identifying consequences to be used in behavioral interventions. Typically, the same functions of behavior (attention, tangible/sensory reinforcement, and escape) that maintain the problem behavior can be used as consequences for the more desirable target behavior or minimization of the problem behavior. For example, a student who is on task 20% of the time could be challenged to increase on-task behavior to 25% or 30% of the time, with the consequence being 5 minutes of escape from work demands (i.e., access to preferred activity). Alternatively, students can be offered a "reinforcer menu" for identification of reinforcers to which the student may respond. The reinforcer menu is a questionnaire that can be completed by the individual whose behavior is targeted for change or by a caregiver. The menu lists preferred activities, edibles and other tangibles, and sensory experiences. A variety of reinforcer menus are available for free online. Additionally, one can simply observe the student to identify activities and objects that the student often accesses for use as potential reinforcers in a behavior intervention plan.

Intervention Design and Implementation

Behavioral interventions involve one or more of the three key elements of reinforcement, extinction, and punishment and range from simple implementations of one of these elements (e.g., positive reinforcement for raising a hand to request to use the restroom) to more complex interventions that may involve all three (e.g., a token economy targeting on-task and pro-social behavior). It is important to understand that the terms *reinforcer, extinction*, and *punishment* are operationally defined very differently from their usual meanings. In the behavioral literature, by definition a *reinforcer* is any stimulus that when presented following a behavior increases the likelihood of the behavior's occurring in the future. A *punishment* is any stimulus that when presented following a behavior decreases the likelihood of that behavior's occurring in the future. Both reinforcement and punishment can be positive or negative, which simply means adding a stimulus or removing a stimulus (not positive or negative in an emotional sense). Thus, yelling at someone could potentially be positive reinforcer or a positive punisher since it involves the application of a stimulus, or it could be a neutral (functionally unrelated) consequence, depending on whether the behavior preceding the yelling is more or less likely to occur in the future. *Extinction* is more related to reinforcement. It is the process by which the reinforcer identified as maintaining the behavior is no longer provided, in an effort to decrease the behavior over time. While some refer to this as "ignoring the behavior," it bears noting that this does not mean ignoring the individual (a potentially punishing or even dangerous situation). A layman's misunderstanding of these terms can severely limit the social validity and often the fidelity and integrity of behavioral interventions and thus should be corrected at the outset.

Interventions should be functionally related to the target behaviors and be feasible and socially valid in the classroom context, the assessment of which requires consultation with the classroom teacher and allied educators. In school settings, the four levels of acceptability of behavior-change interventions, in order of most to least acceptable, are: differential reinforcement (the first choice; it involves providing positive reinforcement for the desired behavior and extinction of the undesired behavior), extinction, negative punishment (e.g., time out), and positive punishment (the least acceptable; an example is physical restraint). Much behavioral change can be achieved by using antecedent manipulations and interventions that involve reinforcement and extinction. Punishment-based interventions should be used as a last resort and should be carefully monitored by the multidisciplinary team and an administrative oversight committee.

Behavior intervention plans should be documented using approved districtwide protocols and forms. Whether the intervention plan is specified as an individual document or as part of an individualized education plan (IEP), 504 plan, or nursing plan likely depends on the nature of the medical condition and the chronicity of the condition. For recommendations on selection, Chesire, Buckley, Leach, Scott, and Scott (2015) is a useful resource.

Measurement, Maintenance, and Generalization

In the design and implementation of behavioral strategies, it is important to give forethought to measurement, maintenance, and generalization. With regard to measurement, it must be decided how and with what frequency the behavior will be observed and measured. Measurement is critical in identifying the extent of the behavior at baseline levels and the response to intervention (positive, neutral, or negative over time). Measurement can be done by an external observer (e.g., teacher or paraprofessional) or many students can be taught to self-monitor (see Handout 11.2 for a measurement template). Once measured behavioral change is occurring in the desired direction, it is important to consider fading supports (if possible) or otherwise maintaining positive response over time (e.g., at 3 months and 6 months after intervention). Once behavioral change is successfully occurring in the desired environment, it is often important that the same change be warranted in other environments (e.g., at home) or with other behavioral change agents (e.g., regular education classroom teacher instead of special education teacher only).

Successful implementation of behavioral interventions requires appropriate assessment, identification, measurement, and maintenance over time. A concerted effort to maintain a collaborative problem-solving team both within the school environment and along with medical personnel and family caregivers is effort very well spent.

CASE EXAMPLE AND DISCUSSION

Sean is a 7-year-old boy who recently began first grade at his neighborhood school. Since infancy, Sean has experienced severe seizures several times daily, which consequently made it very difficult for him to attend classes at the school. He had been placed in a partial day program where he attended school for 2 hours a day, 3 days a week. A consequence of his medical condition and modified school schedule was that he began falling behind in his academic achievement relative to his same-age peers. This year, Sean's school and family decided to attempt to mainstream him into a regular first-grade classroom for a full schedule, 5 days a week.

Before the year began, Sean's teacher was educated about Sean's condition and how to manage his seizures, which averaged two or three during the school day. Sean's classmates appeared to become fearful of Sean and Sean began to appear isolated. As the school year progressed, Sean began to act out, and although his parents supplied the school with Sean's medication, Sean began to protest when it was time to take his medication, complaining that the pills made him feel "yucky" and made him sleepy.

The school psychologist was consulted, and the psychologist completed a functional behavior assessment along with an interview of Sean and his family. It was noted that Sean was having trouble maintaining friendships, and Sean was upset that his medication made him sleepy before recess time later in the day. Sean's parents also informed school personnel that Sean protested about coming to school each morning because he did not like the other children and was feeling bullied.

Sean's parents and teacher discussed behavior-management options. Sean's parents consulted with Sean's pediatrician about changing the time of his medication to after recess so that Sean could participate with his peers. Sean's teacher also became vigilant about times Sean was being harassed or bullied by other children, and she used these moments as teaching moments to facilitate more positive interactions. With the parents' consent, Sean's classmates were also educated about seizures, why Sean has them, and what they can do to support Sean.

Sean's behaviors were monitored daily by his teacher and parents, and weekly by the school psychologist. Biweekly meetings were scheduled for everyone to meet to discuss the behavior intervention program and to make changes as necessary. By the end of 2 months, Sean's teacher reported a significant reduction in Sean's behavioral outbursts, and his parents reported that Sean no longer protested coming to school. The school psychologist noted that Sean's positive peer interactions had also greatly increased. It was decided that the behavioral program would stay in place through the year, parent–teacher contacts would continue as scheduled, and any concerns would be communicated immediately.

Sean is a child with medical needs that affect his behavioral presentation in the classroom and his case example highlights several specific strategies discussed in this chapter. Education of his teacher about Sean's specific medical needs was essential for Sean to be mainstreamed into the classroom. When Sean presented escalating outbursts, the school psychologist was consulted and conducted the FBA. Once patterns of behaviors were identified, a family meeting was scheduled to discuss Sean, and everyone had a chance to share information, concerns, and ideas. In keeping with the principles of the problem-solving skills training (PSST) designed by Greenley and colleagues (2015), a relationship was developed between school and parents, problem-solving steps were identified, a particular problem was selected for intervention, participants were given an assignment to complete with regard to behavior management, and subsequent meetings were scheduled. This team-based, multidisciplinary behavioral approach increased desired behaviors (i.e., positive peer interactions and medication compliance) while reducing undesired behaviors (i.e., behavioral outbursts, isolation, bullying by classmates).

CONCLUSION

This chapter addresses the promotion of adherence and positive health behaviors. It discusses social significance of adherence and increasing positive health behaviors, explores the role of behavioral interventions in schools broadly speaking, and outlines the process for designing behavioral interventions more specifically. Emphasis is given to understanding the challenge faced by educators. A collaborative and interdisciplinary approach for assessment, intervention, and beyond is recommended. Acknowledging the unique role of medical conditions in inciting particular problem behaviors encourages a realistic perspective on achievable outcomes. The chapter highlights the importance of using behavioral language and avoiding colloquial misunderstandings of the terms. Last, the chapter gives guidance on intervention selection in schools. A sample psychosocial interview is provided for reference in behavior intervention planning.

REFERENCES

Burrell, C. D., & Levy, R. A. (1985). Therapeutic consequences of noncompliance. In *Improving medication compliance: Proceedings of a symposium* (pp. 7–16). Reston, VA: National Pharmaceutical Council.

Canto, A. I., Chesire, D. J., Buckley, V. A., Andrews, T. W, & Roehrig, A. D. (2014). Barriers to meeting the needs of students with traumatic brain injuries. *Educational Psychology in Practice, 30*(1), 88–103. doi:10.1080/02667363.2014.883498

Chesire, D. J., Buckley, V. A., Leach, S. L., Scott, R. A., & Scott, K. K. (2015). Navigating the terrain in the identification and program development for children with mild traumatic brain injuries. *School Psychology Forum, 9*(3), 199–213.

Chesire, D. J., Canto, A. I., & Buckley, V. A. (2011). Hospital–school collaboration to serve the needs of children with traumatic brain injury (TBI). *Journal of Applied School Psychology, 27*, 60–76. doi:10.1080/15377903.2011.540513

Greenley, R. N., Gumidayala, A. P., Nguyen, S., Plevinsky, J. M., Poulopoulos, N., Thomason, M. M., . . . Kahn, S. (2015). Can you teach a teen new tricks? Problem solving skills training improves oral medication adherence in pediatric patients with inflammatory bowel disease participating in a randomized trial. *Inflammatory Bowel Diseases, 21*, 2649–2657. doi:10.1097/MIB.0000000000000530

Hilliard, M. E., Powell, P. W. & Anderson, B. J. (2016). Evidence-based behavioral interventions to promote diabetes management in children, adolescents, and families. *American Psychologist, 71*, 590–601. doi:10.1037/a0040359

Kahana, S., Drotar, D., & Frazier, T. (2008). Meta-analysis of psychological interventions to promote adherence to treatment in pediatric chronic health conditions. *Journal of Pediatric Psychology, 33*, 590–611. doi:10.1093/jpepsy/jsm128

Koop, C. E., & Lundberg, G. D. (1992). Violence in America: A public health emergency. *Journal of the American Medical Association, 267*(22), 3075–3076.

Lewis, T. J., Sugai, G., & Colvin, G. (1998). Reducing problem behavior through a school-wide system of effective behavioral support: Investigation of a school-wide social skills training program and contextual interventions. *School Psychology Review, 27*(3), 446–459.

McGrady, M. E., & Hommel, K. A. (2013). Medication adherence and health care utilization in pediatric chronic illness: A systematic review. *Pediatrics, 132*, 730–740. doi:10.1542/peds.2013-1451.

Powell, P. W., & Hilliard, M. E. (2014). Motivational interviewing to promote adherence behaviors in pediatric type 1 diabetes. *Current Diabetes Reports*, *14*, 531. doi:10.1007/s11892-014-0531-z

Rapoff, M. A. (2010). *Adherence to pediatric medical regimens* (2nd ed). New York: NY: Spring Science+Business Media.

Rutherford, R. B., & Nelson, C. M. (1995). Management of aggressive and violent behavior in the schools. *Focus on Exceptional Children*, *27*(6), 1–15.

Santer, M., Ring, N., Yardley, L., Geraghty, A. W. A., & Wyke, S. (2014). Treatment non-adherence in pediatric long-term medical conditions: Systematic review and synthesis of qualitative studies of caregivers' views. *BMC Pediatrics*, *14*, 63. doi:10.1186/1471-2431-14-63

Shaw, S. R., & Páez, D. (2002). Best practices in interdisciplinary service delivery to children with chronic medical issues. In A. Thomas & J. Grimes (Eds.), *Best practices in school psychology* (4th ed., pp. 1473–1483). Washington, DC: National Association of School Psychologists.

Sokol, M., McGuigan, K., Verbrugge, R., & Epstein, R. (2005). Impact of medication adherence on hospitalization and healthcare cost. *Medical Care*, *43*, 521–530. http://www.jstor.org/stable/3768169

Walker, H., Colvin, G., & Ramsey, E. (1996). Antisocial behavior in school: Strategies and best practices. *Behavioral Disorders*, *21*(3), 253–255.

Wu, Y. P., & Hommel, K. A. (2014). Using technology to assess and promote adherence to medical regimens in pediatric chronic illness. *The Journal of Pediatrics*, *164*, 922–927. doi:10.1016/j.jpeds.2013.11.013

Wu, Y. P. & Pai, A. L. H. (2014). Health care provider-delivered adherence promotion interventions: A meta-analysis. *Pediatrics*, *133*, e1698–e1707. doi:10.1542/peds.2013-3639

HANDOUT 11.1.

PSYCHOSOCIAL INTERVIEW TARGETING ADHERENCE

* *This interview can be used to facilitate understanding of the issues that may be affecting adherence. Knowledge of the issues helps to facilitate the design of appropriate behavioral interventions and supports and to identify need for multidisciplinary support (such as help from the school social worker).*

Caregiver characteristics:
- What is the financial impact on the caregiver of treating the child?
- What are the caregiver's beliefs about the nature of the health condition and the effectiveness of the treatment?
- What are the impacts of the child's health condition on other members of the family?
- What are the psychosocial needs of the other members of the family in terms of adapting to the child's health condition?

Psychosocial needs of the child:
- What is the child's ability to understand his or her health condition and how prepared is he or she to take ownership of adherence to treatment?
- What is the child's emotional reaction to the health condition and how does it affect his or her ability to return to the life he or she had before diagnosis?
- How does the child's health condition affect peer relationships?

Educational and school personnel readiness:
- How prepared are teachers and other professionals to monitor the child's health and adherence to treatment?
- What additional training will school personnel require to adequately attend to the child?
- What resources are available to school personnel if they feel overwhelmed or otherwise unable to meet the child's needs?

Specific interventions used previously, and with what effect:
- Behavioral/psychological interventions
- Educational interventions
- Motivational interviewing
- Mobile technologies
- Other interventions

Other Notes/Factors:

HANDOUT 11.2.

OBSERVATION FORM TEMPLATE

Continuous (Event) Recording Data Sheet
(Frequency, Duration, Rate)

Student _____   Target Behavior _____

Observer _____   Date _____

DATE	START TIME (ONSET)	STOP TIME (OFFSET)	FREQUENCY	RATE

Interval Recording Data Sheet
(Interval, Frequency Within Interval)

Student _____   Target Behavior _____

Observer _____   Date _____

10-second intervals

MINUTES OF OBSERVATION	1	2	3	4	5	6
1						
2						
3						
4						
5						
6						
7						
8						
9						
10						
11						
12						
13						
14						
15						

School Reintegration for Children with Chronic Medical Conditions

M. CULLEN GIBBS, ELIZABETH VINCENT,
AND ANA ARENIVAS ■

School reintegration for the student with a chronic medical condition presents many unique challenges. Successful reintegration requires ample preparation and coordination. School personnel, family, and medical providers must work together closely in support of this effort. A student reintegrating into school will have missed instruction during the absence and may also be dealing with significant physical, cognitive, behavioral, and emotional changes that will affect his or her participation in school. The medical providers responsible for the student's care have an important role in helping parents and school personnel understand changes resulting from the medical condition and how the changes may affect the student's participation in school.

Changes experienced by the student frequently require that accommodations and interventions be made available in support of the student's return to school. School personnel must clearly understand the challenges experienced by the student in order to appropriately plan for necessary accommodations and interventions. To appropriately advocate for their child, parents require understanding of the student's needs and of available educational services. Working with the student to identify what to expect upon returning to school and preparing classmates for any changes in the student are also important.

In summary, the process of reintegrating a student into school requires copious and open communication among medical providers, parents, and school personnel, who work as a team in support of the student. This chapter discusses important factors to consider in support of school reintegration for the student with a chronic medical condition.

MEDICAL AND SAFETY ISSUES FOR STUDENTS RETURNING TO SCHOOL

Medical Issues

Following medical illness requiring extended absence from school, students, their families, and their education teams may face a multitude of new routines and daily procedures not previously encountered or imagined. The changes may include management of multiple organ systems and general self-care routines, which may or may not have been problematic prior to the illness.

Many students will return to school with healthcare procedures or medical equipment requiring specialized skill to facilitate. Tasks vary and can include procedures like suctioning mucus from the airway of a student who is unable to independently clear his or her airway. Other activities might include caring for a student who has a special breathing apparatus, inserting a catheter into a child who is unable to urinate, and inserting a feeding tube for nutrition.

Specific procedures may include having a predictable plan in place for administration of medications or insulin, operation of medical equipment, or having a plan of action for emergent events, such as seizure management. Although a designated health professional, such as the school nurse, would be the individual to administer medications, responding to a seizure, for example, may involve any number of unlicensed school personnel. Competency training for these events, as well as for the use of specialized equipment, is key for the skill and comfort of the staff involved.

It is not uncommon for students to require the use of specialized equipment or technologies following their return to school. Mobility challenges often occur and may be related to upper or lower extremity weakness or paralysis. Equipment needed to facilitate mobility includes items like power and manual wheelchairs, scooters, wheeled/rolling walkers, crutches, or canes. In the school, having space for movement, accessing elevators, and knowing where the ramps are located for building entry and exit are important. Mobility and general physical challenges extend into personal care, including toileting and bathroom routines, which may involve many people, depending on the extent of the need. Special equipment or technology may also include an internally placed medical appliance, such as a shunt, nasogastric tube, tracheostomy, and feeding tube, or externally placed equipment, such as a colostomy bag.

Specialized diets are another consideration for students returning to school. At times, children are unable to eat regular meals, and modifications must be made. Common examples include liquid or soft-food diets and substitutions for food allergies. Staff training and assistance are very important for mealtime routines involving these modifications.

Cognitive and physical fatigue are frequently encountered and can make classwork and homework difficult to complete. Decreased physical stamina may be related to increased fatigue. Contributing to these difficulties may be pain associated with the disease or the disease's course, which may make it difficult for the child to consistently focus and work at a regular pace.

Safety Issues

Safety issues arise at various levels in a student's daily routine. The presence of internally placed medical equipment like some of the examples mentioned above introduces choking risks, and meal delivery should be carefully planned to avoid such challenges. For example, although adequate nutrition is ensured by proper feeding practices and routines for a student using a feeding tube or who has swallowing problems, such students are at increased risk for safety issues. If a feeding tube is not handled properly or swallowing and breathing are not monitored well, choking hazards may arise. Therefore, plans are needed for handling equipment related to feeding and respiration. In addition, some students will have specialized, internally placed medical equipment that is sensitive and requires close monitoring (such sensitive equipment includes nasogastric tubes and shunts).

Mobility and transfer assistance also pose safety risks and concerns. When a student needs to move or to change positions and is unable to do so independently, there are several factors to consider. Transfers can take place on the school bus, at home, and in the classroom. Additionally, older students may weigh more and be taller than younger students and thus may require the assistance of more than one person. Having the right type and number of staff available will help to prevent drops and falls. Emergency situations are also sources of safety concern. For example, medical emergencies (e.g., seizures), school facility emergencies (e.g., unplanned fire alarms and other school evacuations), or complications unrelated to the specific medical problem (e.g., possibly related to other medical issues, such as asthma) can present at unexpected times.

Behaviorally, new challenges may be present that require planning for behavioral reinforcement schedules. Together, school staff and parents could be learning new techniques for management of difficult behaviors. Difficult behaviors may include noncompliance related to frustration or aggression related to specific medications, for example. These behaviors not only place the student at risk for self-harm but also place other students, educators, and other personnel at risk. Bullying is a safety issue from mental and physical standpoints, further emphasizing the need for preparedness Overall, safety is relevant not only for the student, but also for staff, which includes any educator or school support staff who are in contact with the student.

For all students, but particularly those who experience chronic medical problems or those who have compromised immunity for any reason, the school setting provides increased opportunities for exposure to infection and communicable diseases (e.g., streptococcal infection, influenza, cold). From a safety standpoint, schools and parents benefit from working together, with school personnel communicating with parents to let them know when there is an infection outbreak. This allows parents to be aware of the risks and to avoid a high-risk situation.

Together, school staff and parents can learn new techniques for safety management. Historically, safety-related skills have been acquired on an individual basis and were tailored to the student's specific needs. Indeed, given the varied needs of each student, there are no universal safety practices; however, the need for staff training and supervision should not be overlooked.

SUPPORTING STUDENTS RETURNING TO SCHOOL

Evan was a middle-school student receiving rehabilitation services after a motor vehicle accident (MVA). He was placed on homebound instruction that involved a transitional plan combining homebound and school-based instruction. The goal was to discontinue homebound services, except for math. In addition, Evan's parents preferred that he return first to noncore classes and gradually add in core classes due to his prior learning differences. Although his parents were empathetic about Evan's self-esteem, the instruction schedule that was developed had varied attendance times that were difficult for Evan's parents to manage, resulting in missed class instruction, disorganization, and difficulty establishing a routine. Evan became frustrated and had difficulty keeping up.

Homebound Services

Depending on the student's medical status, he or she may not immediately return to the brick and mortar of the school building. To keep a student connected, homebound instruction may be the first offering that parents encounter. Homebound services can be general education or special education if a student already had an IEP. In some cases, students receive educational services in the hospital during a prolonged stay. It is important to honestly, directly explain to parents how homebound services are applied in your school district. Furthermore, parents need to understand that the teaching in homebound instruction is not equivalent to instruction in the classroom and the student and parents will shoulder a large part of the responsibility for completing the work.

Accommodations and Interventions

Many medical conditions will alter a student physically, behaviorally, emotionally, or cognitively, resulting in qualification for accommodations under Section 504 of the Rehabilitation Act of 1973 (1977) or under the Individuals with Disabilities Education Act (IDEA; 2004). Parents are often unfamiliar with these laws, but for successful reintegration, it is important to be familiar with the various laws and to guide the parents appropriately. Although laws differ about the level of services provided, a student with a disability is legally required to receive a free appropriate public education (FAPE) and an evaluation for services.

Section 504 of the Rehabilitation Act applies to all federally funded programs and prohibits discrimination against individuals with a documented or recorded physical or mental disability that inhibits the individual in engaging in a major life activity. For students, Section 504 could apply beyond classroom instruction to participation in other school activities (U.S. Department of Education, n.d.).

Furthermore, unlike IDEA, Section 504 does not require an individualized education plan (IEP); however, a binding, documented 504 plan is required that furnishes the student who has a disability with an education analogous to that received by a general education student. Schools are mandated to "provide reasonable accommodations, supports and auxiliary aides to allow the student to participate in the general curriculum" (The Understood Team, n.d.). If an evaluation determines that a student has one of the 13 qualifying conditions under IDEA, the student still receives nondiscrimentation protections under Section 504, but a written IEP with any necessary auxilliary services, including nursing, physcial therapy, occupational therapy, speech therapy, adaptive physical education, paraprofessional aide, and counseling services, is to be developed and agreed upon by the school and parents. Teachers and schools are federally mandated to follow the IEP.

As part of the reintegration process, tranportation to and from school may be a problem. School personnel are advised to consider the following questions:

1. *Is the school building conducive to dropping off and picking up a student in a wheelchair or walker?*
2. *What about the steps and stairs at the entrance to the building?*
3. *Does this student qualify for special education busing or regular busing?*

In some older buildings that have not been modified in accordance with the Americans with Disabilities Act (ADA), the logistics of getting into and out of the building can be stressful for parents and students. Allowing parents to have access to areas that would ease entry decreases the stress. Although it is often preferred that the student return to the same school previously attended, in some cases, students may have to transfer to an alternative location that is compliant with ADA requirements.

Another consideration is to allow students to progressively return to school, in combination with keeping their homebound services. For example, a student may have developed new difficulties (e.g., sensitivity to sound/light, disorientation, cognitive fatigue), and to decrease the student's stress, he or she could benefit from a progressive reintegration approach that, for example, incrementally increases the number of hours in the student's school day until full-time attendance is achieved. Each student needs to be assessed individually.

For elementary school students, parents' assistance in the classroom can be beneficial, especially at the beginning. Parents can be a wonderful resource for the child, the child's classmates, and the teacher, but it is also helpful to promote the student's independence by gradually reducing the parent's role in the classroom.

Keep in mind, it may be a difficult transition for both parent and student. Over the course of the medical crisis, parent and child may have become highly dependent on one another due to fear and changes.

Once the student has returned to school, he or she may continue to require doctor visits, medical procedures, and outside rehabilitation therapy. Through either the student's 504 plan or the special education plan, it is imperative to have a flexible written policy on attendance in order to accommodate outside appointments as well as the potiential for illness or setbacks.

CHANGES IN STUDENTS RETURNING TO SCHOOL

A student returning to school subsequent to treatment for a chronic medical condition may have experienced important changes in behavior and personality, cognition, emotional functioning, and social skills. Changes in functioning may be the direct result of difficulties caused by the medical condition, especially when there is central nervous system (CNS) involvement. Changes may also be secondary to the stress associated with the medical condition and its treatment.

Behavior and Personality Changes

It is well understood that medical conditions involving the CNS frequently affect behavior and personality. CNS conditions that frequently impact children include brain tumors, epilepsy, and traumatic brain injury. The behavior problems that are reported in children with CNS conditions include labile mood, impulsivity, aggression, and difficulty persisting with undesired or difficult tasks (Cohen et al., 2013; Max et al., 2000; Salley et al., 2015).

Behavioral challenges will negatively affect the student's participation in school unless appropriate supports and interventions are put in place. Section 504 accommodations, such as preferential seating, increased structure and routine, and planned breaks from classwork, may be helpful in reducing behavioral difficulties. A functional behavior assessment (FBA) is recommended when a student exhibits significant behavioral difficulties that are unlikely to respond to classroom accommodations alone. Information obtained from the FBA will guide the development and implementation of a behavioral intervention plan to support the student's behavior in school (for more detail, see Chapter 11 of this volume).

Cognitive Changes

Changes in cognitive functioning are also associated with several chronic medical conditions. Difficulties in areas like processing speed, attention, executive function, language, memory, learning, visual motor skills, and intellectual ability are associated with many neurological conditions of childhood, including brain tumor, epilepsy, and multiple sclerosis (Fastenau et al., 2009; Olsson, Perrin, Lundgren, Hjorth, & Johanson, 2014; Suppiej & Cainelli, 2014). Cognitive concerns also occur in children with non-CNS conditions. For instance, Antonini, Beer, Miloh, Dreyer, and Caudle (2017) identified cognitive delays in preschool children undergoing evaluations for liver or heart transplant. Neuropsychological difficulties are also identified in children with certain types of muscular dystrophy (Snow, Anderson, & Jakobson, 2013) as well as early-onset childhood diabetes (Schwartz, Wasserman, Powel, & Axelrad, 2014).

Neuropsychological difficulties contribute to learning problems and poor academic performance. For example, executive function is related to academic achievement in both reading and math (Best, Miller, & Naglieri, 2011). Thus, the presence of neuropsychological difficulties necessitates specialized accommodations and interventions to support the student's academic achievement. Prolonged absences from school also have a negative impact on academic achievement. For example, school absences are associated with reduced academic achievement in children with brain tumor who have undergone bone marrow transplant (Notteghem et al., 2003).

Accommodations and interventions to address the impact of neuropsychological difficulties on academic performance should be based on the results of neuropsychological evaluation that identifies and explains areas of concern. Accommodations, such as breaking assignments down to smaller pieces, extending time for assignment and test completion, and shortened assignments may be necessary to support a child's learning. A child with more significant cognitive difficulties may also require individualized instruction provided by special education support as part of an IEP. The type of individualized instruction needed will be based upon the child's specific needs, but may include modeling, "hands-on" learning, and reducing abstraction by relating new concepts to previously learned information and familiar tasks. The use of outlines and teaching the child problem-solving routines for approaching novel or difficult tasks are frequently helpful, as are strategies to support memory processes, including the storage and retrieval of newly learned information.

Emotional Changes

Children with chronic medical conditions are also vulnerable to emotional difficulties. Significant distress if often associated with the diagnosis and treatment of a chronic medical condition. Potential stressors include uncertainty about diagnosis and outcome, the physical toll of treatment, changes in appearance, and disruption of daily functioning (Rodriguez et al., 2012). These significant stressors result in the child's being vulnerable to emotional difficulties. For instance, children with chronic physical illnesses are known to be at risk for higher levels of depression and anxiety than healthy children (Ferro & Boyle, 2015). Novel anxiety disorders may also arise in children with traumatic brain injury and frequently co-occur with depression (Max et al., 2015).

Emotional difficulties can negatively affect a student's participation in school. For instance, a study by Fröjd et al. (2008) demonstrated that self-reported depression in adolescence is associated with poorer academic performance. Anxiety in children is also associated with poorer school functioning (Mychailyszyn, Méndez, & Kendall, 2010). A school psychologist, counselor, or social worker can meet regularly with the student to discuss situations which may contribute to the student's emotional difficulties, help determine appropriate solutions, and promote the development of more effective coping strategies.

Social Changes

Difficulties with social skills and peer relationships are associated with several chronic medical conditions. The difficulties may include impairments in social perception as well as diminished capacity for establishing and maintaining peer relationships. For instance, Salley et al. (2014) found that survivors of pediatric brain tumor were inaccurate in perceptions of their popularity, leadership, isolation, and victimization in the school setting. Similarly, social difficulties like peer rejection and victimization are reported in children with severe traumatic brain injury (TBI; Yeates et al., 2013). Factors that contribute to social difficulties in brain-injured children include impairments in executive function and theory of mind (Robinson et al., 2014). Regardless of any direct impact of illness on the CNS, the student with a chronic medical condition is often absent due to not feeling well and due to receiving necessary treatment. Being out of school limits the child's opportunities to interact with peers and to develop friendships. Therefore, special effort must be made to monitor the peer relationships of all children with chronic medical conditions.

Special support to help improve social functioning can be provided to the student who is struggling with peer relationships. For example, assigning the student "peer buddies" may be beneficial. Peers serving as buddies should be carefully selected based upon their competence and willingness. The peer buddies can assist the student in initiating and maintaining social interactions with classmates and can serve as models for appropriate social behavior as necessary. Participation in programming to improve interpersonal skills may also be beneficial when the student is struggling to demonstrate socially appropriate behavior.

PREPARING FOR THE RETURN TO SCHOOL

Preparing Classmates

Significant changes may occur in the student who has spent extended time away from school for treatment of a chronic medical condition. Changes in the student's physical appearance, behavior, or cognitive functioning may be confusing for classmates. Confusion and misperception by classmates can make the transition back to school difficult for the student. Therefore, preparing classmates ahead of time for what to expect when the student returns to the classroom is an important component of a successful transition back to school. The benefit of preparing classmates is also supported in the extant literature. An example includes a meta-analytic study completed by Helms et al. (2016) that found peer-supported school re-entry programs improve cancer knowledge in classmates; the increased knowledge was associated with less fear and increased acceptance of the student.

A coordinated effort by parents, educators, and the medical team is helpful when determining what information should be shared with classmates. Enlisting the support of the student's parents in the process is crucial because they have the best understanding of their child and are invaluable sources of information. Some parents may want to personally share information with their child's classmates about what to expect when the child returns to school. Other parents may prefer that a liaison from the child's medical team, such as a social worker or psychologist, share the information. Regardless of who presents the information, it is important that parents are encouraged to provide their input about what to share with classmates. Depending on the child's age and capability, the student may want to personally share information with classmates about his or her medical condition and should be encouraged to do so with the support of parents, school personnel, and the medical team.

Addressing potential misperceptions by classmates about what to expect when the student returns to school is also important. For example, classmates may expect the student to return to school exactly as he or she was before, which will result in considerable confusion if the student returns with significant changes. Classmates may also have misperceptions about the nature of the student's medical condition (e.g., the condition is contagious), which need to be corrected. For this reason, information about the student and the student's medical condition should be explained clearly, using developmentally appropriate language without medical jargon or confusing terms. Encouraging classmates to ask questions is an excellent way to clarify misperceptions and to promote accurate understanding. Many children's books about specific medical conditions are available that may also be helpful to share with classmates.

Preparing School Personnel

Preparing school personnel for supporting the student with a chronic medical condition is a critical component of the return to school. The prospect of managing the educational needs of a student with medical issues can be a daunting for school personnel, who may not have formal training or experience in working with children with medical conditions. A study by Nabors, Little, Akin-Little, and Iobst (2008) found that relatively few regular and special education teachers report high levels of knowledge about, or confidence in, working with children with medical conditions. Thus, it is important to provide teachers with additional education and support to increase their knowledge and confidence in working with students who have chronic medical conditions.

A liaison from the student's medical team can provide important information about the medical condition and the implications for the student's participation in school. Although a meeting to discuss these concerns may be initiated by a parent, the school or medical team representative may also initiate a meeting in consultation with the student's parents. Regardless of who initiates the meeting, it should be scheduled well in advance of the expected date for returning to school to provide ample time to prepare.

It is preferable that the meeting occur in person at the student's school due to the complexity of information to be discussed. All school personnel who may interact with the student should have the opportunity to participate in the meeting. This includes, but is not limited to, administrators, general and special education teachers, the school nurse, and the school counselor. Identifying members of the school staff who are familiar with the medical condition may also be helpful, even if the individuals may not have direct interaction with the student. For instance, there may be individual teachers who have worked with other children with the same or a similar medical condition. School-based occupational, physical, and speech therapists may also be familiar with specific medical conditions.

For the content of the meeting, the presentation of information about the nature of the student's specific medical condition is necessary, but not sufficient, to fully support school personnel. Therefore, school personnel should ensure that they receive other critical information from the medical team representative, such as the student's medical needs, safety issues, and any changes in cognitive, behavioral, emotional, or social functioning. There should be ample opportunity for school personnel to have their questions and concerns addressed.

After the child returns to school, it is important that meetings between school personnel and the medical team liaison occur on a monthly basis for as long as necessary to monitor the reintegration process and proactively address any unforeseen issues. For this reason, it may be helpful for the school to designate a point person, such as a special education coordinator, school counselor, or school psychologist, as liaison between the school and medical team representative to ensure a stable conduit of communication.

Preparing Parents

Parents of a child who has a medical condition, whether it is a TBI, encephalitis, cancer, dysautonomia, or any other number of conditions, can be overwhelmed by the return-to-school process. Over the preceding days or months their thoughts and concerns were about their child's immediate medical conditions. Once the crisis was over and the child was stabilized and was able to return to other aspects of life, parents could start to think about school.

For parents, the process of returning to school can be daunting because, in many cases, the returning student may be performing differently academically or behaviorally than he or she did before the illness/injury. Suddenly, parents are confronted with educational terms and processes that are foreign to them. They may have questions, such as: Will my child be able to learn? Will there be changes in academic settings? How are friends going to relate? What does the future hold? On the other hand, some parents want to quickly get their child back into the same place where he or she left off, and they may not always realize that the child is not capable of functioning at the same level as he or she did before the illness/injury.

Multiple factors contribute to parents' preparation for, and their feelings about, a successful return to school. Providing parents with support and education and addressing their needs promote the student's success. Andersson, Bellon, and Walker (2016) performed a literature review of parents' experience of the return to school after their child's TBI. Although a TBI is a specific medical condition, their review is applicable for working with parents whose child has suffered any medical condition. The authors found that, for parents, the key influencing factors for a child's successful return to school are environment, school, parent, and child. In addition, key interacting factors included information, communication, collaboration, quality of outcomes, conflict, coping, and construction of new roles and identity. Understanding these key factors better prepares parents for the return-to-school process (Andersson et al., 2016).

Parents are often in an emotional, confused, and fatigued state, which may result in an understandable overprotectiveness toward their child. A key element is providing opportunities for parents to feel part of the child's educational program. As discussed earlier, if the child receives services under a Section 504 plan or an IEP, the parent is an integral part of the team. Furthermore, Andersson and colleagues (2016, p. 835) found "that schools showed variations regarding their willingnes and ability to implement agreed or recommended accommodations." The variation occurs for multiple reasons, including lack of education of staff, unwillingness to recognize the effect of the condition, or low expectations (Andersson et al., 2016). Taking time to engage with the parents enhances collaboration on the mutual goal of the student's success in school. Parents are in a position to educate the staff about their child's condition, which will give staff an understanding of the importance of implementing designated accommodations and modifications.

Communication is key to working with parents. Meeting with parents in an informal setting allows parents to express their fears and concerns about their child as well as their goals. For example, for a student who is returning to school with a tracheostomy, it is "important to understand the potential hurdles they face in managing tracheostomies. In particular, school personnel should have the ability to provide basic care for students with tracheostomies" (Patel et al., 2009). Parents want to know that the nursing staff is properly trained. Parents' fears and concerns decrease with positive two-way communication. When staff take time with the parents, they feel more at ease about their child's return to the classroom.

Preparing Students

For the student, return to school can elicit an array of emotions before, during, and after the process. It is important to understand that some students are excited about seeing friends, resuming academics, or completing their senior year. On the other hand, others with chronic health conditions "react to the worries and disruptions the condition presents by becoming depressed or overly anxious" for many reasons, such as loss of friendships, physical changes, fear of the condition getting worse, pain, or disrupted schedules (Children's Hospital of Philadelphia, n.d.). Students have reported more difficulty with the transition when there is decreased awareness of their condition among teachers and staff (Mealings, Douglas, & Olver, 2012). Two cae examples illustrate this:

> **Case 1.** *John had been recovering from a TBI for several months before he went to school with his grandmother in order to sign some papers for re-entry. The school secretary had an opportunity to establish an attitude of acceptance for John, conveying that he was understood and that school would be a safe place. Instead, she asked what was wrong with him. She said, "He looks fine."*

As noted already, students want understanding of their particular circumstances—understanding of their medical condition, their physical, cognitive, behavioral, and emotional changes, and the residual effects of medication.

> **Case 2.** *Sarah, a high school student, returned to school after a TBI without any physical deficits from her experience, although she did have cognitive deficits. Due to her lack of physical impairments, teachers had a difficult time connecting her academic struggles with her TBI. Sarah became so frustrated that she told her mother she wanted to physically injure herself in order to get others to understand her cognitive struggles. Sarah needed an outlet where she could discuss with teachers or the school counselor her experiences in the hospital, the challenges of her return to school, the reactions of her friends, and her academic struggles.*

Allowing students to be involved in their school plan, understanding their needs, following through with accommodations and modifications, and providing reasonable expectations (Mealings et al., 2012) can make students' transitions back to academics successful. Prior to their official return, inviting the student to visit the school can have an instrumental effect on transition. In their review of the literature, Mealings and colleagues (2012) found that "organized transition programs to introduce them to the new structure, such as a visting friends at school before starting, meeting up with teachers or trialing an alternative program before moving" had a positive effect on students' experiences (Mealings et al., 2012). Students with mobility changes, such as using a wheelchair or crutches or simply slower mobility, need to practice navigating through the halls and doorways and using elevators. In addition, students with acquired/traumatic brain injury can have difficulty with orientation to their surroundings and will benefit from walking through the facility to understand where their classes are and how to manage the logistics of moving from one room to another.

CONCLUSION

Successful school reintegration for the student with a chronic medical condition requires ample communication and coordination. The student's medical team has unique and important information about the functional implications of the student's medical condition. The functional implications of a medical condition may directly affect the student's ability to participate in school and include factors like ongoing medical needs, safety issues, and changes that affect learning and behavior. School personnel may be unfamiliar with the student's medical condition and lack the necessary information to support the student in school. Parents are often overwhelmed by managing their child's medical condition and have considerable stress about their child's return to school. Therefore, discussion of the student's return to school should begin in earnest as soon as possible. Through collaboration and working as a team in service of the student, parents, the medical team, and school personnel can lay the groundwork necessary to maximize the student's successful reintegration into school.

REFERENCES

Andersson, K., Bellon, M., & Walker, R. (2016). Parents' experiences of their child's return to school following acquired brain injury (ABI): A systematic review of qualitative studies. *Brain Injury, 30*(7), 829–838.

Antonini, T. N., Beer, S. S., Miloh, T., Dreyer, W. J., & Caudle, S. E. (2017). Neuropsychological functioning in preschool-aged children undergoing evaluation for organ transplant. *The Clinical Neuropsychologist, 31*(2), 352–370.

Best, J. R., Miller, P. H., & Naglieri, J. A. (2011). Relations between executive function and academic achievement from ages 5 to 17 in a large, representative national sample. *Learning and Individual Differences, 21*(4), 327–336.

Children's Hospital of Philadelphia (n.d.). *Conditions and diseases.* Retrieved from http://www.chop.edu/conditions-diseases/depression-and-anxiety-children-chronic-health-conditions

Cohen, R., Senecky, Y., Shuper, A., Inbar, D., Chodick, G., Shalev, V., & Raz, R. (2013). Prevalence of epilepsy and attention-deficit hyperactivity (ADHD) disorder: A population-based study. *Journal of Child Neurology, 28*(1), 120–123.

Fastenau, P. S., Johnson, C. S., Perkins, S. M., Byars, A. W., Austin, J. K., & Dunn, D. W. (2009). Neuropsychological status at seizure onset in children risk factors for early cognitive deficits. *Neurology, 73*(7), 526–534.

Ferro, M. A., & Boyle, M. H. (2015). The impact of chronic physical illness, maternal depressive symptoms, family functioning, and self-esteem on symptoms of anxiety and depression in children. *Journal of Abnormal Child Psychology, 43*(1), 177–187.

Fröjd, S. A., Nissinen, E. S., Pelkonen, M. U., Marttunen, M. J., Koivisto, A. M., & Kaltiala-Heino, R. (2008). Depression and school performance in middle adolescent boys and girls. *Journal of Adolescence, 31*(4), 485–498.

Helms, A. S., Schmiegelow, K., Brok, J., Johansen, C., Thorsteinsson, T., Simovska, V., & Larsen, H. B. (2016). Facilitation of school re-entry and peer acceptance of children with cancer: A review and meta-analysis of intervention studies. *European Journal of Cancer Care, 25*(1), 170–179.

Individuals with Disabilities Education Act, 20 U.S.C. § 1400 (2004)Max, J. E., Koele, S. L., Castillo, C. C., Lindgren, S. D., Arndt, S., Bokura, H., . . . Sato, Y. (2000). Personality change disorder in children and adolescents following traumatic brain injury. *Journal of the International Neuropsychological Society, 6*(03), 279–289.

Max, J. E., Lopez, A., Wilde, E. A., Bigler, E. D., Schachar, R. J., Saunders, A., . . . Levin, H. S. (2015). Anxiety disorders in children and adolescents in the second six months after traumatic brain injury. *Journal of Pediatric Rehabilitation Medicine, 8*(4), 345–355.

Mealings, M., Douglas, J., & Olver, J. (2012). Considering the student perspective in returning to school after TBI: A literature review. *Brain Injury, 26*(10), 1165–1176.

Mychailyszyn, M. P., Méndez, J. L., & Kendall, P. C. (2010). School functioning in youth with and without anxiety disorders: Comparisons by diagnosis and comorbidity. *School Psychology Review, 39*(1), 106.

Nabors, L. A., Little, S. G., Akin-Little, A., & Iobst, E. A. (2008). Teacher knowledge of and confidence in meeting the needs of children with chronic medical conditions: Pediatric psychology's contribution to education. *Psychology in the Schools, 45*(3), 217–226.

Notteghem, P., Soler, C., Dellatolas, G., Kieffer-Renaux, V., Valteau-Couanet, D., Raimondo, G., & Hartmann, O. (2003). Neuropsychological outcome in long-term survivors of a childhood extracranial solid tumor who have undergone autologous bone marrow transplantation. *Bone Marrow Transplantation, 31*(7), 599–606.

Olsson, I. T., Perrin, S., Lundgren, J., Hjorth, L., & Johanson, A. (2014). Long-term cognitive sequelae after pediatric brain tumor related to medical risk factors, age, and sex. *Pediatric Neurology, 51*(4), 515–521.

Patel, M. R., Zdanski, C. J., Abode, K. A., Reilly, C. A., Malinzak, E. B., Stein, J. N., . . . Drake, A. F. (2009). Experience of the school-aged child with tracheostomy. *International Journal of Pediatric Otorhinolaryngology, 73*(7), 975–980.

Rehabilitation Act of 1973, Section 504, P. L. 93–112, 29 U.S.C. § 794 (1977).

Robinson, K. E., Fountain-Zaragoza, S., Dennis, M., Taylor, H. G., Bigler, E. D., Rubin, K., . . . Yeates, K. O. (2014). Executive functions and theory of mind as predictors of social adjustment in childhood traumatic brain injury. *Journal of Neurotrauma, 31*(22), 1835–1842.

Rodriguez, E. M., Dunn, M. J., Zuckerman, T., Vannatta, K., Gerhardt, C. A., & Compas, B. E. (2012). Cancer-related sources of stress for children with cancer and their parents. *Journal of Pediatric Psychology, 37*(2), 185–197.

Salley, C. G., Gerhardt, C. A., Fairclough, D. L., Patenaude, A. F., Kupst, M. J., Barrera, M., & Vannatta, K. (2014). Social self-perception among pediatric brain tumor survivors compared to peers. *Journal of Developmental and Behavioral Pediatrics: JDBP, 35*(7), 427–434.

Salley, C. G., Hewitt, L. L., Patenaude, A. F., Vasey, M. W., Yeates, K. O., Gerhardt, C. A., & Vannatta, K. (2015). Temperament and social behavior in pediatric brain tumor survivors and comparison peers. *Journal of Pediatric Psychology, 40*(3), 297–308.

Schwartz, D. D., Wasserman, R., Powell, P. W., & Axelrad, M. E. (2014). Neurocognitive outcomes in pediatric diabetes: A developmental perspective. *Current Diabetes Reports, 14*(10), 1–10.

Snow, W. M., Anderson, J. E., & Jakobson, L. S. (2013). Neuropsychological and neurobehavioral functioning in Duchenne muscular dystrophy: A review. *Neuroscience & Biobehavioral Reviews, 37*(5), 743–752.

Suppiej, A., & Cainelli, E. (2014). Cognitive dysfunction in pediatric multiple sclerosis. *Neuropsychiatric Disease and Treatment, 10,* 1385.

The Understood Team. (n.d.). *The difference between IEPs and 504 plans.* Retrieved from https://www.understood.org/en/school-learning/special-services/504-plan/the-difference-between-ieps-and-504-plans

U.S. Department of Education. (n.d.). *504 resource guide.* Retrieved from https://www2.ed.gov/about/offices/list/ocr/docs/504-resource-guide-201612.pdf

Yeates, K. O., Gerhardt, C. A., Bigler, E. D., Abildskov, T., Dennis, M., Rubin, K. H., . . . Vannatta, K. (2013). Peer relationships of children with traumatic brain injury. *Journal of the International Neuropsychological Society, 19*(5), 518–527.

13

End-of-Life and Grief Issues in the School Setting

CORTNEY T. ZIMMERMAN, NICOLE M. SCHNEIDER, RYAN M. HILL, AND JULIE B. KAPLOW ∎

Recent estimates suggest that one in seven Americans will experience the death of a parent or sibling before the age of 20 (New York Life, 2010a). Unfortunately, there is also an increasing number of pediatric deaths related to underlying complex chronic health conditions. Feudtner, Christakis, and Connell (2000) noted that over half of reported deaths in children 1 year old and older are attributable to a chronic health condition. Overall, it is undeniable that many individuals will be affected by a death during childhood or adolescence. Therefore, consideration of how to best care for these children and families, as well as their support network, is paramount. The question then becomes: How do school clinicians best assess and support children, families, peers, and staff in these situations? This chapter addresses these areas of concern.

GRIEF

The role of school mental health professionals in assisting children, families, faculty, and staff in the aftermath of a death is complex and multifaceted. School-based clinicians may find themselves acting as caring mentors for students, a sympathetic ear for parents, and as a point of contact for families, faculty, and administrators. Understanding how, when, and to what extent to intervene in support of children, families, and staff starts with an understanding of the prevalence of bereavement, its psychological and behavioral consequences, and developmental manifestations of grief reactions in youth.

Sudden death is the most common form of adversity experienced by adolescent students and has the most potent effects on school performance and behavior, above and beyond any other form of trauma (Oosterhoff, Kaplow, & Layne, 2018). Despite sudden death's prevalence and impact, the majority of bereaved youth will adapt to their situations without serious, lasting clinical impairment. In other words, bereaved youth will typically experience adaptive grief reactions (i.e., individual emotional, cognitive, and behavioral responses to bereavement that contribute to healthy long-term functioning). However, a significant minority of bereaved youth (approximately 10%; Melhem, Porta, Shamseddeen, Walker Payne, & Brent, 2011), appear to experience grief reactions severe enough to produce clinically significant impairment (see Kaplow, Layne, Pynoos, Cohen, & Lieberman, 2012, for a review of maladaptive grief reactions in children and adolescents). In our experience, youth rarely present with entirely maladaptive grief reactions; most youth report some combination of adaptive and maladaptive responses, even when experiencing extreme distress and impairment (Kaplow, Layne, Saltzman, Cozza, & Pynoos, 2013).

Over time, and with appropriate interpersonal and environmental supports, most youth retain their adaptive reactions and discontinue maladaptive grief reactions, returning to a baseline level of functioning. A survey conducted by the New York Life Foundation (2010b) found that most individuals bereaved as children felt that the level of support they received from others tapered off at about 3 months after the death. However, when they were asked how long it took before they were able to "be happy again and move forward after the loss," the mean period of time they reported was over 6 years. These findings indicate a large "grief gap," suggesting that although grief is a normative process, the period of social support most children receive ends prematurely. Therefore, in order to inform treatment and to ensure that the child has the appropriate support for as long as needed, it is imperative to examine the child's understanding of, coping with, and reactions to a death.

UNDERSTANDING OF DEATH BY DEVELOPMENTAL AGE

Broadly, children's awareness and understanding of death largely depend on their developmental age and capacity for abstract thought, as well as their previous experiences with death (Bonoti, Leondari, & Mastora, 2013). In addition, variable individual factors may also ffect coping and adjustment at the end of life (for children with terminal illnesses) and after death (for children coping with the death of others). Early work examining children's developmental changes in understanding death yielded two primary frameworks for conceptualization. One of the earliest frameworks for examination of children's understanding of death proposed that children progress through three phases of understanding: (1) death is not real to them and has lifelike qualities (e.g., sleep); (2) death is personalized or externalized; and (3) children understand that death is internal, universal, unavoidable, and irreversible (Nagy, 1948). A second, well-referenced framework involves a multifaceted understanding of death with four distinct subconcepts: irreversibility, nonfunctionality or finality, inevitability, and causality (Speece & Brent, 1996). Speece and Brent noted that children understand the first three subconcepts of death between ages 5 and 7 years, but they do not fully grasp causality until they are 10 years old. Although these loose frameworks apply, there are individual differences among children and adolescents.

The differences in understanding, even among children at similar developmental stages, may be partially accounted for by previous experiences with death, as well as other less-studied factors, such as how the death was managed by others around the child, the child's personality, and other cultural and familial factors. The research on the impact of previous death experiences had mixed findings. Bonoti and colleagues (2013) found that children with previous death experiences tend to have a more realistic understanding of death than their inexperienced peers. Similarly, other work indicated that children with direct, personal death experiences (Hunter & Smith, 2008) or those who had a long illness or hospitalization themselves, may have an advanced understanding of death. However, other studies indicated that children who lost siblings to trauma-related death were no different in their understanding of death than similar inexperienced peers (Mahon, 1993), and that children who lost loved ones had less accurate death concepts than inexperienced peers (Cotton & Range, 1990). The lack of a coherent conceptualization of the impact of previous death experiences could be due to differences in research factors between studies or in other unmeasured factors; regardless, it is important to consider whether children have had previous death experiences and how the experiences could affect their current understanding.

Given that children and adolescents have varying understanding of death depending upon developmental stage, age, previous death experiences, and potentially a variety of personal factors (e.g., personality, culture), the discussions a clinician may have with children should vary accordingly, with appropriate assessment of, and consideration for, the child's level of understanding.

Preschool-Age Children

Children of preschool age still struggle to understand the concept of death. As mentioned above, they do not fully grasp death's irreversibility, finality, inevitability, and causality (Speece & Brent, 1996). Children at this age may begin to understand death, but they see it as temporary and reversible, and they do not think it can happen to them. They may believe the deceased person is asleep (Nagy, 1948) or will return at some point. This concept is perpetuated by cartoons and other shows where characters unrealistically remain alive and well after events that would be life-ending. As preschoolers grow older, it is also not uncommon for them to exhibit a keen interest in death and dead objects.

Children this age may exhibit regressive behaviors in response to a death (Lyles, 2010); they may become more clingy or dependent, revert to thumb sucking, request to sleep in their parents' bed, or exhibit separation anxiety. They may also become easily irritable, and families may observe an increase in the child's misbehavior at home or in public settings as an outward expression of the child's emotions.

INTERVENTION

It is important to be honest, very clear, and concrete when working with preschoolers. Do not use euphemisms, such as "Johnny has gone to sleep" or even "Amy passed away." Furthermore, dispel the myth that death is a punishment for something someone did. If mood or behavioral concerns are present, the family and other caregivers should maintain boundaries and consequences, and they should encourage positive mood expression. Clinicians can label the children's emotions and teach the children adaptive coping strategies.

School-Age Children

Younger children of school age are quickly moving toward the capacity for abstract thought, and therefore their understanding of death is developing. They begin to understand that death is permanent, although sometimes they still believe it only happens to others (Nagy, 1948). They also develop the capacity for magical thinking, or a belief that thoughts can make accidents, and even death, happen. They may also begin to fear death or to believe that death (or whatever caused the death) is somehow "contagious."

As they grow older, children's understanding of death is increasingly more accurate. Concurrently, children also exhibit more supernatural explanations for death as they age (e.g., they make references to God, Heaven, or the soul; Harris & Giminez, 2005). They understand death, its universality, and its permanence, but they sometimes continue to deny their own mortality. At this stage, they may become more interested in the details of death, and what happens after death, including spiritual explanations.

School-age children may respond to a death by becoming upset, withdrawn, or anxious. They may also exhibit behavioral problems. They may have difficulty sleeping or concentrating, and school may become a challenge for previously well-functioning students. Some children may even report somatic symptoms, such as headaches or stomach pains.

INTERVENTION

Children will need reassurance that not everyone who is sick will die, and they may become concerned about the health of family and friends or their own health. Their magical thinking will need to be dispelled and they may require reassurance that nothing they did caused the death. They will need assistance in expressing their emotions in an adaptive manner.

Adolescents

Early adolescents (12–14 years old) may have a more egocentric focus and wonder how the death will affect them (Serwint, 2007). Adolescents may respond to death by exhibiting school refusal, depression, withdrawal, risky behavior (e.g., drug or alcohol use), oppositional behavior, or somatic symptoms with no known etiology (Christ, Siegel, & Christ, 2002; Robin & Omar, 2014). Middle-to-late adolescents (15–17 years old) may respond to a death similarly to their younger counterparts, contingent upon their developmental age and experiences, or they may respond more similarly to adults. Adolescence is also a developmental stage in which existential or identity distress in response to a death is more common (e.g., "My life isn't worth living now that this person is gone;" Kaplow et al., 2013).

Youth in the later end of adolescence view death abstractly and subjectively; they have an adult understanding of death and typically understand Speece and Brent's (1996) four subconcepts of death. However, because adolescence is also a time of egocentrism and feelings of immortality, they may think of themselves as immortal and view death as something that only happens to others. Some adolescents may have experiences with others who have died, and their understanding then may be influenced by previous experiences, as well as their religious and cultural beliefs.

INTERVENTION

Adolescents will need support in processing the death and understanding how it affects them and others, as well as in developing adaptive coping strategies and positive ways to express their emotions and discuss their concerns. It may also be helpful to encourage them to think of ways that they can carry on the legacy of the person who died (e.g., "I'm going to live the kind of life my Dad would have wanted for me;" Kaplow, Layne, & Pynoos, 2019).

TALKING TO CHILDREN ABOUT DEATH AND DYING

Talking about death and dying is difficult. Talking about it with children—who may have a limited understanding of what death means—can be even more difficult. Therefore, this is an area where school clinicians can intervene to support and guide students and families. Because each family has its own unique values, beliefs, and culture, it is encouraged that clinicians share the best-practice guidelines with parents. Some parents may choose to discuss death and dying differently from the approach that is recommended. As an educator, the school clinician has to balance providing information and recommendations to parents with respecting parents' decisions to talk their children however they deem appropriate. Therefore, in most cases, parents, rather than educators, should be the ones to share information with their children about death and dying. School clinicians can provide resources to parents about how to talk to their children about a death so that the children have the opportunity to ask any questions they may have.

Communication About Death of Others

Although adults often think that not talking to a child about a person's death protects the child, research suggests that honest communication is important. Children should be told the truth about the death of a family member or another person the child knows (Bluebond-Langner, 1994; Kaplow, Howell, & Layne, 2014; Schneider, Steinberg, Grosch, Niedzwicki, & Cline, 2016). This is true regardless of who died—a parent, sibling, extended family member, or peer—and it is true in discussing the child's own death. This guideline appears to transcend cultures as well; studies have shown that when children are not communicated with openly about death and dying, they often feel resentful and angry (Wood, Chase, & Aggleton, 2006). Even children who are very young should be included in conversations about death and dying.

In a study examining disclosure of a parent's impending death to adolescents, Sheehan et al. (2014) found that families tend to disclose to children in one of four ways: (1) measured telling, (2) skirted telling, (3) matter-of-fact telling, and (4) inconsistent telling. Measured telling, the most common style of disclosure (32% of the sample), involves parents' disclosing information in a well-thought-out manner; they considered their child's developmental age, emotional state, timing of conversations, and other pertinent factors. Those who utilized the measured telling disclosure style had multiple conversations with their child, using their child's reactions and responses to inform further conversations. The skirted telling style, utilized by 27% of families in the study, involves families' avoiding straightforward disclosure and "beating around the bush." Matter-of-fact telling involves factual, unemotional, and often brief, day-to-day disclosures about a parent's illness and prognosis. Finally, inconsistent telling is the disclosure style in which disclosures are made in conflicting or confusing ways (such as hinting about death in a joking manner, providing mixed messages about when someone might die). Not surprisingly, families who used measured telling reported consistently high levels of both parent and child satisfaction.

Discussing suicide and death in traumatic circumstances can present bigger challenges. Just as with any death, it is important that information is imparted honestly. In short, depending on the child's developmental stage and understanding, it may be appropriate to explain that the deceased loved one suffered from a mental health concern, as noted in the publicly available brochure by Kaplow, Da Silva, and colleagues (2018). It is helpful to consider that talking about suicide does not make children, adolescents, or adults suicidal. At the same time, however, it is important that suicide not be glamorized (American Foundation for Suicide Prevention/Suicide Prevention Resource Center, 2011).

Communication About the Child's Own Death

Having discussions with children about their high likelihood of death is one of the most difficult conversations imaginable. Again, despite how heartbreaking the idea of this discussion is, it is recommended to be truthful. In a landmark study examining parental satisfaction with prognostic disclosure to children who had a malignant disease, parents who told their children about their impending death unanimously denied regret (Kreicbergs, Valdimarsdottir, Onelov, Henter, & Steineck, 2004). In contrast, just over one fourth of parents who did not disclose this information to their children were found to regret their decisions.

From a child and adolescent's viewpoint, the literature highlights that an overwhelming majority of children (95%) want to be told if they are going to die (Ellis & Leventhal, 1993). This information allows children and adolescents with advanced illnesses (e.g., HIV/AIDS, cancer) to make end-of-life decisions about their preferences and life's legacy (Wiener et al., 2010). The desire to receive honest information echoes findings in adult-focused research, which showed that the majority of patients (86.6%) preferred that their physicians provide them with full disclosure of their prognosis (Marwit & Datson, 2002).

Although existing research highlights the importance of honest communication, in practice, it is hard to do. Kreicbergs et al. (2004) found that only about one third of parents informed their children about their impending death. Older parents were more apt to disclose this information to their children, as were parents with greater levels of education and parents with more children. In general, the older a child is, the more likely a family is to inform him or her about an impending death. However, this association is not perfectly linear; one study indicated that young children (ages 3–6) actually had more information about their imminent death than older children (ages 7–11) did. It was hypothesized that parents find it easier to talk to young children, given their developmental understanding of death and dying (Hernández Núñez-Polo et al., 2009). Others demonstrated that disclosure to older teenagers and young adults (i.e., individuals 16–24 years old) occur slightly less frequently than disclosures to preteens and younger teens (9–15 years old; Kreicbergs et al., 2004). Yet, it is notable that teenagers, as compared to school-age children, more frequently want to make their own decisions about their end-of-life treatment (Ellis & Leventhal, 1993).

Despite the well-established body of research that supports the importance of providing honest disclosure to children, the nature of the conversations—along with adults' misconceptions—often prevents the conversations from occurring. In one study examining parental disclosure about a child's terminal cancer, only about one third (36.1%) of parents indicated that they shared information with their child (van der Geest et al., 2015). Reported barriers include parental inability to share the information, parental desire to protect the child, and lack of opportunity. It is recommended that information be presented in an honest, open, but age and developmentally appropriate manner (see Handout 13.1, from Schneider, Steinberg, & Cline,2016). Although these conversations are difficult, school clinicians, teacers, and administrators are in a unique position to provide support to bereaved and grieving children in the school setting after parental disclosure.

SUPPORTING CHILDREN AND FAMILIES

Given that most youth successfully navigate the difficult experience of bereavement, a school clinician's default plan in the immediate aftermath of a death should be to ensure a supportive and safe school environment for the child, to recognize "red flags" among youth who may be having a more difficult time adjusting, and to provide, or refer youth to, treatment when indicated.

Facilitating a Supportive School Environment

Bereaved children may require a safe place to express their emotions throughout the day, temporary adjustments to their workload, or permission to remove themselves from class when feeling overwhelmed. They may experience loss reminders at school (i.e., cues that evoke memories of the lost person, or that focus attention on the ongoing or future absence of that person), resulting in periods of intense distress (Layne et al., 2006; Pynoos, Steinberg, & Wraith, 1995). Because loss reminders are based on each child's relationship with the deceased, they are unique to the child and may seem unrelated to the outside observer. In fact, people (such as those who look like the deceased or were present at the time of the person's death) tend to be the most potent loss reminders, and encountering loss reminders may lead youth to avoid or to become upset in the presence of certain individuals (Layne, Kaplow, Oosterhoff, Hill, & Pynoos, 2018).

Similarly, if the death occurred under traumatic circumstances (e.g., violent, terrifying, or gruesome circumstances, including being witness to traumatic or very distressing elements of an anticipated death; Kaplow et al., 2014), youth may also experience trauma reminders (i.e., cues that evoke distressing memories of the circumstances of the death). Understanding this phenomenon may help make sense of unexplained outbursts of emotion and may explain youths' responses to certain noises, sounds, or images (e.g., seeing the image of a deceased soldier in a history book may evoke traumatic stress reactions in a child who lost a loved one in the military). Providing support to parents and family may include offering resources on how to talk to children about death, offering psychoeducation on the manifestations and impact of loss or trauma reminders, listening to parents' concerns, and maintaining an open line of communication among children, parents, faculty, and administration.

Risk Screening and Assessment

When children show high levels of functional impairment in important life domains (e.g., school difficulties, withdrawal from peers, family conflict), when moderate impairment persists for at least 6 months after the death has occurred (see Kaplow et al., 2012), or when clinical concern is raised for other reasons (e.g., a student verbalizes suicidal thoughts or desires), an individual evaluation may be needed. Few standardized assessment tools are available to measure childhood bereavement and accompanying grief reactions. One option that is well suited for use in schools is the Persistent Complex Bereavement Disorder (PCBD) Checklist (Kaplow, Layne, et al., 2018; Layne, Kaplow, & Pynoos, 2014). The PCBD Checklist is a youth self-report scale that assesses the proposed criteria for PCBD (American Psychiatric Association, 2013). Designed for youth between the ages of 8 and 18 years, it contains 39 items and requires approximately 5 to 8 minutes to administer. The PCBD Checklist provides a brief assessment of separation distress, identity/existential distress, and circumstance-related distress, consistent with the PCBD criteria as well as multidimensional grief theory (Kaplow et al., 2013; Layne et al., 2014). The relatively brief nature of the PCBD Checklist and the fact that it can be completed independently by children and adolescents makes it ideal for administration in schools, where time is often limited and where parents are infrequently present. In addition to a measure of maladaptive grief, assessment tools that can evaluate trauma exposure and posttraumatic stress symptoms, depressive symptoms, or suicide ideation may also be warranted. For a review of existing grief and posttraumatic stress measures and how to apply the principles of evidence-based assessment to bereavement, see Layne, Kaplow, and Youngstrom (2017).

Psychosocial Treatments for Bereaved Youth

In the event that children report clinically elevated symptoms on screening measures, appropriate treatment or referral options should be presented to families. Whenever possible, providing parents with contact information for specific providers appropriate to the child's needs and the family's resources increases the likelihood that families will connect successfully with mental health services. Although few evidence-based interventions for bereaved youth currently exist (for a review, see Kaplow et al., 2019), a number of school-based interventions are available, and school counselors with a mental health background may wish to seek training in such interventions. For example, multidimensional grief therapy is an evidence-informed, assessment-driven psychosocial treatment for bereaved children 7 to 17 years old who have elevated maladaptive grief reactions; this therapy can be administered individually or in groups (Kaplow et al., 2019). When it is possible to involve parents or caregivers in treatment, the Family

Bereavement Program is a 12-session program that promotes effective parenting and teaches positive coping skills to parents and caregivers after parental bereavement (Sandler et al., 2003). When bereaved youth have previously been exposed to other traumatic events, Trauma and Grief Component Therapy for Adolescents (TGCT-A; Saltzman et al., 2018) may be indicated. TGCT-A is an evidence-based modularized treatment for trauma-exposed or bereaved adolescents that has been delivered in school settings using both group-based and individual formats (Saltzman et al., 2017).

Supporting Peers

The death of a student can have a profound effect on friends, classmates, and the larger school environment. With respect to providing support to peers in the aftermath of a student's death, the same general principles outlined above provide a solid starting point: provide a supportive environment, provide opportunities for students to access counselors, identify peers who may be "at risk" after the death, and promote open communication among students, parents, faculty, and administration. It may also be necessary to invite other school-based mental health professionals, either from neighboring schools or from local mental health agencies, to come to the school and be available to provide additional support in the days after the death. Meetings with counselors and administrators after school provide an opportunity for clinicians to disseminate information to parents, for parents to express concerns, and for the administration to reassure parents that appropriate steps are being taken to provide a safe and supportive learning environment. In some circumstances, additional steps may be warranted. For example, activities to memorialize the deceased, particularly after a sufficient amount of time has passed (see Wardecker, Kaplow, Layne, & Edelstein, 2017), provide opportunities for students to positively reminisce and to express their grief (Kaplow, Layne, et al., 2018). In addition, after a student's suicide, clinicians may consider implementing a postvention strategy, which is typically a series of activities to promote healing and coping after a suicide and to reduce the risk of future suicide-related behaviors among students (e.g., *After a Suicide: A Toolkit for Schools*; American Foundation for Suicide Prevention/Suicide Prevention Resource Center, 2011). Postvention strategies typically include tips for talking about suicide with students and parents, resources for media reporting, suggestions for appropriate memorials, and resources for disseminating educational materials about suicide. Finally, checking in with students periodically can help clinicians identify youth for whom additional assessment and intervention may be needed.

Supporting Faculty and Staff

In the aftermath of a death in the school community, faculty and staff are often adversely affected. In addition to grappling with their own grief reactions, educators may suffer from compassion fatigue or secondary traumatic stress (i.e., being physically, mentally, or emotionally overwhelmed by students' loss experiences). It is important that faculty be aware of the signs and symptoms of compassion fatigue and that they engage in self-care strategies in order to effectively support their bereaved students. Self-care will likely involve the support and encouragement of administrators, who can reinforce the importance of self-care. Grief support groups for faculty and staff may also be particularly useful for facilitating open communication, grief processing, and the establishment of a safe and supportive school environment. Several helpful resources for teachers can be found on the National Child Traumatic Stress Network's website (www.nctsn.org), including self-care strategies and tips for educators.

REVIEW AND CONCLUSIONS

Unfortunately, many children will be exposed to death, and there is evidence that the experience can affect a child in multiple ways. It is imperative to consider how to best support a child or adolescent during bereavement and grief. Clinicians should be cognizant of the fact that multiple factors affect how a child or adolescent will cope with death. Children's developmental age and understanding of the common subconcepts of death (irreversibility, nonfunctionality or finality, inevitability, and causality; Speece & Brent, 1996), as well as their prior experiences with death (Bonoti et al., 2013) and their personality, among other factors, can all influence the grief and bereavement process, including children's outward expressions of grief. Therefore, providers should be mindful of the specific student's understanding and prior experience before moving forward in treatment.

Although talking with a child or adolescent about death is a daunting task for anyone, it is critical; youth also prefer to have these discussions, and they benefit from them. When parents talk to children and adolescents about the death of someone they knew, honesty and openness are essential (Bluebond-Langner, 1994; Kaplow et al., 2014; Schneider et al., 2016; Wood et al., 2006). Children also prefer to have discussions about their own death; terminally ill children and adolescents want to be told if they are going to die (Ellis & Leventhal, 1993), because this knowledge allows them to make end-of-life decisions about their preferences and their life's legacy (Wiener et al., 2010).

Providing a supportive school environment is crucial for those coping with the death of a loved one. Clinicians can provide psychoeducation about the manifestations and impact of loss or trauma reminders, listen to parents' concerns, and maintain an open line of communication. Although few standardized assessment tools are available, the PCBD Checklist (Kaplow, Layne, et al., 2018; Layne et al., 2014) is well suited for use in schools to identify students who are struggling. If youth are significantly struggling with maladaptive and persisting grief reactions, there are a few evidence-based treatments that have been successfully utilized in the school setting (i.e., TGCT-A). In addition to support for the child, peers, and family, school faculty and staff may require assistance with their coping; grief support groups for faculty and staff, or even more individualized resources, may be indicated.

Overall, assessing the child's status, providing a supportive environment, speaking honestly, keeping open lines of communication, and utilizing evidence-based interventions appropriate for the child's developmental age and understanding of death, are all helpful strategies.

REFERENCES

American Foundation for Suicide Prevention/Suicide Prevention Resource Center. (2011). *After a suicide: A toolkit for schools.* Retrieved from www.sprc.org/sites/default/files/migrate/library/AfteraSuicideToolkitforSchools.pdf

American Psychiatric Association. (2013). *Diagnostic and statistical manual of mental disorders* (5th ed.). Arlington, VA: American Psychiatric Association.

Bluebond-Langner, M. (1994). A child's view of death. *Current Paediatrics, 4,* 253–257. doi:10.1016/S0957-5839(05)80068-5

Bonoti, F., Leondari, A., & Mastora, A. (2013). Exploring children's understanding of death: Through drawings and the Death Concept Questionnaire. *Death Studies, 37,* 47–60. doi:10.1080/07481187.2011.623216

Christ, H., Siegel, K., & Christ, A. (2002). Adolescent grief: "It never really hit me . . . until it actually happened." *Journal of the American Medical Association, 288,* 1269–1278.

Cotton, C. R., & Range, L. M. (1990). Children's death concepts: Relationships to cognitive functioning, age, experience with death, fear of death, and hopelessness. *Journal of Clinical Child Psychology, 19,* 123–127.

Ellis, R., & Leventhal, B. (1993). Information needs and decision-making preferences of children with cancer. *Psycho-Oncology, 2*(4), 277–284. doi:10.1002/pon.2960020407

Feudtner, C., Christakis, D. A., & Connell, F. A. (2000). Pediatric deaths attributable to complex chronic health conditions: A population-based study of Washington State, 1980–1997. *Pediatrics, 106* (1), 205–209.

Harris, P., & Gimenez, M. (2005). Children's acceptance of conflicting testimony: The case of death. *Journal of Cognition and Culture, 5*(1–2), 143–164.

Hernández Núñez-Polo, M., Lorenzo González, R., Catá del Palacio, E., López Cabrera, A., Martino Alba, R., Madero López, L., & Pérez Martínez, A. (2009). Talking about death to children with cancer. *Anales de Pediatría, 71*(5), 419–426. doi:10.1016/j.anpedi.2009.08.003

Hunter, S. B., & Smith, D. E. (2008). Predictors of children's understandings of death: Age, cognitive ability, death experience and maternal communicative competence. *Omega, 57,* 143–162.

Kaplow, J. B., Da Silva, L., Hill, R., Mooney, M., Rooney, E., Yudovich, S., . . . King, C. (2018). *Talking to your child about a suicide death: A guide for parents and caregivers.* Retrieved from https://www.texaschildrens.org/sites/default/files/uploads/80810%20Digital%20-%20Talking%20to%20Your%20Child%20About%20a%20Suicide%20Death.pdf-

Kaplow, J. B., Howell, K. H., & Layne, C. M. (2014). Do circumstances of the death matter? Identifying socioenvironmental risks for grief-related psychopathology in bereaved youth. *Journal of Traumatic Stress, 27*(1), 42–49.

Kaplow, J. B., Layne, C. M., Oosterhoff, B., Goldenthal, H., Howell, K., Wamser-Nanney, R.,…Pynoos, R. S. (2018). Validation of the Persistent Complex Bereavement Disorder (PCBD) Checklist: A developmentally-informed assessment tool for bereaved youth. *Journal of Traumatic Stress, 31*(2), 244–254. doi:10.1002/jts.22277

Kaplow, J. B., Layne, C. M., & Pynoos, R. S. (2019). Persistent complex bereavement disorder. In M. Prinstein, E. Youngstrom, E. Mash, & R. Barkley (Eds.), *Treatment of disorders in childhood and adolescence* (4th ed.). New York, NY: Guilford Press.

Kaplow, J. B., Layne, C. M., Pynoos, R. S., Cohen, J., & Lieberman, A. (2012). DSM-V diagnostic criteria for bereavement-related disorders in children and adolescents: Developmental considerations. *Psychiatry, 75*(3), 242–265.

Kaplow, J. B., Layne, C. M., Saltzman, W. R., Cozza, S. J., & Pynoos, R. S. (2013). Using multidimensional grief theory to explore effects of deployment, reintegration, and death on military youth and families. *Clinical Child and Family Psychology Review, 16*(3), 322–340. doi:10.1007/s.10567-013-0143-1

Kreicbergs, U., Valdimarsdottir, U., Onelov, E., Henter, J., & Steineck, G. (2004). Talking about death with children who have severe malignant disease. *The New England Journal of Medicine, 351*(12), 1175–1186. doi:10.1056/NEJMoa040366

Layne, C. M., Kaplow, J. B., Oosterhoff, B., Hill, R. M., & Pynoos, R. S. (2018). The interplay between posttraumatic stress and grief reactions in traumatically bereaved adolescents: When trauma, bereavement, and adolescence converge. *Adolescent Psychiatry, 7*(4), 266–285. doi:10.2174/2210676608666180306162544

Layne, C. M., Kaplow, J. B., & Pynoos, R. S. (2014). Persistent Complex Bereavement Disorder (PCBD) Checklist—Youth Version 1.0. Los Angeles: University of California.

Layne, C. M., Kaplow, J. B., & Youngstrom, E. A. (2017). Applying evidence-based assessment to childhood trauma and bereavement: Concepts, principles, and practices. In M. A. Landolt et al. (Eds.), *Evidence-based treatments for trauma related disorders in children and adolescents*. Cham, Switzerland: Springer International Publishing.

Layne, C. M., Warren, J. S., Saltzman, W. R., Fulton, J. B., Steinberg, A. M., & Pynoos, R. S. (2006). Contextual influences on posttraumatic adjustment: Retraumatization and the roles of revictimization, posttraumatic adversities and distressing reminders. In L. A. Schein, H. I. Spitz, G. M. Burlingame, P. R. Muskin, & S. Vargo (Eds.), *Psychological effects of catastrophic disasters: Group approaches to treatment* (pp. 235–286). New York, NY: Haworth.

Lyles, M. M. (2010). *Children's grief responses*. Information copyrighted by Children's Grief Education Association.

Mahon, M. (1993). Children's concept of death and sibling death from trauma. *Journal of Paediatric Nursing, 8*, 335–344.

Marwit, S. J., & Datson, S. L. (2002). Disclosure preferences about terminal illness: An examination of decision-related factors. *Death Studies, 26*(1), 1–20. doi: 10.1080/07481180210144

Melhem, N. M., Porta, G., Shamseddeen, W., Walker Payne, M., & Brent, D. A. (2011). Grief in children and adolescents bereaved by sudden parental death. *Archives of General Psychiatry, 68*(9), 911–999. doi:10.1001/archgenpsychiatry.2011.101

Nagy, M. (1948). The child's theories concerning death. *Journal of Genetic Psychology, 73*, 3–27.

New York Life. (2010a). *Childhood bereavement survey.* Retrieved from http://www. hellogrief.org/httpwp/wp-content/uploads/2010/03/General-Population-Release-Revised1.pdf.

New York Life. (2010b). *New survey on childhood grief reveals substantial "grief gap."* Retrieved from https://www.newyorklife.com/newsroom/2017/parental-loss-survey/

Oosterhoff, B., Kaplow, J. B., & Layne, C. M. (2018). Links between bereavement due to sudden death and academic functioning: Results from a nationally representative sample of adolescents. *School Psychology Quarterly, 33*(3), 372–380.

Pynoos, R. S., Steinberg, A. M., & Wraith, R. (1995). A developmental model of childhood traumatic stress. In D. Cicchetti & D. J. Cohen (Eds.), *Developmental psychopathology, Volume 2: Risk, disorder, and adaptation* (pp. 72–95). New York, NY: Wiley.

Robin, L., & Omar, H. A. (2014). Adolescent bereavement. In J. Merrick, A. Tenenbaum, & H. A. Omar (Eds.), *School, adolescence, and health issues* (pp. 97–108). Hauppauge, NY: Nova Science Publishers.

Saltzman, W., Layne, C. M., Pynoos, R., Olafson, E., Kaplow, J., & Boat, B. (2017). Trauma and Grief Component Therapy for Adolescents: A modular approach to treating traumatized and bereaved youth. Cambridge, UK: Cambridge University Press.

Sandler, I. N., Ayers, T. S., Wolchik, S. A., Tein, J. Y., Kwok, O. M., Haine, R. A., . . . Griffin, W. A. (2003). The Family Bereavement Program: Efficacy evaluation of a theory-based prevention program for parentally bereaved children and adolescents. *Journal of Consulting and Clinical Psychology, 71*(3), 587–600.

Schneider, N. M., Steinberg, D. M., & Cline, V. D. (2016). *Tough discussions for parents: Tips for talking to children about the death of a family member.* Houston, TX: Authors.

Schneider, N. M., Steinberg, D. M., Grosch, M. C., Niedzwecki, C., & Cline, V. D. (2016). Decisions about discussing traumatic loss with hospitalized pediatric patients: Perspectives from multidisciplinary medical team providers. *Clinical Practice in Pediatric Psychology, 4*(1), 63–73. doi:10.1037/cpp0000130

Serwint, J. (2007). Separation, loss, and bereavement. In R. Kleigman, R. Behrman, H. Jenson, & B. Stranton (Eds.), *Nelson textbook of pediatrics* (18th ed.). Philadelphia, PA: Saunders Elsevier.

Sheehan, D. K., Draucker, C. B., Christ, G. H., Mayo, M. M., Heim, K., & Parish, S. (2014). Telling adolescents a parent is dying. *Journal of Palliative Medicine, 17*(5), 512–520. doi:10.1089/jpm.2013.0344

Speece, M. W., & Brent, S. B. (1996). The development of children's understanding of death. In C. A. Corr & D. M. Corr (Eds.), *Handbook of children's death and bereavement* (pp. 29–50). New York, NY: Springer.

van der Geest, I. M., van den Heuvel-Eibrink, M. M., van Vliet, L. M., Plujm, S. M., Streng, I. C, Michiels, E. M., . . . Darlington, E. (2015) Talking about death with children with incurable cancer: Perspectives from parents. *The Journal of Pediatrics, 167*(6), 1320–1326. doi:10.1016/j.jpeds.2015.08.066

Wardecker, B., Kaplow, J. B., Layne, C. M., & Edelstein, R. (2017). Caregivers' positive emotional expression and children's psychological functioning after parental loss. *Journal of Child and Family Studies, 26*(12), 3490–3501. doi:10.1007/s10826-017-0835-0

Wiener, L., Ballard, E., Brennan, T., Battles, H., Martinez, P., & Pao, M. (2010). How I wish to be remembered: The use of an advance care planning document in adolescent and young adult populations. *Journal of Palliative Medicine, 11*(10), 1309–1313. doi:10.1089/jpm.2008.0126

Wood, K., Chase, E., & Aggleton, P. (2006). "Telling the truth is the best thing": Teenage orphans' experiences of parental AIDS-related illness and bereavement in Zimbabwe. *Social Science & Medicine, S63,* 1923–1933. doi:10.1016/j.socscimed.2006.04.027

HANDOUT 13.1.

TOUGH DISCUSSIONS FOR PARENTS:
TIPS FOR TALKING TO CHILDREN ABOUT THE DEATH OF A FAMILY MEMBER

Having discussions with children about the death of a family member can be extremely hard. We recommend telling your child the truth and leaving the lines of communication open. Below are some tips for how to talk to your child—be truthful, listen, and be compassionate (use TLC). It is also important to engage in self-care before and after you have these difficult conversations with your child.

Be Truthful
- **Be honest.** Telling the truth can be hard, but not telling the basic facts can be confusing and hurtful to a child, particularly because she or he will find out what happened at some point. If a child learns that she or he was lied to, it may be especially damaging.
- **Do not redirect or skirt the issue.** Validation is very important for a child who has experienced loss. Avoiding what is being asked can be frustrating and upsetting for a child.
- **Avoid saying things like "He's in a better place."** While people mean well when they use euphemisms, the euphemisms are not straightforward and might be misunderstood. A child might hear "She's in a better place" or "He did not make it" and think the family member is at work, the park, or anywhere else that is not the hospital. This may further confuse the child.

Listen
- **Follow the child's lead.** Depending on the age and developmental level of your child, the information being delivered can vary. A young child might not understand that death is permanent. A school-age child may be concerned that she or he or others may suddenly die, which may require you to provide reassurance that the child is safe. The child might also exhibit guilt and blame him- or herself for the person's dying by way of magical thinking (e.g., "I kicked my brother Tuesday and that caused Grandma to die on Wednesday"). An adolescent might have a different idea of death, including understanding life it is finite. While truth-telling is important, follow the child's lead about how much information she or he needs to hear (i.e., there is no need to tell children of any age details that they are not seeking). It is easier to deliver extra small bits of information, based on your child's questions, rather than delivering too much information at one time, which cannot be undone.

Be Compassionate
- **Deliver news empathetically.** While we cannot predict when a child might ask tough questions, it is helpful to have a plan for how to deliver

news should questions arise. Some things to consider before having a difficult talk:

- **How to start the conversation.** Try telling your child something like this: "Eva, I need to talk to you about something important. As you know, Grandma was very sick with leukemia . . ."
- **Room environment.** It is helpful to turn off electronics, which can be distracting

- **Normalize.** Your child may experience sadness, anger, confusion, or another feeling. It is also normal not to feel these emotions or to want to play, to watch television, or to do anything else. Kids sometimes will go back and forth between feeling sad, playing, and feeling sad. (Note that often it takes time for children to take in and make sense of information about a death; different children process this information at different rates).
- **Remind the child that this is okay to talk about.** Offer other times to talk about the family member's death. This is an important part of the healing process, because it helps the child to begin grieving. Note that children often bring up topics like death in small chunks, so your child might seem to be done asking you questions, but then later might ask more.

Troubleshooting

You do not have to have all the answers or to be an expert in talking with your child about death.

- **If a child catches you off guard with a tough question and you have difficulty employing TLC, try saying: "That is a great question. I am not sure, but I will find out. We can discuss this in a little bit/tomorrow."** This is helpful because it validates the concern and lets the child know that it will be discussed soon. Follow-through is very important, however, in order to not mislead your child.
- **If you find yourself feeling sad or tearful, that is okay!** By their nature, these conversations are not easy. You can be somewhat open with your child by saying something like, "I am so sad about Dad dying" or "I cried when I first heard the news—it was very difficult." Showing these emotions can actually be helpful in allowing the child to see and understand it is okay to cry. Note that if you find yourself hysterically crying or "falling apart," this is not the best time for you to be involved in a conversation. Engage in self-care first (see "Tips for Self-Care" below) and then come back to the child's concerns, so that your child does not have to support you.
- **If the child continues to ask the same questions repeatedly, it is recommended and encouraged that you continue to repeat the answers.** Difficulty processing information is a normal part of grief. Repeating the answers when the child asks repeated questions is actually part of evidenced-based treatment for children experiencing grief. This can sometimes be very distressing for parents who are repeatedly called upon

to provide the information, but repeating information is a normal part of parenting.

- **If you do not have any idea of what to say, try active listening.** This involves listening to what your child says and repeating paraphrased versions back to the child. For example, if your child says, "I am so angry at my dad for not wearing his seatbelt!" you can respond with, "You feel so mad that your dad wasn't buckled in." This is a simple and effective way to communicate to your child that you are listening.

Tips for Self-Care

Having these discussions can be really hard for anyone, let alone someone who is also experiencing loss. Here are some tips for taking care of yourself before and after you have tough discussions.

- Take a few minutes before or after the discussion and process your feelings; let yourself feel sad or cry if needed.
- Plan to take a break after the conversation—take a brief walk or grab a cup of coffee.
- Engage in something enjoyable or relaxing after having the conversation (e.g., warm bath, comedy movie, exercise).
- **Periodically consider your own level of sadness and coping. It is very typical to need support of your own! Consider reaching out to a friend, adult family member, clergy, or counselor.**

Resource adapted from N. M. Schneider, D. M. Steinberg, & V. D. Cline (2016).

Specific Conditions

The chapters in Section III are dedicated to common groups of medical conditions. Each chapter provides an overview of the condition(s), common school-related concerns, risk and protective factors and cultural considerations, and includes practical strategies, resources, and handouts for the school-based professional. Case examples are used throughout this section to illustrate key concepts and implications for the school setting.

14

Neurodevelopmental Disorders Presenting in Early Childhood

JACK DEMPSEY, AMY K. BARTON, ALLISON G. DEMPSEY, AND STEPHANIE CHAPMAN ■

Neurodevelopmental disorders are a group of disorders that manifest in early childhood and are associated with differences in brain development that result in difficulties with learning, movement, language, or social behaviors. In the *Diagnostic and Statistical Manual of Mental Disorders*, Fifth Edition (DSM-5; American Psychiatric Association, 2013), neurodevelopmental disorders include intellectual disability (ID), communication disorders, learning disorders, autism spectrum disorder (ASD), attention deficit hyperactivity disorder (ADHD), and motor disorders. Medical conditions, such as cerebral palsy (CP), epilepsy, and spina bifida, although not listed in DSM-5, can also be considered neurodevelopmental disorders (Moreno-De-Luca et al., 2013).

Neurodevelopmental disorders often have comorbid symptoms and diagnoses. For example, psychiatric disorders are present in 30% to 50% of children and adolescents with ID (Einfeld, Ellis, & Emerson, 2011). CP, which is defined by impairment in movement and posture, is associated with high rates of ID, learning disabilities, speech and language disorders, ADHD, ASD, epilepsy, visual impairment, and hearing impairment (Moreno-De-Luca, Ledbetter, & Martin, 2012; Odding, Roebroeck, & Stam, 2006). High rates of comorbid symptoms and features indicate that neurodevelopmental disorders should be thought of as different patterns of symptoms or impairments on a common underlying neurodevelopmental continuum, rather than causally and distinct conditions (Moreno-De-Luca et al., 2013).

A complete discussion of neurodevelopmental disorders and the medical conditions associated with them is beyond the scope of this chapter. Therefore, the goal of this chapter is to provide school-based clinicians with a broad overview of the topic, specifically pertaining to the assessment and management of issues within the school setting. To this end, several medical conditions that occur in the fetal and neonatal period that are commonly associated with the presence of neurodevelopmental disorders in early childhood are described: specifically, genetic and congenital anomalies, CP, and preterm birth. Specific medical and neurodevelopmental comorbidities and considerations for assessment and needs identification are discussed for each. The chapter ends with a broad overview of school-based intervention strategies and approaches that are commonly implemented when working with children with these conditions.

GENETIC AND CONGENITAL ANOMALIES

Several medical conditions have a clear and well-established etiological link (i.e., a specific biological cause) that is present during fetal or neonatal development and that underlies the resulting neurodevelopmental disorders. The factors may be teratogenic (exposure-based), genetic, deviation from typical fetal development, or perinatal injury (e.g., stroke, asphyxia). Table 14.1 describes several well-characterized congenital and genetic anomalies occurring in children. It is not meant to be a comprehensive list, nor is it meant to be an exhaustive description of the disorders. The focus of the descriptions is on the medical and neurodevelopmental features associated with the anomalies that could affect the child's functioning in school.

SCHOOL ASSESSMENT CONSIDERATIONS

Because many of the conditions listed in Table 14.1 are associated with ID, assessment batteries will need to include a measure of cognitive functioning (or developmental functioning in the case of young children), as well as measures of functional and adaptive skills and behaviors. Given the increased risk for comorbid neurobehavioral disorders, assessment of social communication behaviors, attention, and other executive function skills may be indicated. It is important to adopt a broad, flexible approach to assessment due to the range of phenotypic expression among children with the disorders. For example, the majority of children with fetal alcohol syndrome (FAS) typically have intelligence quotients (IQs) outside the range of ID, but a substantial minority will meet criteria for ID, and slightly less than one half will meet the criteria for ADHD (Burd, Cotsonas-Hassler, Martsolf, & Kerbeshian, 2003). Children with FAS may also be at greater risk for ASD than their peers (Bishop, Gahagan, & Lord, 2007; Harris, MacKay, & Osborn, 1995). Thus, the school-based clinician should be aware of the possibility of these disorders and should be prepared to redirect the assessment if necessary.

Given the increased risk for comorbid neurodevelopmental disorders associated with genetic and other congenital conditions, parent and teacher interviews, as well as classroom observation of the child, are essential. Interviews and observations will identify red flags, which then can guide selection of

Table 14.1. COMMON MEDICAL CONDITIONS: CAUSES, PHYSICAL FEATURES, AND
ASSOCIATED NEURODEVELOPMENTAL FEATURES AND COMORBIDITIES

Condition	Cause	Physical Features	Common Neurodevelopmental Features and Comorbidities
Fragile X syndrome	Genetic condition		Hyperactivity Aggression in adolescence Stereotypies Autism spectrum disorder
Fetal alcohol syndrome	In utero exposure to alcohol	Characteristic facial features	Learning and intellectual disabilities Executive function deficits Attention and behavioral difficulties Externalizing behaviors Fine motor delays
Down syndrome	Genetic condition	Characteristic facial features Sleep difficulties Frequent ear infections Vision and hearing difficulties	IQ between 40 and 60 Attention and behavioral difficulties Autism spectrum disorder
Prader-Willi syndrome	Genetic condition	Short stature Hypotonia (low muscular tone) Obesity/increased appetite	Fine motor deficits Anxiety related to cognitive rigidity (rituals, restricted interests, hoarding) Irritability Behavioral difficulties Autism spectrum disorder
Spina bifida	Neural tube defect occurring in fetal development	Hydrocephalus (fluid build-up in the brain) with need for a shunt for drainage Bladder and bowel dysfunction	Executive function deficits Attention and behavioral difficulties Learning disability (particularly math) Fine motor delays IQ in low average range (worsening with shunt revisions) Social difficulties
Rett syndrome	Genetic condition occurring almost exclusively in females	Delayed head growth Increased risk for seizures, epilepsy, and scoliosis	Developmental regression in movement, social interaction, and communication starting at 1–4 years and halting at 2–10 years Hyperventilating behaviors Irritability Abnormal hand movements Movement difficulties

assessment materials. If red flags for ID, ASD, ADHD, or language deficits are present, the evaluator can tailor the assessment to allow clear identification of whether the student meets the criteria for a condition. For example, if the student was observed to spend most of his time alone in the classroom and did not interact with any other children during a classroom observation period, the clinician would likely have the parent and teacher fill out rating scales related to ASD symptoms, such as the Social Responsiveness Scale (Constantino & Gruber, 2012), and the clinician might include a direct assessment instrument as well, such as the Autism Diagnostic Observation Schedule (Lord, Rutter, DiLavore, & Risi, 1999).

If it is not possible to rule out ID through interview or observation, it will be necessary to proceed with the assumption that there is a higher than average probability that the child with the genetic or congenital condition has an ID. Based on this assumption, it is essential that the professional select a test of cognitive abilities that has adequate subtest floors, as recommended by Kranzler and Floyd (2013). That is, inadequate subtest floors can bias the estimate of psychometric g (an estimate of overall intelligence).

It is also necessary, when engaging in test selection, for the professional to take into account the higher than average prevalence of fine motor difficulties in children with many of the disorders listed in Table 14.1. That is, intelligence tests should be selected that minimize the influence of access skills (Braden & Elliott, 2003; Phillips, 1994). Fine motor difficulties are unrelated to the construct of intelligence and may interfere with its accurate measurement in tests that have high fine motor input requirements. Thus, it is recommended that the professional avoid using cognitive tests that include subtests requiring extensive fine motor skills, such as rapid movement of manipulatives or drawing increasingly complex geometric designs, particularly during a timed administration.

As described in Table 14.1, many children with congenital and genetic anomalies also exhibit deficits in executive function. Thus, professionals may also need to consider that difficulties related to executive function may interfere with the testing session. To account for such difficulties, it is important to have a planned behavioral system along with tangible reinforcers to ensure the child's best possible effort. Reinforcement does not need to be used if the child is highly motivated and focused, but it should be prepared and available in the event it is needed. Food items are discouraged as rewards due to the possibility of food allergies, dietary restrictions (e.g., gluten-free or casein-free), and choking hazards. A token economy or point system is preferable—the child can earn reward points for compliance and on-task behaviors that can be exchanged at the end of the session for tangible items like stickers or trading cards. Furthermore, students with attention difficulties may need rewards more frequently during the testing session. In cases where a reward system is unsuccessful in obtaining compliance, frequent breaks may be necessary, although it should be noted that some children have difficulty readjusting to the test process after a break.

CEREBRAL PALSY

Unlike medical conditions in which there is a clear etiological link between the condition and neurodevelopmental disorders, CP is often considered to be a neurodevelopmental disorder itself (Moreno-De-Luca et al., 2013). CP is a group of permanent (i.e., incurable) disorders that affect movement, muscle tone, and posture and result in physical activity limitations. CP is attributed to a lesion of the brain that occurs in early development, often prenatally, or at birth (Rosenbaum et al., 2007). CP is the most common motor disorder of childhood (Stanley, Blair, & Alberman, 2000), with over 3 children per 1,000 live births experiencing CP (Christensen et al., 2014). Typical symptoms include floppy or rigid limbs, involuntary motor movements, and exaggerated reflexes (Krigger, 2006). The motor difficulties can cause problems with coordination, stiff muscles, muscle weakness, or paralysis. The severity of CP occurs along a spectrum; some children will display only mild impairments in their gross motor movements, whereas others may have severe impairments that prohibit most volitional movements (both fine motor and gross motor). A majority of children with CP have medical comorbidities, such as epilepsy, low visual acuity, hearing impairments, speech difficulties, chronic pain, bladder incontinence, gastrointestinal and feeding difficulties, and sleep disorders (Odding et al., 2006), although the presence and severity of comorbidities vary greatly as well.

Common Comorbidities

In addition to requiring special consideration due to the direct effects of motor difficulties and comorbid medical conditions, children with CP often require the services of school-based clinicians due to the presence of comorbid neurodevelopmental disorders or mental health symptoms. Approximately 40% of children with CP are at risk of having a comorbid psychological impairment. Of these difficulties, the most commonly reported are related to peer socialization, hyperactivity, and internalizing symptoms of depression and anxiety (Brossard-Racine et al., 2012; Parkes et al., 2008).

Approximately 60% of children with CP have ID, and in 20% of children with CP the comorbid ID is moderate to severe. As a general rule, the level of ID correlates with the level of physical motor impairment, with more severe motor impairment associated with lower IQ and more adaptive functioning deficits (Krigger, 2006). Children with CP have higher rates of ASD than children in the general population as well: estimated rates are 5% to 7% (Christensen et al., 2014; Himmelmann & Uvebrant, 2011). Youth with CP also have a higher risk of learning disorders, and the presence of comorbid conditions, such as ADHD, hearing and visual difficulties, and physical endurance limitations, can further exacerbate learning difficulties (Brossard-Racine et al., 2012; Brunton & Rice, 2012).

School Assessment Considerations

Given the high level of comorbidities associated with CP, children with CP should receive a broad psychoeducational evaluation that enables development of a comprehensive and individualized treatment plan. School-based clinicians should review the child's recent physical evaluation data in order to understand the child's gross and fine motor abilities and to help address functional needs in the classroom. All children with CP should have regular speech/language evaluations, as well as occupational and physical therapy evaluations to identify language, motor, and adaptive needs.

The heterogeneous range of motor, communication, and visual functioning impairments experienced by children with CP precludes a one-size-fits-all approach to assessment and battery selection. Consulting information from recent speech, physical, and occupational therapy evaluations is essential to selection of an appropriate cognitive test. Standardized assessments are typically normed for children with typical physical development and therefore include items that may inaccurately deflate scores of children with CP, as a result of their motor, communication, or visual impairments. Assessment with such an instrument would almost certainly lead to questionable, possibly invalid, results. However, modifying items to make the assessment more appropriate for a certain physical impairment may cause the items to lose standardization, again compromising the overall assessment validity. In their open access review of the literature on intellectual assessment of children with CP, Yin Foo, Guppy, and Johnston (2013) created a clinical reasoning tool to aid the clinician in achieving the best match between the child's physical capabilities and the available IQ tests. In providing recommendations on test selection, the tool considers the child's level of motor involvement and the presence or absence of a communication or visual-perceptual impairment. Use of this tool is highly recommended in conducting intellectual testing of children with CP. For children with severe motor and language delays, direct testing of cognitive skills may not be possible, and a parent report of adaptive and functional skills may be needed instead.

Regarding other aspects of school-based evaluation of children with CP, because children with CP often experience chronic pain, regular assessment of the child's pain experience (e.g., with the Faces pain assessment scale; Hicks, von Baeyer, Spafford, van Korlaar, & Goodenough, 2001) can help identify unmanaged pain for referral back to medical professionals. Similarly, because children with CP often are on complex medication regimens, including medications with sedating properties, school-based clinicians should assess for medication side effects during the day to provide feedback to prescribing physicians. Inattention and hyperactivity should be proactively monitored via teacher observations on narrow-band scales like the Vanderbilt scales (Wolraich, 2003), and ADHD assessment should be conducted if symptoms are identified. Social functioning and risk for social communication developmental delays should be closely monitored, and, if delays are identified, the child should be referred for comprehensive ASD assessment. Finally, because parents of children with CP are at increased risk of depressive symptoms and increased parental stress (Majnemer, Shevell, Law, Poulin, & Rosenbaum, 2012), school-based clinicians may consider at least brief screening of parental distress and family functioning in order to provide necessary referrals to external providers and to determine difficulties in the home that may affect the child's presentation in the school system.

School-Based Interventions

In addition to the intervention strategies described at the end of this chapter, children with CP may need social and emotional interventions as a result of their motor impairments. That is, children with CP are at risk of experiencing bullying or social exclusion (Lindsay & McPherson, 2012a). Schools need to recognize the risk of bullying and intervene proactively. Teachers should be encouraged to model positivity toward children with CP, because teachers' positive attitudes toward children with disabilities have been found to be a protective factor against peer bullying. Teachers need to remain alert to the risk of bullying, to intervene early, and to help the parents and child with strategies for coping when bullying does happen. Teachers can also help students and their families explain CP to peers in order to promote empathetic understanding (Lindsay & McPherson, 2012b).

Like children with other physical disabilities, children with CP often have difficulty participating in leisure and sport activities. Recent reviews indicate that children with CP often are excluded from playground or recess activities (Schenker, Coster, & Parush, 2005), and when they do engage in leisure pursuits, children with CP tend to engage in quiet, nonphysical, and home-based activities (Law et al., 2006). School-based clinicians can work with the teaching team to help identify ways in which children with CP can be included in recess activities. They can also support families by linking them to recreational activities in the community that provide accommodations for children with a disability.

PRETERM BIRTH

Preterm birth occurs when a baby is born before reaching 37 weeks of gestational age. Whereas the previously described conditions are generally considered low-incidence conditions, premature birth occurs at a much higher frequency; in 2016, approximately 1 in 10 infants born in the United States was preterm (Shapiro-Mendoza et al., 2016). The subcategories of preterm birth, based on gestational age, include: moderate to late preterm (32 to < 37 weeks), very preterm (28 to < 32 weeks), and extremely preterm (< 28 weeks). Premature infants may also be classified by weight independent of gestational age, including: low birth weight (LBW: < 5lbs, 8 oz.), very low birth weight (VLBW: < 3 lbs, 5 oz.), or extremely low birth weight (ELBW: < 2 lbs, 3 oz.). Significant brain developmental occurs in the second and third trimesters of pregnancy and pre-term birth may disrupt optimal neural development, as well as increase the risk for neural injury. Thus, lower gestational age and lower birthweight are related to an increased likelihood of neurodevelopmental and behavioral comorbidities and other medical complications (Kerstjens, Winter, Bocca-Tjeertes, Bos, & Reijneveld, 2012).

Common Comorbidities

Some of the major medical complications that occur in children born preterm include pulmonary complications (e.g., need for oxygen supplementation and/ or ventilator support), gastrointestinal complications (e.g., feeding difficulties, need for G-tubes, short gut due to necrotizing enterocolitis), neurological complications (e.g., seizures, white matter loss, intracranial hemorrhage), neuromuscular complications (e.g., CP, hypotonia, developmental coordination disorder), reduced height and build, cardiac complications, and hearing and vision problems. Although medical complications are more common among children born before 32 weeks, late-preterm birth is associated with significant increases in persistent asthma and numbers of acute respiratory visits compared with full-term birth (Goyal, Fiks, & Lorch, 2011). Children who experience neurological complications associated with prematurity, such as intraventricular hemorrhage (IVH) or periventricular leukomalacia (PVL), are at greatly increased likelihood of having CP and other neurodevelopmental complications (Tran, Gray, & O'Callaghan, 2005; Vincer et al., 2006).

In addition to medical complications that may directly cause neurodevelopmental delays, children born preterm without identified medical complications remain at increased likelihood of having difficulties in cognition, learning, social communication, and behavioral functioning. Some of the difficulties may be evident in the early childhood period, whereas others are detected at school age. Preterm birth is a clear predictor of difficulties with early school performance in mathematics, reading, and language arts (Richards, Chapple-McGruder, Williams, & Kramer, 2015). Children born extremely preterm are also more likely to have an ID (Marlow, Wolke, Bracewell, & Samara, 2005) or ASD (Johnson et al., 2010).

Compared to children born full-term, children born very preterm are at an increased risk of pervasive emotional problems, inattention, hyperactivity, behavioral dysregulation, and other problems with executive functioning (Bora, Pritchard, Moor, Austin, & Woodward, 2011). Parent reports indicate that, even in early childhood, children who are born at low birthweights or very preterm have more trouble starting activities, generating new ideas and strategies, holding information in mind, planning a sequence of actions in advance, and organizing information and thoughts (Anderson, 2004). Subsequently, children born preterm are at much higher risk of receiving a diagnosis of ADHD than their peers. Preterm birth is also associated with increased rates of parenting stress (Polic et al., 2016), which in turn may affect parenting behaviors, resulting in more emotional and behavioral difficulties in childhood and beyond. Therefore, consideration of the family system is important when assessing a child born preterm.

School Assessment Considerations

Gathering background information on the student is always crucial in completing a psychoeducational evaluation. Obtaining the pregnancy and delivery history (obstetric history) is especially important for children born preterm. In addition to evaluating the child's early developmental milestones and reviewing the therapeutic history, diagnosticians and school psychologists may need to ask specific questions about each condition a child born preterm may face. For example, they may need to enquire about neurological complications, feeding difficulties, and other complications the child may currently have or may have experienced in the past. This information is important because it helps the professional understand the level of risk and anticipate ongoing challenges in the future. Specifically, if a child born preterm has more physical difficulties, he or she may miss more school for doctor's appointments and medical procedures, and specific medical complications are associated with increased risk for a range of neurodevelopmental and learning outcomes. Additionally, asking about hearing and vision difficulties is critical. If the child has not previously received hearing and vision testing, this is recommended prior to completion of any formal neurodevelopmental testing.

Because children born preterm are at an increased risk for many developmental delays, behavioral and emotional deficits, and problems with learning and academic achievement, a broad approach to assessment is necessary. Furthermore, because many of the school-related difficulties that are common in children born preterm are not evident until school age, broad assessment is recommended both in early childhood and when the child is in elementary school. Thus, many of the recommendations for assessment of children with congenital and genetic anomalies also apply to children born preterm with regard to the need to account for the increased likelihood of ASD, ADHD, or ID. Specifically, assessment should consider a child's language, motor (gross and fine), behavioral, emotional, social, cognitive, adaptive, and academic functioning, in addition to consideration of ongoing medical complications. (For a review and recommendations on approaches to assessment of children born preterm, see Dempsey et al., 2015.)

Case Example

Charlie is a 6-year-old male in first grade who was referred to the school psychologist for testing due to concerns about behavioral difficulties in the classroom. Through interview with his parents, the clinician learned that Charlie was born at 25 weeks' gestational age (approximately 4 months early) and was in the neonatal intensive care unit (NICU) for 6 months after birth. Because his lungs had not had time to adequately develop, Charlie was placed on a mechanical ventilator to support his breathing for the first 4 months of his life, and he eventually went home with ox-ygen supplementation through a nasal cannula for his first year. Charlie experienced several complications during his NICU stay, including treatment for a small hole in his heart, a mild bleed in his brain, and feeding difficulties that eventually required surgical insertion of a tube in his stomach so his parents could feed him (the tube was ultimately removed when Charlie was 18 months old). Charlie was followed in a neonatal follow-up specialty clinic until age 2 years and had a formal developmental assessment at 2 years that indicated mild delays in language and fine motor skills. At that time, Charlie was referred to the state's early intervention agency, and he quali-fied for occupational and speech therapy, which he received until he was 2½ years old, but they were discontinued when his family moved to a new state and he no longer qualified for services under the new state's eligibility criteria. Charlie's parents were not concerned because they had previously (and inaccurately) been told that children born preterm displayed delays early on but usually "caught up" to their peers.

Charlie's parents enrolled him in a neighborhood early childhood learning center/day care when they moved. However, after 6 months, the center told the family that they would need to find a new center because Charlie's behavior was too disruptive and he was "not a good listener." The family arranged for Charlie to be enrolled in a home-based day care run by a neighbor. At age 5, he was enrolled in a half-day kindergarten program. Teachers in the program reported that he displayed difficult behaviors in the classroom, was often out of his seat, engaged in behavioral outbursts when frus-trated, and had trouble with learning letter sounds and early numeracy skills. They suggested that Charlie repeat kindergarten, but his parents declined due to concerns that it could cause social problems for him. When Charlie transitioned to first grade, his disruptive behaviors in the classroom worsened and he continued to struggle in reading and math. His peers commented about his behavioral difficulties and occa-sionally complained that he bothered them when they were trying to do their work.

The school psychologist completed a comprehensive assessment that included observations of Charlie in his classroom, in the lunch room, and in physical education class; interviews of his parents and teachers; questionnaires about his emotional and behavioral functioning and social behaviors; and direct testing of Charlie's language, motor, cognitive, and academic skills. Results indicated that Charlie displayed sig-nificant difficulties with his fine motor skills that made writing challenging for him. He also displayed delays in both receptive and expressive communication, as well as problems with inattention, impulsive behaviors, and behavioral dysregulation that were exacerbated when he was frustrated. Charlie's cognitive function was in the low-average range and he displayed deficits in his basic reading and math skills. With the permission of his parents, results were discussed with his pediatrician, who diagnosed him with ADHD and developmental coordination disorder. Charlie was prescribed a small dose of a nonstimulant medication to treat symptoms of ADHD, and he was referred to a child psychologist for behavioral intervention/parent management training. The school-based clinician worked collaboratively with the psychologist to implement behavioral interventions in the classroom. Charlie also received an IEP that allowed him to have speech therapy, occupational therapy, extra *support from a learning specialist, social skills training in a group setting with the school counselor, and classroom-based accommodations, such as preferential seating and reduced length of assignments.*

SCHOOL-BASED INTERVENTION FOR NEURODEVELOPMENTAL DISORDERS

Given the phenotypic variability both among and within medical conditions associated with neurodevelopmental disorders, it is not advisable to define one-size-fits-all strategies for intervention or remediation. Thus, comprehensive assessment to identify a child's specific needs and targets for intervention is critical. The school-based professional is probably well versed in the therapies available to support development of language, motor, and adaptive skills, as well as general learning and behavioral supports for children who present with difficulties. Therefore, the review of interventions here focuses on specific strategies for improving services for children with neurodevelopmental conditions resulting from medical diagnoses and complications in early childhood.

Communication About Developmental Expectations

Because cognitive delays are common in children with neurodevelopmental disorders, communication about the child's developmental skill level is important. Particularly for children with moderate to severe intellectual delays, it is important to inform those working closest with the children (e.g., parents, teachers, paraprofessionals) about the child's developmental level, so they can appropriately conceptualize the needs and abilities of the child, as well as expectations for behavior. For teachers, the information not only informs instructional planning, curricular modifications, and teaching style, but also can be especially helpful in formulating more appropriate behavioral expectations. For example, a child with a chronological age of 10 years who is functioning at a 4-year-old level developmentally is expected to display more hyperactive/impulsive behavior and to have temper tantrums (especially in response to verbal correction). However, if it is not clearly communicated that the teacher should judge the child's behavior according to his developmental level, rather than his chronological age, the behavior could seem highly aberrant and could lead to referral for unnecessary psychotropic medications.

Facilitating Access to Outside Services

As already mentioned, many children with complex medical disorders in the fetal and neonatal period are at increased risk for neurodevelopmental disorders, such as ASD, ADHD, and ID. In many cases, a school psychologist or other school-based clinician may be the first to identify the presence of one of these disorders, as symptoms may not be detected until the child presents in the formal school setting (either in preschool or at school age). Thus, the school-based clinician may be the first to discuss the symptoms and diagnosis with the family and will be the first to facilitate access to treatment. Although the child will likely be eligible for many school-based services, additional services outside the school system (e.g., private therapy) are often recommended to promote child development and adaptive and behavioral functioning across settings. Thus, close communication and collaboration with the child's primary medical provider (with parental consent) is critical.

Additionally, knowledge of resources for which the student may be eligible and may benefit from (e.g., waiver programs for group housing) will be critical in ensuring an at-risk student receives the best care possible. For example, even if the primary care physician (PCP) provides a student with a diagnosis of ASD based on the school psychologist's recommendation, the PCP may not know where to refer the child for receipt of needed services. To become more familiar with the available resources (and to educate families about them), the school-based clinician is encouraged to reach out to the social workers associated with the department of developmental-behavioral pediatrics at the nearest children's hospital. These professionals have a wealth of knowledge about the services that are available to children with neurodevelopmental disorders like ASD and ID and how to access them. Many social workers are able to send clinicians the same information packets that they provide to families in the clinic, allowing the clinician to direct a family to needed resources as much as 1 year earlier than would occur if the family waited to be seen in the specialty clinic. It is important, though, to inform families that many services may not be available to them without a formal diagnosis from a medical provider, such as the child's pediatrician.

Communication with the Pediatrician

Prior to communicating with the student's physician, it is essential to obtain consent from the student's parent or legal guardian. The school-based clinician can explain to the parent that:

1. The results of evaluation are sufficient to allow the school to begin providing the student with the necessary supports in the school setting.
2. Many of the treatment and support services that the child would benefit from accessing outside of the school are available only after a physician or clinical psychologist confirms that the child meets medical diagnostic criteria for ASD, ADHD, or (in some cases) ID.
3. Allowing direct communication between the school-based clinician and the child's PCP makes it possible to obtain a diagnosis and to avoid wasting weeks or months on a waitlist for evaluation at a specialty center.

For children with ASD, accessing home-based treatment services, such as applied behavior analysis (ABA), often requires a medical (DSM-5) diagnosis of ASD rather than an educational classification of ASD. Obviously, there is substantial overlap of the criteria for medical diagnosis and those for educational classification of the disorder, with most children who meet the criteria for one also meeting the criteria for the other. Thus, clearly communicating with the child's PCP that the child was given the classification of ASD and expressing the opinion that the child also meets medical diagnostic criteria for ASD may result in the PCP's providing the child with the medical diagnosis required for access to ABA or other early intensive intervention services.

Without clear communication with the child's PCP to obtain a diagnosis, the child is often referred to a large autism center for specialists to ascertain whether the child meets DSM-5 criteria. The majority of autism centers, particularly in larger cities, have waitlists that range from months to years, which can result in a substantial delay between the child's first being identified and then receiving services. Notably, simply sending the PCP a dense and technical final evaluation report will probably not achieve the aforementioned goal. Given the extremely high workloads in most pediatric practices, which results in limited time for pediatricians to review documentation from external professionals, such as school psychologists, clear and concise communication is essential. The school psychologist should provide the physician with a simple, one-page letter or summary of the evaluation and recommendations (in addition to the full report). It is important that the summary concisely explain that the child was evaluated for eligibility for school services according to educational classification, which does not always align with the DSM-5 (medical) criteria for a disorder. Thus, specifically listing the symptoms that were observed and their overlap with DSM-5 symptoms may be helpful.

Similarly, if a child displays symptoms of ADHD, it is often beyond the scope of the school-based clinician's role to diagnose the disorder; instead, the clinician can describe the symptoms that interfere with the child's educational functioning and communicate the symptoms to the child's medical provider so that the physician can make an official diagnosis. As in the case of a child displaying symptoms of autism, when communicating assessment results to the pediatrician of a child displaying symptoms consistent with ADHD, a one-page summary, submitted in conjunction with the full report, is likely to be more useful to the pediatrician in making an appropriate diagnostic decision. For the child with ADHD, the benefit of this process is twofold. Having a medical diagnosis of ADHD allows the child access to medication for symptom management, when appropriate, and allows the child to receive classroom accommodations and modifications to better support learning through either a Section 504 plan or an other health impairment (OHI) designation.

REFERENCES

American Psychiatric Association. (2013). *Diagnostic and statistical manual of mental disorders* (5th ed.). Arlington, VA: American Psychiatric Association.

Anderson, P. J. (2004). Executive functioning in school-aged children who were born very preterm or with extremely low birth weight in the 1990s. *Pediatrics, 114*(1), 50–57. doi:10.1542/peds.114.1.50

Bishop, S., Gahagan, S., & Lord, C. (2007). Re-examining the core features of autism: A comparison of autism spectrum disorder and fetal alcohol spectrum disorder. *Journal of Child Psychology and Psychiatry, 48*(11), 1111–1121.

Bora, S., Pritchard, V. E., Moor, S., Austin, N. C., & Woodward, L. J. (2011). Emotional and behavioural adjustment of children born very preterm at early school age. *Journal of Paediatrics and Child Health, 47*(12), 863–869. doi:10.1111/j.1440-1754.2011.02105.x

Braden, J., & Elliott, S. (2003). Accommodations on the Stanford-Binet Intelligence Scales, Fifth Edition. In *Standford-Binet Intelligence Scales* (5th ed.), *Assessment Service Bulletin Number 2*. Itasca, IL: Riverside Publishing.

Brossard-Racine, M., Hall, N., Majnemer, A., Shevell, M. I., Law, M., Poulin, C., & Rosenbaum, P. (2012). Behavioural problems in school age children with cerebral palsy. *European Journal of Paediatric Neurology, 16*(1), 35–41.

Brunton, L. K., & Rice, C. L. (2012). Fatigue in cerebral palsy: A critical review. *Developmental Neurorehabilitation, 15*(1), 54–62.

Burd, L., Cotsonas-Hassler, T. M., Martsolf, J. T., & Kerbeshian, J. (2003). Recognition and management of fetal alcohol syndrome. *Neurotoxicology and Teratology, 25*(6), 681–688.

Christensen, D., Van Naarden Braun, K., Doernberg, N. S., Maenner, M. J., Arneson, C. L., Durkin, M. S., . . . Fitzgerald, R. (2014). Prevalence of cerebral palsy, co-occurring autism spectrum disorders, and motor functioning—Autism and Developmental Disabilities Monitoring Network, USA, 2008. *Developmental Medicine & Child Neurology, 56*(1), 59–65.

Constantino, J. N., & Gruber, C. P. (2012). *Social Responsiveness Scale (SRS)*. Torrance, CA: Western Psychological Services.

Dempsey, A. G., Keller-Margulis, M., Mire, S., Abrahamson, C., Dutt, S., Llorens, A., & Payan, A. (2015). School-aged children born preterm: Review of functioning across multiple domains and guidelines for assessment. *Advances in School Mental Health Promotion, 8*, 17–28.

Einfeld, S. L., Ellis, L. A., & Emerson, E. (2011). Comorbidity of intellectual disability and mental disorder in children and adolescents: A systematic review. *Journal of Intellectual and Developmental Disability, 36*(2), 137–143.

Goyal, N. K., Fiks, A. G., & Lorch, S. A. (2011). Association of late-preterm birth with asthma in young children: Practice-based study. *Pediatrics, 128*(4), e830–e838. doi:10.1542/peds.2011-0809

Harris, S. R., MacKay, L. L., & Osborn, J. A. (1995). Autistic behaviors in offspring of mothers abusing alcohol and other drugs: a series of case reports. *Alcoholism: Clinical and Experimental Research, 19*(3), 660–665.

Hicks, C. L., von Baeyer, C. L., Spafford, P. A., van Korlaar, I., & Goodenough, B. (2001). The Faces Pain Scale–Revised: Toward a common metric in pediatric pain measurement. *Pain, 93*(2), 173–183.

Himmelmann, K., & Uvebrant, P. (2011). Function and neuroimaging in cerebral palsy: A population-based study. *Developmental Medicine & Child Neurology, 53*(6), 516–521.

Johnson, S., Hollis, C., Kochhar, P., Hennessy, E., Wolke, D., & Marlow, N. (2010). Autism spectrum disorders in extremely preterm children. *The Journal of Pediatrics, 156*(4), 525–531. doi:10.1016/j.jpeds.2009.10.041

Kerstjens, J. M., Winter, A. F., Bocca-Tjeertes, I., Bos, A. F., & Reijneveld, S. A. (2012). Risk of developmental delay increases exponentially as gestational age of preterm infants decreases: A cohort study at age 4 years. *Developmental Medicine & Child Neurology, 54*(12), 1096–1101.

Kranzler, J. H., & Floyd, R. G. (2013). *Assessing intelligence in children and adolescents: A practical guide*: New York, NY: Guilford Press.

Krigger, K. W. (2006). Cerebral palsy: An overview. *American Family Physician, 73*(1), 91–100.

Law, M., King, G., King, S., Kertoy, M., Hurley, P., Rosenbaum, P., . . . Hanna, S. (2006). Patterns of participation in recreational and leisure activities among children with complex physical disabilities. *Developmental Medicine and Child Neurology, 48*(5), 337–342.

Lindsay, S., & McPherson, A. C. (2012a). Experiences of social exclusion and bullying at school among children and youth with cerebral palsy. *Disability and Rehabilitation, 34*(2), 101–109.

Lindsay, S., & McPherson, A. C. (2012b). Strategies for improving disability awareness and social inclusion of children and young people with cerebral palsy. *Child: Care, Health and Development, 38*(6), 809–816.

Lord, C., Rutter, M., DiLavore, P. C., & Risi, S. (1999). *Autism diagnostic observation schedule*. Los Angeles, CA: Western Psychological Services.

Majnemer, A., Shevell, M., Law, M., Poulin, C., & Rosenbaum, P. (2012). Indicators of distress in families of children with cerebral palsy. *Disability and Rehabilitation, 34*(14), 1202–1207.

Marlow, N., Wolke, D., Bracewell, M. A., & Samara, M. (2005). Neurologic and developmental disability at six years of age after extremely preterm birth. *New England Journal of Medicine, 352*(1), 9–19. doi:10.1056/nejmoa041367

Moreno-De-Luca, A., Ledbetter, D. H., & Martin, C. L. (2012). Genetic insights into the causes and classification of the cerebral palsies. *The Lancet Neurology, 11*(3), 283–292.

Moreno-De-Luca, A., Myers, S. M., Challman, T. D., Moreno-De-Luca, D., Evans, D. W., & Ledbetter, D. H. (2013). Developmental brain dysfunction: Revival and expansion of old concepts based on new genetic evidence. *The Lancet Neurology, 12*(4), 406–414.

Odding, E., Roebroeck, M. E., & Stam, H. J. (2006). The epidemiology of cerebral palsy: incidence, impairments and risk factors. *Disability and Rehabilitation, 28*(4), 183–191.

Parkes, J., White-Koning, M., Dickinson, H. O., Thyen, U., Arnaud, C., Beckung, E., . . . Colver, A. (2008). Psychological problems in children with cerebral palsy: A cross-sectional European study. *Journal of Child Psychology and Psychiatry, 49*(4), 405–413. doi:10.1111/j.1469-7610.2007.01845.x

Phillips, S. E. (1994). High-stakes testing accommodations: Validity versus disabled rights. *Applied Measurement in Education, 7*(2), 93–120.

Polic, B., Bubic, A., Mestrovic, J., Markic, J., Kovacevic, T., Juric, M., . . . Kolcic, I. (2016). Late preterm birth is a strong predictor of maternal stress later in life: Retrospective cohort study in school-aged children. *Journal of Paediatrics and Child Health, 52*(6), 608–613. doi:10.1111/jpc.13167

Richards, J. L., Chapple-McGruder, T., Williams, B. L., & Kramer, M. R. (2015). Does neighborhood deprivation modify the effect of preterm birth on children's first grade academic performance? *Social Science & Medicine, 132*, 122–131. doi:10.1016/j.socscimed.2015.03.032

Rosenbaum, P., Paneth, N., Leviton, A., Goldstein, M., Bax, M., Damiano, D., . . . Jacobsson, B. (2007). A report: The definition and classification of cerebral palsy April 2006. *Developmental Medicine & Child Neurology, 109*(Suppl. 109), 8–14.

Schenker, R., Coster, W., & Parush, S. (2005). Participation and activity performance of students with cerebral palsy within the school environment. *Disability and Rehabilitation, 27*(10), 539–552. doi:10.1080/09638280400018437

Shapiro-Mendoza, C. K., Barfield, W. D., Henderson, Z., James, A., Howse, J. L., Iksander, J., & Thorpe, P. G. (2016). CDC grand rounds: Public health strategies to prevent preterm birth. *Morbidity and Mortality Weekly Report, 65*, 826–830. doi:10.15585/mmwr.mm6532a4

Stanley, F. J., Blair, E., & Alberman, E. (2000). *Cerebral palsies: Epidemiology and causal pathways.* London: Mac Keith Press.

Tran, U., Gray, P. H., & O'Callaghan, M. J. (2005). Neonatal antecedents for cerebral palsy in extremely preterm babies and interaction with maternal factors. *Early Human Development, 81*(6), 555–561. doi:10.1016/j.earlhumdev.2004.12.009

Vincer, M. J., Allen, A. C., Joseph, K. S., Stinson, D. A., Scott, H., & Wood, E. (2006). Increasing prevalence of cerebral palsy among very preterm infants: A population-based study. *Pediatrics, 118*(6), e1621–e1626. doi:10.1542/peds.2006-1522

Wolraich, M. L. (2003). Psychometric properties of the Vanderbilt ADHD diagnostic parent rating scale in a referred population. *Journal of Pediatric Psychology, 28*(8), 559–568. doi:10.1093/jpepsy/jsg046

Yin Foo, R., Guppy, M., & Johnston, L. M. (2013). Intelligence assessments for children with cerebral palsy: A systematic review. *Developmental Medicine & Child Neurology, 55*(10), 911–918.

15

Gastrointestinal Disorders

RACHEL FEIN, AMY GOETZ, AND SHANNON MCKEE ■

Gastrointestinal (GI) disorders are a range of disorders that may affect children and adolescents with varying symptoms and levels of severity, and that have implications for presentation and interventions in the school setting. GI disorders result from disruptions to any part of the gastrointestinal tract and include disorders with organic causes, such as celiac disease (CD) and inflammatory bowel disease (IBD; Satherly, Howard, & Higgs, 2015). The symptoms associated with these disorders include, but are not limited to, nausea, bloating, constipation, diarrhea, changes in weight, and abdominal pain (Satherly et al., 2015). Additionally, GI disorders with non-organic origins are known as functional GI disorders (Satherly et al., 2015), and they include irritable bowel syndrome (IBS), encopresis, and constipation. The most common GI disorders among pediatric and school-age populations include CD, IBD, encopresis, and constipation. A description of each of the disorders is provided, followed by an overview of school-related issues, including treatment for specific GI disorders, barriers to adherence, behavioral and emotional functioning, academics, and how schools can assist students with GI disorders.

CELIAC DISEASE

CD is an autoimmune disorder that occurs in genetically predisposed individuals, and symptoms are caused by the ingestion of gluten, a protein found in wheat, barley, and rye (Porto, 2017; Saps, Adams, Bonilla, & Nichols-Vinueza, 2013). In individuals with CD, ingestion of gluten causes inflammation of the small intestine and interferes with the absorption of dietary nutrients (Porto, 2017; Saps et al., 2013). CD has been found to be the most common autoimmune inherited disease, with a prevalence of 1% to 2% in the general population and 0.3% to 2.9% in pediatric populations (Ludvigson & Green, 2011). Individuals with CD react to the ingestion of gluten with a number of symptoms. The symptoms exist on a clinical spectrum and, depending on the individual, include gastrointestinal (e.g., nutrient malabsorption, chronic diarrhea, abdominal pain, vomiting), nutritional (e.g., failure to thrive, stunted growth, weight loss, obesity), autoimmune (e.g., type 1 diabetes, hypo- and hyperthyroidism), skeletal (e.g., osteoporosis), dermatological (e.g., dermatitis herpetiformis, eczema), neurological (e.g., epilepsy, migraines), and psychological symptoms (e.g., adjustment disorder, mood disorder, anxiety, inattention; The Celiac Disease Program at Children's National Health System & The Celiac Disease Foundation, n.d.; Porto, 2017; Saps et al., 2013; Skjerning, Mahony, Husby, & Dunn-Galvin, 2014). Some studies indicate that as many as 41% of individuals with CD do not display any symptoms (Fasano et al., 2003).

Treatment

The only treatment for CD is strict lifelong adherence to a gluten-free diet (GFD), which involves eliminating all forms of wheat, rye, and barley from the diet (The Celiac Disease Program at Children's National Health System & The Celiac Disease Foundation, n.d.; Porto, 2017; Saps et al., 2013). Patients who strictly follow the GFD can begin to experience relief of symptoms within 1 week, although it often takes 6 to 12 months for the small intestine to heal in pediatric populations (The Celiac Disease Program at Children's National Health System & The Celiac Disease Foundation, n.d.; Porto, 2017). Medication is normally not required; however, treatment sometimes includes use of anti-inflammatory medication along with the GFD (The Celiac Disease Program at Children's National Health System & The Celiac Disease Foundation, n.d.).

Barriers to Treatment Adherence

Despite the fact that the treatment for CD (i.e., GFD) is relatively well known, there are several barriers to treatment adherence, including familial constraints, general misunderstanding about the diagnosis of CD, and lack of GFD resources (Bacigalupe & Plocha, 2015). Many families report that going completely gluten-free at home is a burden, meaning that family members who do not have CD are required to maintain a GFD at home (Bacigalupe & Plocha, 2015). Other families report general misunderstanding about what it means to have CD or to maintain a GFD (Bacigalupe & Plocha, 2015). For instance, students with CD may exhibit physical symptoms due to cross-contamination. In other words, if the gluten-free food or nonfood product touches food or another nonfood product containing gluten (e.g., Play-Doh) and the student subsequently ingests the food or nonfood product, he or she may experience severe physical symptoms. Furthermore, many people are unaware of the presence of gluten in foods and nonfood products (e.g., over-the-counter medications, cosmetics, toothpaste, and mouthwash; Bacigalupe & Plocha, 2015). Additionally, many people are unaware of the consequences of ingesting gluten, which range from mild abdominal pain to the development of epilepsy (Bacigalupe & Plocha, 2015; The Celiac Disease Program at Children's National Health System & The Celiac Disease Foundation, n.d.). Therefore, the onus of educating family, friends, and teachers is often placed on the child with CD and the child's family.

Behavioral and Emotional Functioning

Researchers have determined that more than 20% of patients with CD develop neurological or psychological symptoms that impair their daily functioning (Skjerning et al., 2014). Specifically, Butwicka and colleagues (2017) discovered that children with CD are at increased risk for mood disorders, anxiety disorders, eating disorders, behavioral disorders, attention deficit hyperactivity disorder, and intellectual disability. They concluded that a history of previous psychiatric disorders is more common in patients with CD, but the association is statistically significant only for eating disorders and behavioral disorders. Other researchers suggested that the most common psychological disorders among children with CD are major depressive disorder, dysthymic disorders, and adjustment disorders (e.g., difficulty coping with a new diagnosis or adherence to a GFD), although the prevalence of the disorders varied between 10% and 80% (van Hees, Van der Does, & Giltay, 2013).

Academic and Social Functioning

Like other chronic health conditions, CD may disrupt a student's academic and social functioning. With regard to school, some students with CD are distracted by their physical symptoms (e.g., abdominal pain, headaches), whereas others experience "brain fog," fatigue, poor memory, slow processing, and inattention (Chick, 2014). Further, physical symptoms related to CD may cause frequent absenteeism, resulting in poor academic performance (Chick, 2014). Socially, many students with CD report feelings of social isolation, including feeling left out, embarrassed, or different from their peers as a result of their chronic health condition (Addolorato et al., 2008). For instance, children and adolescents with CD often are unable to eat the same food as their peers at social gatherings (e.g., school lunch, parties, sleepovers, camp, dances, restaurants, friends' homes), resulting in their either being socially excluded or choosing to avoid social situations altogether (Addolorato et al., 2008). Furthermore, a GFD requires constant meal planning, resulting in a lack of social spontaneity. Adhering to a GFD may also draw unwanted attention (e.g., frequent questions about diet, symptoms, and diagnosis, teasing, or bullying) from peers. Last, the diagnosis of CD may contribute to challenges in family functioning. For instance, adhering to a GFD requires families to spend an excessive amount of time attending to and discussing grocery shopping, meal planning in different contexts, choosing restaurants that are GFD-friendly, and deciding if the entire family should follow a GFD.

Cultural Considerations

The importance of cultural considerations in pediatric chronic health conditions has been well established; however, research specifically addressing the interaction between CD and culture is scarce. In Western countries, CD is estimated to occur in approximately 1% of the population (Krigel et al., 2016). Although CD has been found to be most common in Caucasian individuals, studies have found that patients who are black or Hispanic are less likely to undergo a biopsy after an upper endoscopy, suggesting that CD may be underdiagnosed in these populations (Krigel et al., 2016). Further, CD is now being diagnosed at higher rates among individuals from the Punjabi region of India, as well as among Ashkenazi Jews (Krigel et al., 2016). Research on the sex distribution of CD suggests that the disease affects adult males and females equally; however, studies examining children in the United States have found females are more likely be diagnosed with CD than males (Liu et al., 2014). In other cultural considerations, it has been found that the increased financial burden of GFD creates additional challenges. For instance, many stores do not carry gluten-free items, forcing families to shop in specialty grocery stores or to purchase gluten-free food and nonfood items online (Isaac, Wu, Mager, & Turner, 2016). Because a GFD requires ample planning, many families from low-income backgrounds, single-family homes, or families who work multiple jobs do not have time to adequately plan meals, shop for groceries, or contact manufacturers about ingredients. Furthermore, a GFD may conflict with the culture and customs of families who typically serve food or dishes containing gluten. For instance, soy sauce, which is commonly used in Chinese and Japanese dishes, contains gluten. Sociocultural and language barriers can also lead to adherence concerns (Isaac et al., 2016). Specifically, families from culturally and linguistically diverse backgrounds may not fully understand or accept the extent to which gluten must be avoided (Isaac et al., 2016). Therefore, providers, including physicians and school personnel, should ensure that they are effectively communicating with parents and students using appropriate means.

School Personnel

With regard to school, it is crucial that students with CD and their parents advocate for supports within school settings. However, school personnel serve an equally important role in helping students with CD successfully function within the school environment. Before the student with CD starts the school year, adequate staff training regarding the diagnosis of CD (e.g., causes, symptoms, treatment), the GFD (e.g., approved foods and nonfood items, cross-contamination), and the legal obligations of meeting the needs of children with the disease is absolutely necessary (Chick, 2014; Wright, 2004). Schools are encouraged to be in contact with the student's medical team (e.g., physicians, pediatric psychologist, dietitian, social worker, etc.) in order to ensure that they have the appropriate information related to CD and to the unique needs of the student.

School personnel are encouraged to develop formal safety protocols to prevent cross-contamination of gluten-free food and nonfood items (Chick, 2014). Examples include requiring hand-washing after snacks and meals for all teachers and children in the same classroom as a student with CD, using a separate microwave to heat up gluten-free food brought from home, having a separate food preparation area in the cafeteria kitchen, using placemats to put gluten-free food on (instead of requiring students with CD to sit a separate table in the cafeteria), and not permitting homemade goods in the classroom of a student with CD. Further, gluten-free meal options should be available to students with CD for breakfast and lunch and should match what their peers are eating (Chick, 2014).

Additionally, school personnel can contribute to the positive adjustment of students with CD by creating a safe social environment. For example, teachers and school staff should allow students their privacy; however, they should also offer them an opportunity to share information about their experience with CD with other students in their classroom through a brief presentation or a handout. In order to avoid feelings of social isolation or exclusion, schools should give advance notice (e.g., at least a week) to students with CD and their families about class parties, cooking projects, field trips, or any school-related events that potentially involve food (Chick, 2014).

If a diagnosis of CD causes a student to have an educational need, then the student may meet the special education eligibility of other health impairment and should receive modifications to the general education curriculum under the Individuals with Disabilities Education Improvement Act (IDEIA; Wright, 2004). However, more often than not, students with CD many not exhibit an educational need, but they will require accommodations to gain access to the general educational curriculum and school in general. The accommodations fall under the purview of Section 504 of the Rehabilitation Act of 1973 and may include previously suggested supports (e.g., gluten-free school lunches, gluten-free classroom supplies, unrestricted access to bathroom and school nurse) as well as additional supports, including, but not limited to, delayed start of school days, excused absences for doctor appointments, and extended time for assignments (see Table 15.1 for a comprehensive list of possible accommodations).

Case Example

Joey is a 14-year-old Hispanic male who was recently diagnosed with CD. Joey initially adjusted well to his diagnosis; however, managing his physical symptoms (abdominal pain, diarrhea, and headaches) and adhering to his GFD have been a challenge. Joey frequently needs to use the restroom throughout the day and often leaves school early due to his ongoing symptoms. Furthermore, he continues to miss his favorite foods (e.g., pizza), and he continues to eat favorite foods containing gluten. Prior to his diagnosis, Joey generally performed well academically, participated in the gifted and talented program, and maintained mostly A's across subjects. However, after his CD diagnosis, Joey's grades declined. Per teacher report, Joey has not been consistently

Table 15.1. SECTION 504 ACCOMMODATIONS FOR GI DISORDERS

Celiac disease	• All staff members involved in child's care or education are trained in the management of celiac disease • Staff members involved in child's care are provided with a list of prohibited foods for the child • Specific staff member is designated for cleaning lunch tables to prevent cross-contamination • Student has unlimited bathroom access • Snack bag is available at school with allergen-friendly snacks • Student and family receive advance notification of food-related instruction or events • Student and staff have access to hand sanitizer and cleaning materials to prevent cross-contamination • Student will need access to hand-washing facilities after handling art projects or products that contain gluten, such as Play-Doh or papier-mâché • Separate food preparation station in the kitchen cafeteria, including separate microwave, is used • Gluten-free cafeteria meals (breakfast and lunch) are available • Emergency plan is in place
Inflammatory bowel disease	• Student has unlimited restroom access • Student is allowed to lie down in nurse's office if necessary during the school day • Stop-the-clock-testing: When taking an exam, the student may need to take a break due to pain or bowel urgency. The student's test time will be extended by the amount of time that the student is away from the exam. • Student has ability to hydrate • Student has access to personal supply bag with small snacks, wet wipes, etc. • Extended time for testing is allowed • Options are available for student to make up class time and assignments that were missed for medical appointments and illness without penalty • Tutoring is available after a specific period of absence due to disease flare up • Full participation in extracurricular activities is allowed even after classroom absences • Alternate seating placement is used in classroom • Adjustment of class schedules is possible • Copies of class notes are provided by teacher or selected peer • Use of aids, such as tape recorders, is allowed

Table 15.1. CONTINUED

Constipation and encopresis	• Medicaltreatment regimen is followed • Toileting schedule is followed during the school day • Student is allowed unlimited restroom access and private bathroom privileges as needed • Student has a change of clothes and wipes available • Student is monitored for signs and symptoms of constipation • Plan for a consistent response to events is in place • Student is observed for consistent trigger events

turning in homework, and he has been tardy to class. Further, his teachers previously described him as a "dream student;" however, within the past month they have reported that he exhibits inattention and has started "having an attitude." Although Joey has a best friend and several close friends from his baseball team, he has been less interested in seeing his friends and often avoids social situations, including lunch at school or spending time at his friends' houses after baseball practice. Additionally, Joey's parents reported that he has been eating less, has had trouble falling asleep, and has been quite moody. Based on these concerns, Joey's parents contacted the school psychologist to see how they, along with his school, can best assist him. Of note, Joey speaks both English and Spanish fluently, but his parents speak only Spanish.

The school psychologist scheduled a meeting with Joey's parents to develop a 504 plan. As part of the meeting, Joey's parents provided the school with documentation from his physician about his diagnosis, and they signed a consent form authorizing the school to communicate with the Joey's medical team (pediatric psychologist and dietitian). The school provided an in-person interpreter in order to ensure that Joey's parents could communicate with school personnel as well as understand what was being discussed. Given the physical symptoms associated with Joey's CD, the school decided to provide Joey with unrestricted access to the restroom and school nurse, and they seated him near the classroom exit to avoid disruption of classroom activities and unwanted attention from peers. Furthermore, due to his frequent bathroom breaks throughout the day, Joey was given a hall pass, which allows him a few extra minutes to arrive at class. In response to concerns about his GFD adherence, Joey's school began to offer gluten-free breakfast and lunch options in the cafeteria. Since he plays on the school's baseball team, gluten-free drinks and snacks were made available at baseball games as well. Due to mood and behavior concerns (e.g., problems with sleep, eating, and attitude, and avoiding friends), the school determined that the school psychologist or school counselor will meet with Joey regularly to assess symptoms of depression and anxiety and to provide intervention as necessary. Each of these accommodations was written into his 504 plan, and Joey's school and parents will continue to assess and update his plan as needed.

INFLAMMATORY BOWEL DISEASE

IBD includes two disorders that affect the digestive tract at distinct anatomical locations: Crohn's disease and ulcerative colitis (Molodecky et al., 2012). Both disorders are marked by gastrointestinal inflammation and unpredictable periods of relapse and remission (Molodecky et al., 2012). Crohn's disease involves inflammation at any location in the digestive tract from the mouth to the anus. Ulcerative colitis is characterized by inflammation that is confined to the large intestine. Furthermore, ulcerative colitis generally affects the inner layer of the intestinal tract, whereas Crohn's disease can affect multiple intestinal layers. Common symptoms of both conditions include abdominal pain or cramps, persistent diarrhea, rectal bleeding, rectal urgency, weight loss, delayed growth, and fatigue. The prevalence of Crohn's disease and ulcerative colitis has grown considerably in developed regions, including Europe and North America (Molodecky et al., 2012), and Caucasians are more likely to be diagnosed with IBD than black or Hispanic individuals (Malaty, Fan, Opekun, Thibodeaux, & Ferry, 2010). Approximately 20% to 30% of patients with IBD experience onset of symptoms before they are 20 years old (Baldassano & Piccoli, 1999).

Treatment

Management of IBD symptoms is complex, depending on multiple medications as well as dietary modifications, and in cases where medical management is insufficient, surgical intervention is often indicated. First-line therapy includes corticosteroids, which serve to decrease inflammation in the digestive tract, reduce symptoms, and induce remission (Conrad & Rosh, 2017). Chronic corticosteroid use may delay growth and affect sleep, mood, and behavior (Mrakotsky et al., 2013). As a result, other immunomodulators are often necessary for long-term treatment of IBD (Thomas & Lodhia, 2014). In addition to medical management, dietary modifications are often needed to relieve symptoms of IBD. Although the Crohn's and Colitis Foundation of America (The Celiac Disease Program at Children's National Health System & The Celiac Disease Foundation, n.d.) does not promote any specific diet or dietary modifications, some foods may cause gastrointestinal discomfort, particularly during a disease flare-up (e.g., spicy food, dairy products). It may be necessary to remove these foods from the child's diet during periods of active disease. Despite the lack of specific nutritional recommendations, enteral nutrition (use of a feeding tube) has demonstrated some benefit in promoting remission (Gupta et al., 2013). It should be noted that, except for total colectomy (i.e., complete removal of the colon) in ulcerative colitis, treatment methods are not curative.

Barriers to Treatment Adherence

Adolescents with IBD report common barriers to adherence, including forgetting to take medication, being away from home, medication interference with activity, and difficulty swallowing pills (Gray, Denson, Baldassano, & Hommel, 2011; Hommel & Baldassano, 2010). A recent systematic review revealed that nonadherence to oral medication in IBD is prevalent and may range between 2% and 93% of patients with a diagnosis of IBD (Spekhorst, Hummel, Benninga, van Rheenen, & Kindermann, 2016). This large variation may reflect investigator-based differences in the definition of adherence, as well as the wide range of available therapies. Moreover, a relationship has been shown between emotional functioning, barriers to adherence, and actual adherence, such that adherence is lower among adolescents with a high level of barriers and elevated negative affect (Gray et al., 2011).

Behavioral and Emotional Functioning

Both Crohn's disease and ulcerative colitis are marked by an unpredictable disease course, in addition to symptoms that affect the major life activity of toileting. Furthermore, the medications designed to manage symptoms often have troubling side effects, such as sleep difficulties and emotional lability (Mrakotsky et al., 2013), in addition to causing cushingoid features (e.g., facial puffiness) and weight gain. Research has shown that children with IBD are at greater risk for general emotional difficulties, such as anxiety and depression (Mackner & Crandall, 2007). Fear and worry may be related to the waxing and waning course of the disease, bathroom use, and medication side effects (Conrad & Rosh, 2017). As in many pediatric chronic health conditions, children may have difficulty identifying and expressing their fears (e.g., heightened possibility of cancer, need for surgical intervention) and adolescents may be reluctant to express their concerns due to feelings of embarrassment and shame.

Academic and Social Functioning

Academic and social difficulties are important to consider within the context of IBD. Research has demonstrated that children with IBD may be frequently absent from school (Mackner, Bickmeier, & Crandall, 2012; Moody, Eaden, & Mayberry, 1999). IBD may also reduce the extent of their participation in the classroom. For example, secondary disease-related complications (e.g., anemia, nutritional deficiency) may impair cognitive functioning (Thayu & Mamula, 2005) and lead to poor school functioning. Further, the fatigue associated with IBD may promote difficulties in initiating and sustaining attention in the classroom, as well as preclude participation in certain activities. Finally, children and adolescents may not want their friends to be aware of their illness due to the potential stigma associated with bowel concerns.

Cultural Considerations

Some research suggests that psychosocial factors have an influence on IBD. Cross-cultural differences in the experience of a specific disease are common, and they may be related to race, ethnicity, gender, socioeconomic status, age, family heritage, family structure, values, beliefs about the healthcare system, and other important factors. In a study investigating black and white adult patients with Crohn's disease, black patients were likely to experience greater disease-related disability, including difficulty affording healthcare costs and greater impact of IBD on their jobs (Straus, Eisen, Sandler, Murray et al., 2000). The study's authors attributed these findings to possible differences in socioeconomic status. One systematic review found racially and socioeconomically based disparities in medical and surgical care for IBD, which suggests distinct barriers in access to, and accessibility of, effective diagnosis and treatment (Sewell & Velayos, 2013). Furthermore, black children with IBD were found to be older at the time of diagnosis and symptom onset, and they evidenced a greater incidence of Crohn's disease than children who were not black (White et al., 2008). Taken together, these data may indicate specific racial and socioeconomic vulnerabilities in healthcare delivery.

School Personnel

Children and adolescents benefit from having a formal mechanism that outlines necessary accommodations that may arise due to symptoms of IBD (see Table 15.1). There is a need for open and frequent communication between home and school, because the healthcare needs of children with IBD may change over time and because of the variability in the illness process. Children with IBD may require accommodations throughout the school day that incorporate medication administration and monitoring, dietary adaptations or modifications, and personal care.

Many public schools require that the school nurse dispense medications; if the child must go to another area of the school to take medication, it should be accomplished in a manner that minimizes disruptions (e.g., the process should not cause the child to be late and should prevent undue attention to the child). It is important to note that adolescents may periodically refuse to take their medications. The refusal is often related to medication side effects or the current disease state (e.g., when their symptoms subside, they may think they "do not need to take" the medication). Should this occur, it is important to involve a trusted teacher or other school personnel to speak directly with the child, as well as to inform the parent or guardian of the child. Other accommodations throughout the day may reflect dietary needs and areas of personal assistance. For example, dietary accommodations may include elimination of specific foods, monitoring dietary and fluid requirements, adjusting the food intake schedule, and provision of frequent meals and snacks. Allowing cheduled and frequent restroom breaks, ensuring access to a private restroom, and availability of an extra set of clothing are also important.

In addition to accommodations that may be included in a child's formal 504 plan, school personnel share an important responsibility in assessing the child for distress, given the child spends most of the day in the school setting. As indicated, children with IBD may be vulnerable to a host of social, academic, emotional, and behavioral difficulties. For a child with a chronic medical condition that involves bowel dysfunction, it is important for the school to attend to possible social withdrawal, interpersonal difficulty, challenges with school avoidance, and difficulty participating in previously enjoyed activities. Should such difficulties significantly affect the child's life or cause distress, referral to a mental health professional should be considered.

Case Example

Mary is a 14-year-old Caucasian female who was recently diagnosed with Crohn's disease. The course of her illness has been unpredictable and marked by symptoms that wax and wane, including abdominal pain, chronic diarrhea, flatulence, and rectal bleeding. Per the recommendation of her pediatric gastroenterologist, she was placed on a course of high-dose corticosteroids, which had side effects that included excessive weight gain and acne. Her daily treatment plan includes administration of several medications, consumption of small and frequent meals, and achievement of hydration goals. Since her diagnosis, Mary has missed multiple weeks of school due to illness, medical appointments, and hospitalization, as well as side effects from her medication. Mary has also been experiencing significant fatigue, body image concerns, and reluctance to return to school due to her "bathroom symptoms."

Mary's parents and medical team collaborated with personnel from Mary's school to devise a 504 plan to optimize her success in the classroom as she transitions back to her neighborhood school. Given the core gastrointestinal symptoms associated with her diagnosis, she was provided unrestricted access to the restroom and was seated near the classroom exit so that she can leave in an expedient manner and not disrupt other students or attract unnecessary or undue attention. Due to Mary's fatigue and her low activity tolerance, realistic goals were set to manage her energy level and endurance, as well as to encourage rest periods during physical education class and throughout her school day. Further, in Mary's plan, she is permitted access to nutritious snacks during the day. The school also wants to assess the impact of Mary's illness on her performance and hopes to ensure a smooth transition back to school. School personnel, including the guidance counselor, will periodically check in with Mary to assesher for symptoms of anxiety and depression and to connect her to resources if necessary. Mary, her parents, and her medical team, as well as her school, will continue to assess and update her plan as the need arises or her medical condition changes.

CONSTIPATION AND ENCOPRESIS

Encopresis is repeated fecal soiling in inappropriate places (e.g., in clothing, on the floor) by a child at least 4 years old (American Psychiatric Association, 2013). The soiling is either intentional or involuntary and is not better accounted for by another medical condition (e.g., Hirschsprung disease, anorectal malformation). Furthermore, intentional soiling may reflect other externalizing psychopathology, such as oppositional defiant disorder (American Psychiatric Association, 2013). Most often, the passage of fecal material into the underwear, diaper, or pull-up is involuntary and is a result of chronic constipation and painful defecation (Loening-Baucke, 1993; Partin, Hamill, Fischel, & Partin, 1992). Healthcare providers frequently define constipation based on objective markers, such as stool frequency (e.g., the passage of large and/or hardened stools fewer than three times per week, Sulphen, Borowitz, Hutchison, & Cox, 1995). In addition to the frequency and consistency of stools, other symptoms of constipation include withholding, straining, pain with passage of a bowel movement, feelings of incomplete evacuation, and fecal incontinence.

Chronic constipation often results from withholding stool due to painful or distressing experiences with previous defecation. As stool is retained, the fecal matter becomes hardened, large, and difficult to pass; this can lead to secondary complications, including abdominal pain and distension, nausea, vomiting, and loss of appetite. With chronic constipation, the child may develop acquired megacolon, wherein the walls of the rectum dilate to accommodate the large stool burden. When the colon is dilated, the child ultimately has reduced sensitivity to the urge to defecate (Loening-Baucke, 1993). Overflow incontinence may then occur when new, soft stool collects around the large mass of hardened, retained stool and then leaks into the child's underwear, diaper, or pull-up. Because of stool retention, the rectum absorbs the water from the fecal mass (water normally leads stools to be soft and easy to evacuate) and the retained stools become more difficult to pass.

Encopresis tends to be a common concern among preschool and school-age children. The prevalence of constipation in youth ranges from 0.7% to 29.6% (Mugie, Benninga, & Di Lorenzo, 2011; van den Berg, Benninga, & Di Lorenzo, 2006), and encopresis is more common in males (American Psychiatric Association, 2013; van der Wal, Benninga, & Hirasing, 2005).

Treatment

Treatment may entail several components, including psychoeducation, medical management and disimpaction, and conditioning of normal bowel habits. Education should include information on the prevalence and etiology of constipation, in addition to the cycle by which constipation may be perpetuated. Additional information regarding the normal frequency of bowel movements and nutritional guidance (e.g., fiber intake, hydration goals) is also helpful. Common (problematic) beliefs and myths related to incontinence should be discussed and debunked (e.g., the child's fecal incontinence is not a result of willful behavior, stooling is not the parent's fault).

The second step in treatment is to reduce or eliminate the large amount of stool that is retained in the colon (Loening-Baucke, 1993). If the stool burden is not evacuated or disimpacted, the chronic constipation is unlikely to resolve. A primary care physician or pediatric gastroenterologist is typically trained to manage the clean-out procedure. Once the colon is disimpacted, incorporation of a daily maintenance regimen is vital to prevent the reaccumulation of stool, as well as to allow the colon time to resume normal tone and size. The child may continue to require the use of oral medications (e.g., stool softener, laxatives), suppositories, and dietary modifications (e.g., increased fiber, increased fluid intake) to establish typical bowel habits.

Behavioral interventions are designed to manage contingencies and to reduce the level of distress surrounding toileting, as well as promote normal bowel habits (Freeman, Riley, Duke, & Fu, 2014). First-line behavioral interventions for constipation and encopresis may incorporate appropriate toilet sittings, increasing dietary fiber and fluid intake, and adherence to medical management (Howe & Walker, 1992; Stark, Owens-Stively, Spirito, Lewis, & Guevremont, 1990. The child's parents are also encouraged to monitor scheduled toilet sittings (see Handout 15.1), daily bowel movements (including the consistency of stools), fecal soiling (see Handout 15.2), and medication use. Intervention may additionally focus on emotional concerns related to toileting. For example, a child who experienced large and painful stools may become fearful and avoidant of the toilet and may refuse to sit. Therefore, behavioral goals and graded exposure assignments may be developed to increase approach behavior and to extinguish fears, thereby promoting adaptive toileting efforts.

Emotional and Behavioral Functioning

Children with encopresis are reported to have more symptoms of emotional distress than children without toileting concerns (Cox, Morris, Borowitz, & Sutphen, 2002; Joinson, Heron, Butler, von Fontard, & Avon Longitudinal Study of Parents and Children Study Team, 2006). They are also rated by their teachers as more aggressive than children without encopresis (Cox et al., 2002). Identified risk factors for toileting problems include delayed development, difficult temperament, and maternal anxiety or depression (Joinson et al., 2008). Furthermore, soiling may confer greater risk, because the combination of fecal incontinence and constipation decreases quality of life more than constipation alone (Kovacic et al., 2015). In general, difficulties with bowel habits may be associated with several areas of psychosocial concern.

Academic and Social Functioning

Children with encopresis have greater problems with inattention and social interactions, and poorer school performance than children without these
concerns (Cox et al., 2002; Joinson et al., 2006). Furthermore, affected children
score lower on academic measures of spelling, arithmetic, and reading compared
to their healthy peers (Cox et al., 2002; Stern, Lowitz, Prince, Altshuler, & Stroh,
1988). With overflow incontinence, children frequently are unable to detect the
smell or tactile sensation of soiled underwear because of habituation. Therefore,
children are frequently teased by their peers and family for being unable to detect
the fecal matter. Furthermore, children are often subject to blame and punishment related to soiling; it is common for children to hide underwear and pull-ups
in an attempt to conceal the problem.

Cultural Considerations

Specific psychosocial and environmental variables are associated with problematic bowel habits, constipation, and fecal incontinence. For example, straining
and a lower frequency of stooling are more common in girls (Wald et al., 2009),
and having a first-degree relative with constipation may confer greater risk for
a child to have toileting difficulties (Dehghani et al., 2015; Ostwani et al., 2010).
Additionally, certain parental child-rearing attitudes (i.e., a high level of overprotectiveness and self-pity; van Dijk, de Vries, Last, Benninga, & Grootenhuis,
2015), patterns of dietary intake (e.g., consumption of fast food; Tam et al., 2012),
and fewer hours of sleep (Tam et al., 2012) are associated with constipation and
incontinence. Moreover, parents often adopt a negative or punitive response to
fecal soiling and may blame and shame the child for a problem that is uninten-
tional (Friman, Hofstadter, & Jones, 2006).

School Personnel

Encopresis may quickly become emotionally and social challenging for a child,
particularly as the child grows older. The development and implementation of
a formal school plan to manage concerns related to encopresis is important.
Accommodations that the school may implement include complying with a
toileting schedule throughout the day in an unhurried and private environment. It may also be important for the family to leave personal care items (e.g.,
clothing changes, wipes, bags to store soiled items) at the school should the
child soil. A health plan may include medication administration, and the school
nurse may serve the important role of ensuring their delivery to the child. Given

that some medications for restoring proper bowel habits can promote frequent trips to the bathroom (e.g., laxatives), the school nurse may wish to educate teachers about management of such a situation. The school also serves an important function in being able to monitor a child's current intake of foods that promote elimination patterns (e.g., fiber, vegetables) and potentially to optimize that intake.

Case Example

Brian is a typically developing 7-year-old African American male who has been resistant to toilet training for stool from a young age. Following a painful bowel movement years earlier, he has been avoidant of the toilet and prefers to stool while crouching in his bedroom closet. Although he avoids the toilet for bowel movements, he does urinate in the toilet. He stools about once per week and is often seen clutching his stomach just prior to stooling. Brian is currently enrolled in the second grade and his school is unaware of his toileting problem. He has recently had several episodes in school where he was surrounded by the smell of foul fecal material, was sent to the office, and his parents were called to pick him up from the school. Brian's parents are frustrated and cannot understand why— despite their giving him a daily stool softener—he cannot produce a bowel movement in the toilet.

The school nurse was alerted to the situation and placed a call to Brian's parents to discuss management of the situation across contexts. The nurse discussed medical and behavioral treatment of encopresis and overflow incontinence, in addition to the underlying etiology of the problems, constipation. Brian's parents, the school nurse, and the school psychologist worked together to develop a 504 plan for when Brian soils his underwear at school (e.g., Brian goes to the nurse's office for clean-up and a change of clothes, he places his soiled clothes in a plastic bag, and then he returns to class). The nurse also discussed long-term goals for continence, including contacting his pediatrician and/or pediatric gastroenterologist to begin appropriate medical management and oversight. The school nurse additionally informed Brian's parents that the accommodations in his current 504 plan could be modified and changed depending upon Brain's health status and current healthcare needs.

CLINICAL ASSESSMENT

Due to the increased risk for mood and behavioral concerns among students with GI disorders, it is recommended that school professionals routinely screen students with these chronic health conditions for social and emotional concerns using well-established assessment measures, including the Pediatric Symptom Checklist (PSC; Jellinek et al., 1988) or Behavior Assessment System for Children, Third Edition (BASC-3; Reynolds & Kamphaus, 2015). Both measures can be used to assess mental health concerns from the perspective of parents; the BASC-3 also offers measures that can be completed by the teacher and student (depending on the age of the student). In addition to using these broadband measures, school psychologists and school counselors are encouraged to routinely assess students with GI disorders for mental health concerns by engaging students and parents in a structured interview process. However, when working with students with a chronic health condition like CD, IBD, encopresis, or constipation, it is recommended that school psychologists and school counselors ask questions that directly target concerns related to the condition (see Box 15.1), such as knowledge of the condition, quality of life, social and school functioning, family functioning, adherence, and psychological functioning.

Box 15.1.

QUESTIONS TO ASK STUDENTS AND PARENTS AS PART OF CLINICAL ASSESSMENT

Knowledge of Condition
- When were you first diagnosed with ____?
- How do you refer to your diagnosis?
- What do you know about your diagnosis of ____?
- How do you explain it to other people?
- What caused it?

Quality of Life

- What has been different about your life since receiving your diagnosis?
  - Home?
  - School?
  - Friends?
  - Extracurricular activities?
  - Food?
  - Medicine?
- What has been difficult since receiving the diagnosis?
- If you could change anything about your life, what would you change?
  - Diagnosis?
  - Diet?
  - Home/family?
  - School?
  - Friends?

Social and School Functioning
- Who knows about your diagnosis?
  - Friends?
  - Teachers?
  - Coaches?
- How have people reacted to the diagnosis? Has their behavior changed or stayed the same?
- Does having _____ interfere with socializing with peers?
- Are there activity limitations due to _____?
- How has school attendance been affected?
- How have academics been affected?
- If there was something you wish others could know about your diagnosis, what would that be?

Family Functioning

- Do your siblings/parents understand what _____ is?
- How have they treated you since learning about your diagnosis?

Adherence
- What do you need to do to manage your _____?
- Who is responsible for ensuring that you _____?

Mood

- Any changes in mood?
- How do you feel most of the time?
- What are some things that make you feel sad?
- What are some thing that you worry about?
- When was the last time you felt happy?
- How is your energy level?
- What do you like to do for fun? When was the last time you were interested in doing those things?
- When was the last time you saw your friends?
- When you feel down or worried, what do you do to help yourself feel better?
- Suicide risk assessment: Have you ever been so sad that you have thought about killing yourself?

Behavior

- Any changes in behavior?
- Any concerns about staying focused or getting distracted easily?
- Any concerns about staying seated or talking too much?
- Any concerns about impulsivity?
- Any concerns about following instructions or listening?

Sleep

- Any changes in sleep?
- When do you go to sleep?
- Do you ever have trouble falling asleep?
- What do you do to help you fall asleep?
- Do you ever have trouble staying asleep?
- What do you do to help you go back to sleep?
- Where do you sleep?
- When do you wake up?

Eating

- Any changes in appetite or weight?
- When do you typically eat?
- What do you typically eat?
- Where do you typically eat?
- Who is typically around you when you are eating?

Toileting

- Any changes in toileting habits?
- How often are you using the toilet?
- Any accidents during the day? If so, how many?
- Any pain when you stool?

FACILITATORS OF TREATMENT ADHERENCE

Although there are unique barriers to treatment adherence for each GI disorder, there are several facilitators to treatment adherence, including developmentally appropriate psychoeducation about the disorder, planning ahead, social supports, addressing emotional and behavioral concerns, and advocating for academic supports. In terms of psychoeducation about the disorder, it is paramount that students with GI disorders receive developmentally appropriate psychoeducation; however, it is equally imperative that the important people in the student's life (e.g., family members, peers, teachers) also receive accurate information about the disorder. In fact, much of psychoeducation involves dispelling myths about causes, symptoms, and treatment of the disorder and providing appropriate resources to all parties involved

Families are also encouraged to be proactive. For children with CD, this includes calling manufacturers about ingredients in store-bought items, finding out what will be served at a party or is available at a restaurant, or bringing gluten-free food to social situations (Chick, 2014). For families of children with IBD, encopresis, or constipation, planning may include locating the nearest bathroom in different environments, setting reminders to take medication, and establishing toileting schedules. Social supports are also helpful when it comes to treatment adherence. Specifically, having the support of a student's school (e.g., teachers, principal, nurse, school psychologist) and the student's community (e.g., sports team, Scout Troop, religious organization), as well as group support (e.g., support groups for the medical condition), is critical to adherence (Chick, 2014).

Another facilitator of treatment adherence for children and adolescents who experience GI disorders is addressing the emotional and behavioral concerns that arise in response to a diagnosis and symptoms. An evidence-based approach to addressing these concerns is cognitive-behavioral therapy (CBT), which is based on the idea that maladaptive thoughts cause psychological symptoms (e.g., feeling anxious or depressed), which in turn cause or exacerbate physical symptoms and increase safety or avoidant behaviors (Palsson & Whitehead, 2013; White, 2011). The crux of CBT is changing maladaptive thinking patterns and increasing healthy behavioral patterns. CBT often involves use of relaxation strategies, behavioral strategies, and cognitive strategies to address both psychological and physical symptoms that develop (Palsson & Whitehead, 2013; White, 2011). Relaxation strategies may include diaphragmatic breathing, guided imagery, and progressive muscle relaxation. Behavioral strategies include both behavioral activation (i.e., increasing engagement in preferred activities) and exposures (i.e., gradual exposure to a feared or avoided stimulus or situation). Last, cognitive strategies involve challenging cognitive distortions (e.g., catastrophizing) through increasing awareness of the association among stressors, thoughts, and physical symptoms and subsequently adopting effective coping strategies to manage life stressors and the associated gastrointestinal symptoms (Palsson & Whitehead, 2013; White, 2011).

LEGAL AND ETHICAL CONCERNS

Serving students with GI disorders presents several legal and ethical concerns for schools. As noted earlier, students with GI disorders who demonstrate an educational need may be eligible to receive services under the special education category of other health impairment. Therefore, an admission, review, and dismissal (ARD) or individualized education plan (IEP) committee will be formed to develop an IEP to meet the student's educational needs by ensuring free and appropriate public education (FAPE) in the least restrictive environment (LRE). In contrast, if a student has a disability but does not demonstrate an educational need, he or she may qualify for Section 504 services, which ensure that students with GI disorders are integrated into the mainstream to the fullest extent possible. However, the laws in place that govern meeting the needs of students with chronic health conditions do not provide concrete examples of how to meet those needs, leaving ample room for interpretation among schools, families, and the legal system (Chick, 2014).

In general, most schools do not have formal protocols for effectively serving students with chronic health conditions, let alone GI disorders. Therefore, school personnel often have to scramble to develop a plan and offer accommodations when a student receives a diagnosis. For instance, most schools do not have procedures for managing cross-contamination of items for students with CD. Further, if cross-contamination does occur, it is unclear if the school is liable (Chick, 2014). Additionally, it is not certain if schools are legally required to pay for gluten-free school meals for students with CD or the extent of the options that they must provide, or if families are required to provide their own food (Chick, 2014). Other issues that span the scope of GI disorders include concerns related to missing school for doctor's appointments or illness and the subsequent consequences. For example, although school districts have an overarching policy on truancy, individual schools tend to respond to students' missing school for medical appointments on a case-by-case basis.

Moreover, issues of students' privacy and violations of the Family Educational Rights and Privacy Act of 1974 (FERPA) or the Health Insurance Portability and Accountability Act of 1996 (HIPAA) arise when working with students with chronic health conditions. For instance, information related to the student's condition, including the diagnosis, symptoms, and treatment should be shared only at the discretion of the student's guardians. Unfortunately, in school settings, private information may be unintentionally shared with other students and school staff. To that end, there are several ways to avoid miscommunications between school personnel and parents, as shown in Table 15.2. Last, like students with other types of chronic health conditions, students with GI disorders are faced with determining whose responsibility it is to ensure adherence (e.g., the student takes his or her scheduled medications, goes to the bathroom at appropriate times, or eats at appropriate times during the school day). Overall, it is imperative that school personnel have a strong working knowledge of the law as well as foundational procedures in place to effectively serve students with GI disorders.

USEFUL RESOURCES

- Crohn's and Colitis Foundation of America: www.crohnscolitisfoundation.org
- GatroKids: www.gikids.org
- University of Michigan Health System: Practice Guide for Constipation & Soiling in Children: www.med.umich.edu/1info/FHP/practiceguides/newconstipation.html
- Pediatric IBD Foundation: www.pedsibd.org
- Crohn's & Colitis Foundation of America (Just Like Me: Teens with IBD): http://www.justlikemeibd.org

Table 15.2. POTENTIAL CHALLENGES OF WORKING WITH STUDENTS WITH
GI DISORDERS

Challenges	Solutions
Communication between school and parents	• Use appropriate medical terminology to discuss the student's disorder or health concerns. • Avoid using slang or insensitive terminology when talking about symptoms or student behaviors that are related to the medical condition. • School staff should be aware of, educated about, and sensitive to the student's conditions, needs, and treatment plans, and staff members should be cognizant of the individual impact and chronicity of the student's disorder.
Communication between school and medical teams	• Receive written consent from the student's parents to have communication with the student's medical providers and team. • Respect professional boundaries and respective expertise. • Provide open communication with medical teams regarding student's current symptoms and behaviors related to his or her condition. • Maintain ongoing data collection regarding student behaviors and symptoms that could assist the medical team with future treatment planning. • Work together to make sure that all parties involved in a child's care understand the need for consistency in the behavioral schedule across multiple settings.
Gathering information to establish educational plan	• Share reports and records between school and medical teams. • Monitor and collect data regarding the child's symptoms and difficulties functioning within the school environment. • Ensure that all school staff understand the accommodations and treatment plan, and reasonable goals are set for the student.
Frequent student absences due to medical appointments	• Work with the family to determine if the student is well enough to return to school or if in-home or hospital tutoring services are needed. • Work with teachers to determine if alternate assignments or activities are appropriate.

REFERENCES

Addolorato, G., Mirijello, A., D'Angelo, C., Leggio, L., Ferrulli, A., Vonghia, L., . . . Gasbarrini, G. (2008). Social phobia in coelic disease. *Scandinavian Journal of Gastroenterology, 43*, 410–415.

American Psychiatric Association. (2013). *Diagnostic and statistical manual of mental disorders* (5th ed., DSM-5®). Arlington, VA: American Psychiatric Publishing.

Bacigalupe, G., & Plocha, A. (2015). Celiac is a social disease: Family challenges and strategies. *Families, Systems, & Health, 33*(1), 46–54.

Baldassano, R. N., & Piccoli, D. A. (1999). Inflammatory bowel disease in pediatric and adolescent patients. *Gastroenterology Clinics, 28*(2), 445–458.

Butwicka, A., Lichtenstein, P., Frisen, L., Almqvist, C., Larsson, H., & Ludvigsson, J. F. (2017). Celiac disease is associated with childhood psychiatric disorders: A population-based study. *The Journal of Pediatrics, 184*, 87–94.

Crohn's and Colitis Foundation (n.d.). Retrieved from http://www. crohnscolitisfoundation.org/

The Celiac Disease Program at Children's National Health System and The Celiac Disease Foundation. (n.d.). *Celiac disease and gluten-related conditions psychological health manual.* Retrieved from https://celiac.org/for-professionals/psychological-health-training-program/healthmanual/

Chick, K. A. (2014). Focus on inclusive education: The educational and social challenges of children with celiac disease: What educators should know. *Childhood Education, 90*(1), 71–74. doi:10.1080/00094056.2014.872520

Conrad, M. A., & Rosh, J. R. (2017). Pediatric inflammatory bowel disease. *Pediatric Clinics of North America, 64*(3), 577–591.

Cox, D. J., Morris, J. B., Jr., Borowitz, S. M., & Sutphen, J. L. (2002). Psychological differences between children with and without chronic encopresis. *Journal of Pediatric Psychology, 27*(7), 585–591.

Dehghani, S. M., Moravej, H., Rajaei, E., & Javaherizadeh, H. (2015). Evaluation of familial aggregation, vegetable consumption, legumes consumption, and physical activity on functional constipation in families of children with functional constipation versus children without constipation. *Przeglad Gastroenterologiczny, 10*(2), 89–93.

Family Educational Rights and Privacy Act of 1974, 20 U.S.C. § 1232 (1974). Retrieved from https://ed.gov/policy/gen/guid/fpco/ferpa/index.html

Fasano, A., Berti, I., Gerarduzzi, T., Not, T., Colletti, R., Drago, S., . . . Horvath, K. (2003). Prevalence of celiac disease in at-risk and not-at risk groups in the United States. *Archives of Internal, 163*(3), 286–292.

Freeman, K. A., Riley, A., Duke, D. C., & Fu, R. (2014). Systematic review and meta-analysis of behavioral interventions for fecal incontinence with constipation. *Journal of Pediatric Psychology, 39*(8), 887–902.

Friman, P. D., Hofstadter, K. L., & Jones, K. M. (2006). A biobehavioral approach to the treatment of functional encopresis in children, *Journal of Early and Intensive Behavior Intervention, 3*(3), 263–272.

Gray, W. N., Denson, L. A., Baldassano, R. N., & Hommel, K. A. (2011). Treatment adherence in adolescents with inflammatory bowel disease: The collective impact of barriers to adherence and anxiety/depressive symptoms. *Journal of Pediatric Psychology, 37*(3), 282–291.

Gupta, K., Noble, A., Kachelries, K. E., Albenberg, L., Kelsen, J. R., Grossman, A. B., & Baldassano, R. N. (2013). A novel enteral nutrition protocol for the treatment of pediatric Crohn's disease. *Inflammatory Bowel Diseases, 19*(7), 1374–1378.

United States. (1996). *The Health Insurance Portability and Accountability Act (HIPAA)*. Washington, D.C.: U.S. Department of Labor, Employee Benefits Secruity Administration.

Hommel, K. A., & Baldassano, R. N. (2010). Brief report: Barriers to treatment adherence in pediatric inflammatory bowel disease. *Journal of Pediatric Psychology, 35*(9), 1005–1010.

Howe, A. C., & Walker, C. E. (1992). Behavioral management of toilet training, enuresis, and encopresis. *Pediatric Clinics of North America, 39*(3), 413–432.

Isaac, D. M., Wu, J., Mager, D. R., & Turner, J. M. (2016). Managing the pediatric patient with celiac disease: A multidisciplinary approach. *Journal of Multidisciplinary Healthcare, 9*, 529–536.

Jellinek, M. S., Murphy, M., Robinson, J., Feins, A., Lamb, S., & Fenton, T. (1988). Pediatric Symptom Checklist: Screening school-age children for psychosocial dysfunction. *The Journal of Pediatrics, 112*(2), 201–209.

Joinson, C., Heron, J., Butler, U., von Gontard, A., & Avon Longitudinal Study of Parents and Children Study Team. (2006). Psychological differences between children with and without soiling problems. *Pediatrics, 117*(5), 1575–1584.

Joinson, C., Heron, J., von Gontard, A., Butler, U., Golding, J., & Emond, A. (2008). Early childhood risk factors associated with daytime wetting and soiling in school-age children. *Journal of Pediatric Psychology, 33*(7), 739–750.

Kovacic, K., Sood, M. R., Mugie, S., Di Lorenzo, C., Nurko, S., Heinz, N., . . . Silverman, A. H. (2015). A multicenter study on childhood constipation and fecal incontinence: Effects on quality of life. *The Journal of Pediatrics, 166*(6), 1482–1487.

Krigel, A., Turner, K. O., Makharia, G. K., Green, P. H. R., Genta, R. M., & Lebwohl, B. (2016). Ethnic variations in duodenal villous atrophy consistent with celiac disease in the united states. *Clinical Gastroenterology and Hepatology,14*, 1105–1111.

Liu, E., Lee, H. S., Aronsson, C. A., Hagopian, W. A., Koletzko, S., Rewers, M., . . . Agardh, D. (2014). Risk of pediatric celiac disease according to HLA haplotype and country. *New England Journal of Medicine, 371*, 42–49.

Loening-Baucke, V. (1993). Chronic constipation in children. *Gastroenterology, 105*(5), 1557–1564.

Ludvigsson, J. F., & Green, P. H. (2011). Clinical management of coeliac disease. *Journal of Internal Medicine, 269*, 560–571.

Mackner, L. M., Bickmeier, R. M., & Crandall, W. V. (2012). Academic achievement, attendance, and school-related quality of life in pediatric inflammatory bowel disease. *Journal of Developmental & Behavioral Pediatrics, 33*(2), 106–111.

Mackner, L. M., & Crandall, W. V. (2007). Psychological factors affecting pediatric inflammatory bowel disease. *Current Opinion in Pediatrics, 19*(5), 548–552.

Malaty, H. M., Fan, X., Opekun, A. R., Thibodeaux, C., & Ferry, G. D. (2010). Rising incidence of inflammatory bowel disease among children: A 12-year study. *Journal of Pediatric Gastroenterology and Nutrition, 50*(1), 27–31.

Molodecky, N. A., Soon, S., Rabi, D. M., Ghali, W. A., Ferris, M., Chernoff, G., . . . Kaplan, G. G. (2012). Increasing incidence and prevalence of the inflammatory bowel diseases with time, based on systematic review. *Gastroenterology, 142*(1), 46–54.

Moody, G., Eaden, J. A., & Mayberry, J. F. (1999). Social implications of childhood Crohn's disease. *Journal of Pediatric Gastroenterology and Nutrition. 28*(4), S43–50.

Mrakotsky, C., Forbes, P. W., Bernstein, J. H., Grand, R. J., Bousvaros, A., Szigethy, E., & Waber, D. P. (2013). Acute cognitive and behavioral effects of systemic corticosteroids in children treated for inflammatory bowel disease. *Journal of the International Neuropsychological Society, 19*(1), 96–109.

Mugie, S. M., Benninga, M. A., & Di Lorenzo, C. (2011). Epidemiology of constipation in children and adults: A systematic review. *Best Practice & Research Clinical Gastroenterology, 25*(1), 3–18.

Ostwani, W., Dolan, J., & .Elitsur, Y. (2010). Familial clustering of habitual constipation: A prospective study in children from West Virginia. *Journal of Pediatric Gastroenterology and Nutrition, 50*, 287–289.

Palsson, O. S., & Whitehead, W. E. (2013). Psychological treatments in functional GI disorders: A primer for the gastroenterologist. *Clinical Gastroenterology and Hepatology, 11*(3), 208–216.

Partin, J. C., Hamill, S. K., Fischel, J. E., & Partin, J. S. (1992). Painful defecation and fecal soiling in children. *Pediatrics, 89*(6), 1007–1009.

Porto, A. (2017). *Celiac disease in children & teens.* Retrieved from https://www.healthychildren.org/English/health-Issues/conditions/abdominal/Pages/Celiac-Disease.aspx

Reynolds, C. R., & Kamphaus, R. W. (2015). *Behavior assessment system for children* (3rd ed.). Bloomington, MN: Pearson.

Saps, M., Adams, P., Bonilla, S., & Nichols-Vinueza, D. (2013). Abdominal pain and functional GI disorders in children with celiac disease. *The Journal of Pediatrics, 162*(3), 505–509.

Satherly, R., Howard, R., & Higgs, S. (2015). Disordered eating practices in GI disorders. *Appetite, 84*, 240–250.

Section 504 of the Rehabilitation Act of 1973, 34 C. F. R. Part 104.

Sewell, J. L., & Velayos, F. S. (2013). Systematic review: The role of race and socioeconomic factors on IBD healthcare delivery and effectiveness. *Inflammatory Bowel Disease, 19*(3), 627–643.

Skjerning, H., Mahony, R. O., Husby, S., & DunnGalvin, A. (2014). Health-related quality of life in children and adolescents with celiac disease: Patient-driven data from focus group interviews. *Quality of Life Research, 23*, 1883–1894.

Spekhorst, L. M., Hummel, T. Z., Benninga, M. A., van Rheenen, P. F., & Kindermann, A. (2016). Adherence to oral maintenance treatment in adolescents with inflammatory bowel disease. *Journal of Pediatric Gastroenterology and Nutrition, 62*(2), 264–270.

Stark, L. J., Owens-Stively, J., Spirito, A., Lewis, A., & Guevremont, D. (1990). Group behavioral treatment of retentive encopresis. *Journal of Pediatric Psychology, 15*(5), 659–671.

Stern, H. P., Lowitz, G. H., Prince, M. T., Altshuler, L., & Stroh, S. E. (1988). The incidence of cognitive dysfunction in an encopretic population in children. *Neurotoxicology, 9*, 351–357.

Straus, W. L, Eisen, G. M, Sandler, R. S., Murray, S. C., & Sessions, J. T. (2000). Crohn's disease: Does race matter? The Mid-Atlantic Crohn's Disease Study Group. *American Journal of Gastroenterology, 95*, 479–483.

Sutphen, J. L., Borowitz, S. M., Hutchison, R. L., & Cox, D. J. (1995). Long-term follow-up of medically treated childhood constipation. *Clinical Pediatrics, 34*(11), 576–580.

Tam, Y. H., Li, A. M., So, H. K., Shit, K. Y., Pang, K. K., Wong, Y. S., . . . Lee, K. H. (2012). Socioenvironmental factors associated with constipation in Hong Kong children and Rome III criteria. *Journal of Pediatric Gastroenterology and Nutrition, 55*(1), 56–61.

Thayu, M., & Mamula, P. (2005). Treatment of iron deficiency anemia in pediatric inflammatory bowel disease. *Current Treatment Options in Gastroenterology, 8*(5), 411–417.

Thomas, A., & Lodhia, N. (2014). Advanced therapy for inflammatory bowel disease: A guide for the primary care physician. *Journal of the American Board of Family Medicine, 27*(3), 411–420.

van den Berg, M. M., Benninga, M. A., & Di Lorenzo, C. (2006). Epidemiology of childhood constipation: A systematic review. *American Journal of Gastroenterology, 101*(10), 2401–2409.

van der Wal, M. F., Benninga, M. A., & Hirasing, R. A. (2005). The prevalence of encopresis in a multicultural population. *Journal of Pediatric Gastroenterology and Nutrition, 40*(3), 345–348.

van Dijk, M., de Vries, G. J., Last, B. F., Benninga, M. A., & Grootenhuis, M. A. (2015). Parental child-rearing attitudes are associated with functional constipation in childhood. *Archives of Disease in Childhood, 100*, 329–333.

van Hees, N. J., Van der Does, W., & Giltay, E. J. (2013). Coeliac disease, diet adherence and depressive symptoms. *Journal of Psychosomatic Research, 74*, 155–60.

Wald, E. R., Di Lorenzo, C., Cipriani, L., Colborn, D. K., Burgers, R., & Wald, A. (2009). Bowel habits and toileting training in a diverse population of children. *Journal of Pediatric Gastroenterology and Nutrition, 48*(3), 294–298.

White, C. A. (2011). *Cognitive behaviour therapy for chronic medical problems: A guide to assessment and treatment in practice.* Chichester, UK: John Wiley & Sons.

White, J. M., O'Connor, S., Winter, H. S., Heyman, M. B., Kirschner, B. S., Ferry, G. D., . . . Gold, B. D. (2008). Inflammatory bowel disease in African American children compared with other racial/ethnic groups in a multicenter registry. *Clinical Gastroenterology and Hepatology, 6*(12), 1361–1369.

Wright, P. (2004). The Individuals with Disabilities Education Improvement Act of 2004: Overview, explanation, and comparison. Retrieved from www.wrightslaw.com

SAMPLE TOILETING SCHEDULE

		MONDAY	TUESDAY	WEDNESDAY	THURSDAY	FRIDAY	SATURDAY	SUNDAY
Morning								
Sent to Toilet (Time)								
Pants:	Dry (D)							
	Wet (W)							
	Stool, small (S)							
	Stool, large (L)							
Toilet:	Urine (U)							
	Stools (S)							
Midday								
Sent to Toilet (Time)								
Pants:	Dry (D)							
	Wet (W)							
	Stool, small (S)							
	Stool, large (L)							
Toilet:	Urine (U)							
	Stools (S)							
Evening								
Sent to Toilet (Time)								
Pants:	Dry (D)							
	Wet (W)							
	Stool, small (S)							
	Stool, large (L)							
Toilet:	Urine (U)							
	Stools (S)							

HANDOUT 15.2.

SAMPLE ENCOPRESIS BEHAVIORAL CHART

Directions: When your child has a bowel movement, urinates, or practices sitting:

- Put time of day in the Time column
- Add the letter codes to the Time column

DAY	TIME	TIME	TIME	TIME	TIME	TIME	TIME	TIME
Sunday Example:	9 AM BMB, UB	12 PM PS, UT	2 PM BMP, UP					
Monday								
Tuesday								
Wednesday								
Thursday								
Friday								
Saturday								

BMT: bowel movement in toilet; BMP: bowel movement in pants; BMB: bowel movement in bed; PS: practice sit; UT: urinated in toilet; UP: urinated in pants; UB: urinated in bed.

16

Neurological Disorders

DAVID L. WODRICH, RANDA G. JARRAR,
AND MICHAEL M. ETZL, JR. ∎

Neurological conditions (illnesses and diseases) are critically important in school success. This is true, of course, because the human central nervous system (CNS) supports all the attentional, perceptual, cognitive, memory-related, affective, and interpersonal capabilities that students depend upon for school success. This chapter covers two educationally relevant neurological conditions: epilepsy and pediatric cancers that either directly or indirectly affect the CNS, which are just two of many neurological conditions. These two conditions nonetheless illustrate several principles broadly important to all neurological conditions at school. The chapter covers a brief overview of each condition, a concise explanation of a model concerned with pediatric illnesses at school, how epilepsy and cancer express themselves in terms of the model, and interventions for both conditions. Finally, there are website links to educator-friendly resources.

Pediatric epilepsy and cancer share common factors related to school success. Both engender fear and anxiety, especially among classmates and teachers (Wodrich, Jarrar, Buchhalter, Levy, & Gay, 2011). Both involve a risk of social stigma as well as potential embarrassment and bullying (Austin & Caplan, 2007). Too often, both are associated with CNS effects that cause struggles with essential school tasks, or at least their quick and easy execution. But the two also differ. The pathology of epilepsy is confined to the brain. Cancer, however, may originate outside the brain (as in the case of leukemia), although its treatment has important CNS implications. Life-saving cancer treatment, not the cancer itself, often causes school problems (Khan et al., 2014), whereas in epilepsy it is CNS anomalies unrelated to treatment that can cause neurocognitive and school problems (Fastenau, Shen, Dunn, & Austin, 2008). Both epilepsy and pediatric cancer, as they relate to neurological functioning, are described in detail in this chapter.

THE P-CSI MODEL

To make sense of these two conditions (and many others) at school, a comprehensive model (referred to here as the Model) has been presented by Wodrich (2014, in press). The Model is called P-CSI because it concerns pediatric illnesses (P), challenges (C), strengths and supports (S), and impacts (I), as shown in Figure 16.1. The Model proposes that stakeholders must have an understanding of basic medical facts about any particular student's condition (e.g., epilepsy, cancer, asthma, hemophilia) before it is possible to rationally address schooling. Even more critical, however, is to understand the array of challenges caused by each unique condition (see Table 16.1). The Model argues that the number and severity of illness-related challenges confronting each student best predict his or her risk of actual school problems. In other words, a condition like epilepsy might cause challenges ranging from numerous and severe in one student to very few and largely inconsequential in another. Furthermore, the degree to which genuine academic problems (e.g., poor work productivity, limited academic and cognitive progress, interpersonal struggles, spotty attendance) materialize is buffered by each student's collection of strengths and supports (see Figure 16.1). Using the Model as a template, the chapter begins with a brief overview of epilepsy, followed by coverage of each prospective epilepsy-related challenge. The same sequence is then followed for cancer. Then potential interventions for both conditions are addressed within the list of potential strengths and supports. The chapter concludes with a list of website links and resources.

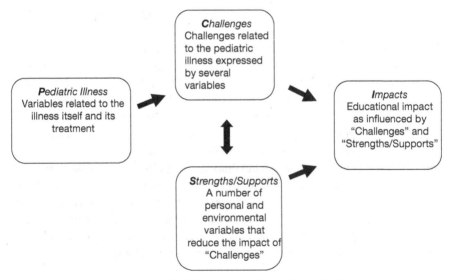

Figure 16.1. Graphic of Model of P-CSI Approach (from Wodrich 2014; in press).

Table 16.1. Sources of Educational Challenges and Mitigating
Strengths and Supports

Challenges	Strengths and Supports

• Direct neurocognitive effects
• Indirect neurocognitive effects
• Somatic effects
• Psychiatric conditions associated with illness
• Worry about upcoming treatments
• Pessimism about the future
• Academic frustration
• Anxious classmates
• Overly protective classmates
• Uninformed teachers
• Unsure or anxious teachers
	• Cognitive reserves and
	  premorbid intellectual strengths
	• Emotional resilience
	• Access to effective health care
	• Effective home-school-clinic
	  communication
	• Instructional supports at school
	• Instructional supports extending
	  to home
	• Social supports at school
	• Social supports at home

EPILEPSY

Epilepsy is defined as recurrent, unprovoked seizures. Not a singular "disease," epilepsy is instead the result of a heterogeneous set of conditions. The International League Against Epilepsy has recently updated its nomenclature and schema for epilepsy classification (for details, see www.ilae.org/Visitors/Centre/documents/ClassificationSeizureILAE-2016.pdf). Although there is no need to learn all the epilepsy subclassifications, two concepts are especially worth recognizing. The first is focal versus generalized epilepsy; the second concerns children with epilepsy (CWE) whose epilepsy has a known, underlying cause versus epilepsy without a known cause. Regarding the first distinction, focal epilepsy denotes seizures that start in a single region of the brain only; generalized epilepsy involves bilateral networks at seizure onset. As one might expect, focal seizures (and their localized electrical disturbances) result in circumscribed overt seizure expressions (e.g., isolated motor movements; limited sensory or cognitive symptoms). Furthermore, focal seizures may be less obvious to classmates and teachers. In contrast, generalized seizures are often conspicuous and may involve loss of bodily control. The second important distinction is epilepsy of unknown etiology versus epilepsy with a known etiology (as part of a more pervasive condition, such as having a genetic disorder or metabolic disturbance). For example, CWE who have a genetic disorder like tuberous sclerosis complex are quite likely to have epilepsy, along with intellectual disability and physical symptoms or signs (e.g., skin lesions). The same genetic anomaly that produces lesions on their skin may produce lesions in the brain, causing both neurocognitive deficits and seizures. Obviously, these CWE are likely to present differently at school than counterparts with epilepsy of unknown etiology.

To some extent, the nature of a student's epilepsy predicts treatment. For example, some antiepileptic drugs (AEDs), are better for focal epilepsy and others are better for generalized epilepsy. AEDs are the most common treatment for epilepsy and are effective in approximately 70% of CWE (Sarhan, Walker, & Selai, 2015). Occasionally, multiple AEDs are needed. Even so, many CWE still experience breakthrough seizures. When AEDs alone prove ineffective, alternative treatments may be required, such as a restrictive diet high in fat (ketogenic diet), surgical implantation of an electrical stimulator on the vagus nerve or the brain, or rarely, surgical excision of a seizure focus. From these facts alone, it is easy to anticipate that an array of challenges might threaten the child's school success.

Epilepsy and Its Educational Challenges

Like any condition affecting the brain, epilepsy is associated with (direct) neurocognitive effects (i.e., those arising directly from the medical condition itself). Critically, most of these effects matter at school. For example, on average, CWE underperform across cognitive domains in comparison to healthy agemates (Fastenau et al., 2008). The dimensions include low verbal and full-scale IQ scores and substandard learning in comparison to typical peers (Rantanen, Nieminen, & Eriksson, 2010). Also, instances of low IQ seem to be disproportionately common—25% of CWE have been found to have full-scale IQs less than 80 (Berg et al., 2008). These stark cumulative numbers, however, ignore epilepsy's remarkable heterogeneity. Subcategories reveal a somewhat different picture.

When comparing CWE whose epilepsy is of unknown etiology with CWE whose epilepsy has a known etiology, for example, one finds that, in the latter group, intellectual disabilities are nearly five times more common (54.5% vs. 10.7%) and speech-language impairments are nearly three times more common (10.0% vs. 3.6%; Wodrich, Kaplan, & Deering, 2006). This makes intuitive sense because the known etiologies include complex syndromes, such as tuberous sclerosis complex or Angelman syndrome. Still, epilepsy of unknown etiology sometimes involves direct neurocognitive challenges. As a case in point, Hermann and colleagues (2016) found that although 44% of youth with new-onset epilepsy of unknown etiology demonstrated unremarkable neuropsychological profiles, another 44% evidenced mild, but wide-ranging, impairments (i.e., verbal, perceptual, speed, attention, executive function). Critically, 12% of these youth expressed impairments across all dimensions assessed, as well as coexisting and severe attentional impairments.

Other subdistinctions also matter. For example, epilepsy of the focal type might be expected to incur risk for neurocognitive deficits that are circumscribed and correspond to the brain location involved. Indeed, CWE whose seizures have right hemisphere foci, on average, perform worse on face recognition and dot location tasks than counterparts with left hemisphere foci (Kibby et al., 2014). Similarly, frontal foci do in fact predict executive dysfunction, and temporal foci predict auditory and memory problems (Lin; Mula, & Hermann, 2012). Thus, part of epilepsy's educational impact seems to depend on the location of the seizure focus, but these associations are generalizations only and exceptions abound.

Epilepsy, perhaps uniquely among neurological conditions, sometimes confers school-relevant direct neurocognitive effects that are transitory in nature. Consider that the acute electrical disturbance that defines a seizure sometimes stops (i.e., the overt seizure is over) while the brain has not yet returned to normal (i.e., nonseizure) status. (Because a seizure is referred to as an ictus, the term *postictal* is used to describe the period of time after a seizure.) There are sometimes postictal neurocognitive effects that are hard to characterize. Also, postictal effects vary; some CWE readily resume learning without delay, whereas others confront seconds or minutes of mental slowing, foggy attention, and suboptimal memory. Moreover, postitcal effects differ from student to student depending on the severity of the seizure, the extent of brain involvement, seizure duration, and seizure frequency (which can range from one a year to many per hour).

Indirect neurocognitive effects represent important educational challenges for some CWE. This is particularly true for children prescribed AEDs. Many of the skills involved in generic learning disabilities (e.g., processing speed, sustained memory, new learning) are also sometimes affected by AEDs (Bromley, Leeman, Baker, & Meador, 2011). Even broad indicators of cognition, such as IQ, seem affected, as a multicenter study from Europe showed. When a group of CWE underwent surgery (to reduce seizure frequency and thus to reduce or stop AED use), on average, modest postoperative IQ improvement was detected and 23% improved by 10 or more IQ points (Boshuisen et al., 2015). Most psychologists would agree that a 10-point IQ boost facilitates classroom learning. Furthermore, as a rule of thumb, addition of a second or third AED boosts neurocognitive risk. This is meaningful because studies find rates of polytherapy (more than one AED) exceed 25% both in community settings (Reilly et al., 2015) and in specialized centers (Wodrich et al., 2006).

Somatic effects (e.g., nausea, malaise), especially common in some illnesses, can also appear as medication side effects among CWE. When present, these effects can contribute to poor focus in class or to missed instruction.

Psychiatric conditions are among the best-documented comorbidities of childhood epilepsy, affecting 37% in one study (Davies, Heyman, & Goodman, 2003) and 30% to 40% in another (Lossius, Clench-Aas, van Roy, Mowinckel, & Gjerstad, 2006). Compared to healthy peers, CWE experience elevated rates of internalizing psychopathology (e.g., 4 times more depression than in unaffected children; 5.7 times more anxiety) as well as externalizing psychopathology (e.g., 5.3 times more conduct disorder; Russ, Larson, & Halfon, 2012). Attention deficit hyperactivity disorder (ADHD) may be diagnosable in nearly one fourth of CWE (Cohen et al., 2013; Russ et al., 2012). Seemingly related, executive dysfunction is common in CWE and appears to contribute to the expression of psychopathology (as broadly defined; Alfstad et al., 2016).

Although common, psychiatric disorders among CWE are without a fully understood cause. One possibility is that all CWE have some dysfunction in the brain, but for some, only seizures appear; for others, the dysfunction causes both seizures and emotional and behavioral symptoms. The excitatory and inhibitory neurotransmitter systems responsible for modulating the brain's electrical activity are disordered in CWE (this is why they seize) and the very same under-lying neurotransmitter disorder may predispose CWE to psychiatric conditions. Alternatively, the profound social and educational consequences of living with epilepsy may constitute the primary cause (or contributor) to psychiatric morbidity. And, of course, it is likely that both CNS and environmental factors interact and contribute jointly to the overt emotional and behavioral problems sometimes seen in CWE. No matter their etiology, psychiatric conditions pose challenges to learning and school adjustment.

Worry about upcoming treatment, common to some pediatric illness, is rarely consequential for CWE, although the topic seems to lack empirical research. In general, clinic checkups are not especially stressful, and complicated medical procedures or hospital stays are not typical. Possibly more problematic is pessimism about the future, as might occur, for example, when a high school student confronts recurrent breakthrough seizures despite careful management of AEDs. Understandably, the student may come to doubt her prospects for post-high-school education, vocational success, or independent living. Pessimism, often disproportionate to clinical realities, is not restricted to teens. Qualitative studies suggest that even young CWE feel apprehension about transitioning to independent living (Moffat, Dorris, Connor, & Espie, 2009), although the topic remains understudied.

Academic frustration is another challenge facing CWE. As already mentioned, direct and indirect neurocognitive effects are abundant and are likely to provoke academic problems. Like their classmates without epilepsy, CWE are prone to act out or give up when dealing with general cognitive limitations, slowed processing speed, or memory deficits. Additionally, these problems are sometimes exacerbated by classmates' reactions. Witnessing a seizure can prove frightening and confusing to classmates. For CWE with conspicuous seizures (e.g., generalized tonic-clonic seizures) social problems are likely to arise. Accordingly, CWE sometimes avoid school as a strategy to sidestep the embarrassment of having a dreaded seizure occur at school. Anxious classmates, especially if they have witnessed a seizure first-hand, represent an obvious potential social burden for CWE. Teasing and bullying are a possibility, as is less malicious, but still potentially ruinous, social shunning. Paradoxically, classmates sometimes respond with approach (rather than avoidance), which might take the form of overly protective classmates' treating the child with epilepsy as "the class pet" rather than a peer. Although generally it is beneficial, compassionate support can be so overdone that it inadvertently distorts important classmate-to-classmate relations.

A final challenge for CWE is encounters with either uninformed or unsure teachers. Research findings that cut across different settings and teachers' backgrounds (e.g., elementary vs. high school, regular education vs. special education, currently teaching a child with epilepsy vs. not now doing so) confirms a dearth of epilepsy knowledge among teachers (Wodrich et al., 2011). Even among those currently teaching a child with epilepsy, some knowledge gaps are striking (fewer than 7% knew that CWE have an elevated risk of depressive feelings; fewer than 15% knew about the risk of attention problems). The same teachers expressed considerable uncertainty about successfully managing the educational and social needs of CWE, with concern about recognizing classroom instructional barriers and spotting AED side effects in class topping the list of things engendering their lack of confidence.

CANCERS AFFECTING THE CNS

Basic facts about pediatric cancer, including epidemiology and treatment, are covered elsewhere (see Chapter 21 of this book). This chapter addresses brain tumors and leukemia (two conditions often affecting the CNS), within the framework of the Model.

Pediatric brain tumors are a heterogeneous group of both benign and malignant neoplasms. Direct neurocognitive effects depend on tumor location within the brain, tumor type, degree of malignancy, and age of the patient. Some of the presenting symptoms (which may remain permanent) include: headaches, vomiting, problems with balance and coordination, lethargy, seizures, decreased vision, precocious puberty, and poor academic performance. The indirect neurocognitive effects (late effects) are usually treatment-related. Therapy is dictated by tumor type, tumor location, presence of metastasis, and especially the age of the patient. Therapy may include biopsy, surgical resection, radiation, chemotherapy, hematologic stem cell transplantation, or individualized combinations of treatments. Radiation is frequently required to cure many types of brain tumor and it can prove the most devastating to the child's neurocognitive development. Young children's brains are still growing and myelinating, heightening their sensitivity to radiation effects. The late effects of radiation can progress for up to 5 years after the treatment and they tend to be permanent. The most important considerations are the area of the brain radiated, the volume of radiation, the dose of radiation, and the age of the patient.

Leukemias are cancers of white blood cells and are named for the type of white blood cell that becomes malignant. Leukemias originate in bone marrow cells and interfere with the production of normal white blood cells, red blood cells, and platelets. They then travel throughout the body in the blood, sometimes invading the CNS. Acute lymphoblastic leukemia (ALL), the most common leukemia, rarely has direct neurocognitive effects. Treatment consists of aggressive combinations of oral, intravenous, and intrathecal (medicine introduced into the cerebrospinal fluid and CNS via a spinal tap) agents. A minority of cases require cranial radiation and hematopoietic stem cell transplantation (which involves the administration of very high doses of chemotherapy that destroy bone marrow cells followed by the infusion of healthy blood stem cells to repopulate the marrow). The indirect neurocognitive effects are usually treatment-related, especially with cranial radiation and intrathecal chemotherapy. Like children with brain tumors (CWBT), children with leukemia (CWL) experience dose- and age-related late effects of cranial radiation.

Cancer and Its Educational Challenges

As suggested above, sometimes a brain tumor causes direct neurocognitive effects (effects attributable to the illness itself) as it grows. On the other hand, leukemia seldom presents with neurocognitive effects at the time of diagnosis.

The treatment-associated indirect neurocognitive effects (late effects), however, can prove most important regarding schooling. First, for CWBT, even full-scale IQ is a consideration. For example, de Ruiter, van Mourik, Schouten-van Meeteren, Grootenhuis, and Oosterlaan (2013) conducted a meta-analysis summarizing 21 studies that used Wechsler IQ tests. They found a nearly 12-point full-scale IQ decrement among CWBT (age range 6–16 years and at least 2 years after treatment). Several factors predicted lower IQ—treatment with radiation, chemotherapy, and a longer time since diagnosis and treatment (which meant the children were younger when treated and sufficient time had passed so that late effects had become fully manifest). Other studies echo the findings of IQ decrements over time; children younger at time of treatment demonstrate the greatest neurocognitive effects (Merchant, Conklin, Wu, Lustig, & Xiong, 2009). Perhaps equally important, skills like working memory, processing speed, executive function (de Ruiter et al., 2017), and attention (but not impulse control) also are compromised (de Ruiter et al., 2013).

Late effects are often less problematic among CWL. For one thing, only about 20% of CWL now require cranial radiation, and, as fewer pediatric patients receive cranial radiation, researchers document reduced rates of neurocognitive problems (Richards, Pui, & Gayon, 2013). CWL who need only intravenously delivered chemotherapy fare better, but they may not escape late effects completely. For example, one recent study found vulnerability to verbal working memory decline among children receiving no cranial radiation, and the younger the child at treatment, the more marked, on average, the decline (Insel et al., 2017). All age groups, however, had declines in verbal working memory. Critically, verbal working memory changes were associated with posttreatment reading and calculation skills. Furthermore, spatial memory declines were less common, but, when present, they were associated with posttreatment math skills. In another study (Jacola et al., 2016), among chemotherapy-only CWL (teenagers), academic problems were a risk (i.e., they were evident at twice the rate found among healthy siblings). Although CWL experienced only a modestly elevated risk of inattention-hyperactivity problems, the risk grew with increased doses of medication (methotrexate). It is easy to envision how this host of neurocognitive effects threatens school success, but strengths and supports can help mitigate their pernicious effects.

Unlike CWE, CWBT and CWL are at risk of troubling somatic effects. These effects are classically related to treatment and can include nausea, vomiting, pain, weakness, fatigue, severe mouth sores, bleeding, infections, hospitalization for fever when the white blood cell count is low, and recovery from anesthesia for bone marrow and lumbar puncture procedures. Somatic effects represent an educational challenge when they prevent a student from deploying all of his or her attention and effort toward schoolwork or when they prevent a student from coming to school at all. That is, classroom productivity and attendance problems may result from somatic effects unless these effects are buffered.

Psychiatric conditions, not surprisingly, are common among CWBT and CWL. For example, a recent review found that approximately 57% of CWBT experienced at least one diagnosable psychiatric condition (Zyrianova, Alexander, & Faruqui, 2016), with internalizing diagnoses predominating. Similarly, Pastore and colleagues (2013) confirmed internalizing problems (e.g., anxiety, depression) among 77.8% of a preschool group with various brain lesions. By the same token, adolescents with brain tumors commonly had internalizing problems and at a rate surpassing the rate for externalizing conditions (48.4% to 11.8%; Poggi et al., 2005). Other studies, however, suggest lower rates of problems (Shah et al., 2015). Methodological differences from study to study (e.g., precise diagnoses investigated, manner of treatment, measurement of outcomes, etc.) likely drive the differences in findings.

CWL also are at risk, as exemplified when a radiation-free group was studied 1 month after treatment and was found to still encounter elevated anxiety and depression rates (approximately 25%; Kunin-Batson et al., 2016). Equally important, immediate posttreatment indicators of anxiety and depression predicted a quadrupled risk of anxiety or depression persisting long after treatment ceased.

Because CWBT and CWL confront intensive and protracted treatment, both groups worry about upcoming treatments and may experience pessimism. Specifically, cancer treatment may involve repeated infusion of nausea-inducing medications, irradiation delivered under unnerving circumstances (e.g., in a confined space with restricted ability to move), or even surgery. Additionally, the life-threatening element of pediatric cancer can cause patients and families to worry about the future. If neurocognitive late effects appear, of course, there is even more to worry the student. These challenges can sap a student's motivation and diminish all stakeholders' (teachers, parents, students) expectations for school success.

Academic frustration is the logical consequence of the many challenges cited in this section (see Table 16.1). In general the challenges are greater for CWBT than for CWL, probably in part because of neurocognitive effects, although documentation of this supposition awaits empirical research. Furthermore, discrepancies between expectations and performance, rather than performance alone, cause frustration. It is understandable that a student who appears different physically, or who may die, causes anxiety among classmates. Perhaps this is why CWBT are found to be more socially isolated and to receive fewer friendship nominations than healthy classmates (Vannatta, Gartstein, Short, & Noll, 1998). Like CWE, CWBT and CWL may also encounter overly protective classmates and the prospect of being treated as class pets.

It is easy to see that if teachers are unsure, anxious, or uninformed about epilepsy, which is relatively common and sometimes educationally inconsequential, then cancer will provoke even greater challenges for educators. Although only a few teachers may have previously taught a student with cancer, most teachers have at least one acquaintance who has died from cancer, usually an adult who had a poor prognosis. Thus, it is understandable when teachers are anxious about teaching a student with cancer. One study found that just 17.5% of teachers said they were very well informed about cancer and only 35.5% claimed a reasonably high level of confidence that they could meet the social needs of a student with cancer (Nabors, Little, Akin-Little, & Iobst, 2008). In reality, however, most students with cancer become long-term survivors, cured of their cancer. Thus, teachers' prospective anxiety and lack of knowledge represent clear challenges that must be addressed to maximize school success for CWBT and CWL.

PLANNING AND INTERVENING VIA STRENGTHS AND SUPPORTS

It is clear that many students with medical and neurological conditions encounter school problems. How might these be prevented? How might those whose problems are already evident be helped? According to the Model, the logical way is to capitalize on students' strengths and to offer them targeted supports (see Table 16.1). In other words, working systematically via strengths and supports is advised. For this to be effective, however, each student's challenges and his or her strengths are typically assessed. In other words, school-based professionals (e.g., school psychologists, school nurses, special educators) working in concert with clinic-based professionals, formulate referral questions using the bullet-pointed items from Table 16.1 and then proceed with data collection. This typically includes record review, interview of stakeholders, classroom observations, and psychometric testing, if needed. The resulting information is then a springboard to understanding each student's status regarding challenges and strengths and supports, which permits development of individualized modifications and interventions.

Students who possess cognitive reserves and premorbid intellectual strengths on average fare better than their less-able counterparts. This is especially relevant for CWBT and CWL facing chemotherapy or radiation regimens likely to cause long-term cognitive decline (i.e., late effects). Two students, one with a full-scale IQ of 120 and the other with a full-scale IQ of 80, face divergent long-term prospects when treatment with radiation and intrathecal medication is considered. Contemplation of pretreatment cognitive differences, however, may miss the point that cognitive resources can sometimes be enhanced. For example, Conklin and colleagues (2015) reported that a computer-based intervention boosted working memory, processing speed, and executive function for CWBT and CWL (at least 1 year posttreatment when enrolled) compared to children in a control group. The same study found pre–post functional MRI changes paralleling the treatment-induced cognitive improvements, prompting speculation that neural plasticity was greater than previously assumed. More research is clearly needed regarding how much cognitive training programs benefit bottom-line school success. At present, cognitive interventions seem to be tied to clinics and rehabilitation centers. It is understandable that school districts are unlikely to apply an intervention that fits the needs of just a few students, that has technical and specialized application, and that still lacks compelling documentation of its potential effectiveness.

Like cognitive reserves, emotional resilience is arguably an antidote to a host of the challenges cited above. Resilience is sometimes conceptualized as a part of temperament, suggesting that it is constitutional and relatively fixed. But emotional resilience, such as making proper attributions and avoiding overfocus on negative possibilities, is malleable. Thus, behavioral cognitive interventions might be used with some students with cancer (Williams, Davis, Hancock, & Phipps, 2010). Working with a psychologist in a clinic or at a school site, a CWBT or a CWL might develop skills to help identify faulty cognitions or to block recurring negative thoughts. The same is true for youngsters with assorted neurological conditions, although the cognitive-based programs' elements would likely need to vary from youngster to youngster (reflecting different attributes and coping styles) and from diagnosis to diagnosis (reflecting common themes of, for instance, living with epilepsy or cancer).

Children with all neurological conditions, especially CWE, CWBT, and CWL, must have access to effective health care. It is axiomatic that a well-controlled illness (a byproduct of effective health care) represents a strength that minimizes school problems. Consider seizure control. The number of seizures per month is strongly associated with good attendance ($r = .83$), as well as high-stakes test scores in math ($r = .57$), writing ($r = .47$), and reading ($r = .44$; Bohac & Wodrich, 2012).

In general, stakeholders should advocate for care in specialized settings. Although a pediatrician or family doctor can manage AEDs, they are unlikely to know the clinical subtleties of their use, especially pertaining to side effects that may arise at school. As well, CWL can be treated by a solo-practice oncologist but he or she almost certainly would lack the systematic support regarding nutrition, family support, or school liaison found at most specialized children's hospitals. This is presumably why the American Cancer Society advocates treatment at children's cancer centers staffed by multidisciplinary teams. Treatment in such centers allows teams to distribute responsibility, including the important family and educational elements that typically accompany treatment. In truth, the complexity of the diseases, the explosion of new information, and access to the latest treatments means that the days of solo or small private practice pediatric hematologist/oncologists, outside of a pediatric medical center, are essentially gone. Fortunately, almost all patients nationwide are now treated with at least some elements of clinic-based psychosocial support.

Although effective home–school–clinic communication is generally improved with specialized care, maximizing this important support is not always simple for CWE or CWBT and CWL when emotional, interpersonal, and neurocognitive challenges are involved. A way to support students is via a school reintegration plan after hospitalization. One program that has been studied is called the Back on Track Program, which has elements aiming to "foster collaboration between the families of children and young people with cancer, their schools, and the hospital and health networks supporting them" (St. Leger & Campbell, 2007, p. 119). But research suggests that even highly structured programs supported by sophisticated elements (e.g., virtual classroom, templates for communication) remain difficult to implement when a student has complex cancer-associated needs. One possible solution is to give liaison responsibilities to school professionals free of teaching duties (e.g., school nurse, school psychologist, school counselor, school social worker). School psychologists, for example, are trained in consultation skills that might be used for CWBT (Schmitt, 2011). The psychologists know how to identify problems, seek acceptable solutions, and monitor whether the solutions actually alleviate the problem. A method for school psychologists to execute this role has been previously described (Wodrich, in press; Wodrich & Cunningham, 2008). Research is needed, however, to confirm stakeholders' acceptance of, as well as the bottom-line effectiveness of, liaison/consultative services for children with neurological conditions.

Case Example

Briana's case illustrates the advantages of effective home–school–clinic collaboration. Briana, a teenager with focal epilepsy, had been treated with a single AED. In the fall semester, however, she began to struggle emotionally and academically, and she experienced three seizures at school. Consequently, her epileptologist (neurologist specializing in epilepsy) added a second AED, which curtailed nearly all seizures. As the second AED was adjusted upward, however, subtle cognitive side effects emerged (e.g., Briana told the school nurse about problems with notetaking and difficulty listening closely in two morning classes). Following a special services referral, Briana underwent psychometric testing and several classroom observations before she was considered for either a special education designation in the category of other health impairment (OHI) or an accommodation plan based on Section 504 of the Americans with Disabilities Act. In lieu of a formal IEP (individualized education plan, which would be OHI-related) or a formal accommodation plan (504-related), a simpler solution was formulated in discussion among Briana's parent, her physician, and the school psychologist. It was agreed that subsequent AED changes would prompt repeated classroom observations by the school psychologist (and tabulation of updated teacher checklists) as a way to monitor potential side effects. Because testing detected no meaningful cognitive difficulty, information processing problems, or academic deficits, it was agreed that, if an IEP or 504 plan was needed, it would include Briana's receiving class notes directly from her teachers (precluding in-class notetaking), a schedule change to move her away from lecture-style classes (reducing listening demands), and the option to take examinations during afternoons (the time of maximum alertness). Another fact turned up during the meeting—several teachers were never informed that Briana had seizures, what they might look like, or that she could be experiencing AED side effects. Briana consented to have information shared with each of her teachers. This practice is consistent with research that shows that withholding an epilepsy diagnosis from classroom teachers causes them to mistake epilepsy-related classroom behaviors for other problems (e.g., laziness, lack of parental support, ADHD; Wodrich, 2005). In addition to a meeting with Briana and the school nurse to share her diagnosis and to answer questions about epilepsy at school, each teacher was provided a link to a teacher-friendly website about epilepsy, www.edmedkids.arizona.edu.

Instructional supports at school start with an informed teacher. It is hard for teachers to support a student about whom critical facts are lacking. Research seems to concur. Bohac and Wodrich (2012) found that teachers' attitudes toward persons with epilepsy, as measured by a psychometric tool, predicted students' academic performance (high-stake test scores) better than some medical variables (e.g., seizure frequency). Thus, pediatric psychologists specializing in epilepsy often call for psychoeducation (providing stakeholders with facts and supports) as a cornerstone intervention (Guildfoyle et al., 2017). As shown in the case of Briana, an IEP or Section 504 plan may be needed. Besides specifying direct academic instruction (e.g., in reading or math), an IEP or 504 plan often details instructional modifications of the type familiar to teachers. For example, regarding those with language deficits, Titus and Thio (2009) proposed extended time for verbal responses, limiting oral examinations and presentations, and tweaking verbal material and instructions. The authors also described ways to minimize the consequences of memory problems by assisting students with information capture, as memory encoding is often more of a problem than memory consolidation and retrieval. Attention and executive problems that are often associated with underlying neural dysfunction or appear with the use of AEDs may require redirection, cuing, one-on-one instruction, decomposing assignments into smaller steps, or alternative examination formats. Parallel instructional supports may help to mitigate against academic frustration for CWBT or CWL when general cognitive or selective memory problems are present.

Instructional support extending to home is ideal. For example, a parent willing to practice subtraction with his second-grader after school (during a seizure-free interval that is also free of postictal effects) can be invaluable. This is true even when the student's day is spent with a knowledgeable, confident teacher executing a well-crafted IEP. Likewise, an older sister who tutors a sister with a brain tumor at home where she might feel especially safe (e.g., with no risk of classmates' teasing) can make the difference between academic success and failure. Of course, support at home is a strength that is able to reduce (or occasionally to eliminate) a host of challenges, not just academic frustration. More broadly, family members who convey a strong ethic for school engagement and classroom success transmit these values to the children. Similarly, a home environment that communicates an intention to collaborate with school goes a long way toward supporting a student with any neurological condition. Early, repeated, respectful, and two-way communication with parents is recommended to shore up supports and strengths that many students with neurological conditions need if they are to continue with regular school attendance and uninterrupted academic progress.

Social supports at school are documented elements in successful return to school by students with cancer (McLoone, Wakefield, Bulow, Fleming, & Cohn, 2011). To minimize the risk of social problems of CWBT and to capitalize on supports, Devine et al. (2016) outlined a 5- to 8-session program delivered at school by peer leaders. Group meetings (which include but do not identify CWBT) emphasize skills like tolerating differences, including others in games and social situations, initiating and responding during child-to-child interactions, methods for sustaining engagement, and conflict resolution. Although still under development, this intervention is shown to increase nominations for friendship among CWBT, as well as to reduce classwide levels of victimization and rejection. It is logical that problems arising from anxious or overly protective classmates of CWE might be reduced by similar programs. Programs like this seem especially germane because research (Hamiwka et al., 2009) found that 42% of CWE had been victims of bullying, double the rate for both healthy controls and students with a non-neurological chronic illness (e.g., chronic kidney disease). Smaller-scale qualitative studies also confirm that CWBT experience bullying (Vance, Eiser, & Horne, 2004). Thus, social skill development programs that teach concrete ways to act appropriately, especially toward CWE, CWBT, and CWL, may be an important support.

Taking steps to improve social supports at home also seems to matter. For example, among CWE, higher levels of family cohesion are associated with lower levels of stigma plus better quality of life for the child (Mendes, Crespo, & Austin, 2017). This makes sense. Families who work together and make judgments about how to allocate resources and when to deploy supports to meet various members' needs are also likely to do the same when the child with epilepsy confronts challenges. Research that includes mothers and fathers of pediatric cancer patients also confirms parents' vulnerability and, in turn, the contribution of their ill child's adjustment status to their adjustment (Robinson, Gerhardt, Vannatta, & Noll, 2007). Although parents' adjustment and its relationship to child adjustment is complex, the findings nonetheless suggest that assessment, or at least informal judgments, about how parents are dealing with their ill child may need to be considered. Seeking support for parents, so they can in turn support their child, may be necessary.

CONCLUSION

Students with neurological and medical conditions affecting the CNS, exemplified here by CWE, CWBT, and CWL, confront an array of educational challenges. The challenges are often most conspicuously neurocognitive, but they can extend to less obvious challenges, such as classmates' reactions as well as teachers' knowledge and confidence. Helping these students is possible by working logically to consider the list of potential challenges facing students, to assess each challenge, and then to formulat interventions that capitalize on strengths and supports. When all stakeholders—parents, teachers, medical professionals, and the student—work together, the prospect for attaining a school experience filled with success is maximized.

RESOURCES

- American Cancer Society—Children Diagnosed with Cancer: Returning to School: https://www.cancer.org/treatment/children-and-cancer/when-your-child-has-cancer/returning-to-school.html
- Children's Oncology Group: www.curesearch.org (an excellent site for nonphysicians)
- EdMedKids: www.edmedkids.arizona.edu (facts and supporting documents for teachers of students with epilepsy or cancer)
- Epilepsy Foundation: http://www.epilepsy.com/ (general link with many important facts)
- Epilepsy Foundation—What Can Parents Do to Prepare for School? http://www.epilepsy.com/article/2014/8/what-can-parents-do-prepare-school

REFERENCES

Alfstad, K. A., Torgersen, H., van Roy, B., Hessen, E., Hansen, B. H., Henning, O., . . . Lossius, M. I. (2016). Psychiatric comorbidity in children and youth with epilepsy: An association with executive dysfunction? *Epilepsy & Behavior, 56*, 88–94. doi:10.1016/j.yebeh.2016.01.007

Austin, J. K., & Caplan, R. (2007). Behavioral and psychiatric comorbities in pediatric epilepsy: Toward and integrative model. *Epilepsia, 48*, 1639–1651. doi:10.1111/j.1528-1167.2007.01154.x

Berg, A. T., Langfitt, J. T., Testa, F. M., Levy, S. R., DiMario, F., Westervelt, M., & Kulas, J. (2008). Global cognitive function in children with epilepsy: A community-based study. *Epilepsia, 49*, 608–614. doi:10.1016/j.yebeh.200807.007

Bohac, G., & Wodrich, D. L. (2012). A model-based approach to understanding school status of students with epilepsy. *Epilepsy & Behavior, 27*, 4–8. doi:10.1016/yebeh.2012.12.012

Boshuisen, K., Schooneveld, M. M. J., Uiterwaal, C. S. P. M., Cross, J. H., Harrison, S., Polster, T., . . . Braun, K. P. J. (2015). Intelligence quotient improves after anti-epileptic drug withdrawal following pediatric epilepsy surgery. *Annals of Neurology, 78*, 104–114. doi:10.1002/ana.24427

Bromley, R. L., Leeman, B. A., Baker, G. A., & Meador, K. J. (2011). Cognitive and neurodevelopmental effects of antiepileptic drugs, *Epilepsy & Behavior, 22*, 9–16. doi:10.1016/j.yebeh.2011.04.009

Cohen, R., Senecky, Y., Shuper, A., Inbar, D., Chodick, G., Shalev, V., & Raz, R. (2013). Prevalence of epilepsy and attention-deficit hyperactivity (ADHD) disorder: A population-based study. *Journal of Child Neurology, 28,* 120–123. doi:10.1177/0883073812440327.

Conklin, H. M., Ogg, R. J., Ashford, J. M., Scoggins, M. A., Zou, P., Clark, K. N. . . . Zhang, H. (2015). Computerized cognitive training for amelioration of cognitive late effects among childhood cancer survivors: A randomized controlled trial. *Journal of Clinical Oncology, 33,* 3894–3902. doi:10.1200/JCO:201561.6672

Davies, S., Heyman, I., & Goodman, R. (2003). A population survey of mental health problems in children with epilepsy. *Developmental Medicine and Child Neurology, 45,* 292–295.

de Ruiter, M. A., Grootenhuis, M. A., van Mourik, R., Maurice-Stam, H., Breteler, M. H. M., Gidding, C., & Oosterlaan, J. (2017). Time to performance weaknesses on computerized tasks in pediatric brain tumor survivors: A comparison with sibling controls. *Child Neuropsychology, 23,* 208–227. doi:10.1080/09297049.2015.1108395

de Ruiter, M. A., van Mourik, R., Schouten-van Meeteren, A. Y. N., Grootenhuis, M. A., & Oosterlaan, J. (2013). Neurocognitive consequences of a pediatric brain tumor and its treatment: A meta-analysis. *Developmental Medicine and Child Neurology, 55,* 408–417. doi:10.1111/dmcn.1020

Devine, K. A., Bukowski, W. M., Sahler, O. J. Z., Ohman-Strickland, P. Smith, T. H., Lown, E. A., . . . Noll, R. B. (2016). Social competence in childhood brain tumor survivors: Feasibility and preliminary outcomes of a peer-mediated intervention. *Journal of Developmental and Behavioral Pediatrics, 37,* 475–482. doi:10.1097/DBP00000000000000315

Fastenau, P. S., Shen, J., Dunn, D. W., & Austin, J. K. (2008). Academic underachievement among children with epilepsy. *Journal of Learning Disabilities, 41,* 195–207. doi:10117/002219408317548

Guildfoyle, S. M., Wagner, J. I., Modi, A. C., Junger, K. F., Barrett, L. E., Risen, A. C., . . . Weyand, C. (2017). Pediatric epilepsy and behavioral health: The state of the literature and directions for evidence-based interprofessional care, training, and research. *Clinical Practice in Pediatric Psychology, 5,* 79–90. doi:10.1037/cpp0000169.

Hamiwka, L. D., Yu, C. G., Hamiwka, L. A., Sherman, E. M. S, Anderson, B., & Wirrell, E. (2009). Are children with epilepsy a greater risk for bullying than their peers? *Epilepsy & Behavior 15,* 500–505. doi:10.1016/j.yebeh.2009.06.015

Hermann, B. P., Zhao, Q., Jackson, D. C., Jones, J. E., Dabbs, K., Almane, D., . . . Rathouz, P. J. (2016). Cognitive phenotypes in childhood idiopathic epilepsies. *Epilepsy & Behavior, 61,* 269–274 doi.org/10.1016/j.yebeh.2016.05.013

Insel, K. C., Hockenberry, M. J., Harris, L. L., Koerner, K. M., Lu, Z., Adkins, K. B., . . . Moore, I. M. (2017). Declines noted in cognitive processes and associated achievement among children with leukemia. *Oncology Nursing Forum, 44,* 503–511. doi:10.1188/17.ONF.503-511

Jacola, L. M., Edelstein, K., Lui, W., Pui, C. H., Hayashi, R., Kadan-Lottick, N. S., . . . Krull, K. R. (2016). Cognitive, behavior, and academic functioning in adolescent and young adult surviviors of childhood acute lymphoblastic leukaemia: A report from the Childhood Cancer Survivor Study. *Lancet Psychiatry, 3,* 965–972. doi:10.1016/S2215-0366

Khan, R. B., Hudson, M. M., Ledet, D. S., Morris, E. B., Pui, C., Howard, S. C., . . . Ness, K. K. (2014). Neurologic morbidity and quality of life in survivors of childhood acute lymphoblastic leukemia: A prospective cross-sectional study. *Journal of Cancer Survival, 8,* 688–696. doi:10.1007/s11764-014-0375-1

Kibby, M. Y., Cohen, M. J., Lee, S. E., Stanford, L., Park, Y. D., & Strickland, S. M. (2014). There are laterality effects in memory functioning in children/adolescents with focal epilepsy. *Developmental Neuropsychology, 39,* 569–584. doi:10.1080/87565641.2014.962695.

Kunin-Batson, A. S., Lu, X., Balsamo, L. Graber, K., Devidas, M., Hunger, S. P., ... Kadan-Lottick, N. S. (2016). Prevalence and predictors of anxiety and depression after completion of chemotherapy for childhood acute lymphoblastic leukemia: A prospective longitudinal study. *Cancer, 122,* 1608–1717.

Lin, J. J., Mula, M., & Hermann, B. P. (2012). Uncovering the neurobehavioural comorbidities of epilepsy over the lifespan. *Lancet, 380,* 1180–1192. doi:10.1016/SO140-6736(12)61455-X

Lossius, M. I., Clench-Aas, J., van Roy, B., Mowinckel, P., & Gjerstad, L. (2006). Psychiatric symptoms in adolescents with epilepsy in junior high school in Norway: A population survey. *Epilepsy and Behavior, 9,* 286–292. doi:10.1016/j.yebeh.2006.06.018.

McLoone, J. K., Wakefield, C. E., Bulow, P., Fleming, C., & Cohn, R. J. (2011). Returning to school after adolescent cancer: A qualitative examination of Australian survivors' and their families' perspectives. *Journal of Adolescent and Young Adult Oncology, 1,* 87–94. doi:10.1089/jayao.2011.0006

Mendes, T. P, Crespo, C. A., & Austin, J. K. (2017). Family cohesion, stigma, and quality of life in dyads of children with epilepsy and their parents. *Journal of Pediatric Psychology, 46,* 689–699. doi:10.1093/jpepsy/jsw105

Merchant, T. E., Conklin, H. M., Wu, S. J., Listig, R. H., & Xiong, X. (2009). Late effects of conformal radiation therapy for pediatric patients with low-grade glioma: Prospective evaluation of cognitive, endocrine, and hearing deficits. *Journal of Clinical Oncology, 27,* 3691–3697. doi:10.1200/JCO.2008.21.2738

Moffat, C., Dorris, L., Connor, L., & Espie, C. A. (2009). The impact of childhood epilepsy on quality of life: A qualitative investigation using focus group methods to obtain children's perspectives on living with epilepsy. *Epilepsy & Behavior, 14,* 179–189. doi:10.1016/jbeh.2008.09.025.

Nabors, L. A., Little, S. G., Akin-Little, A., & Iobst, E. A. (2008). Teacher knowledge and confidence in meeting the needs of children with chronic medical conditions: Pediatric psychology's contribution to education. *Psychology in the Schools, 45,* 217–226. doi:10.1002/pits. 20292.

Pastore, V., Colombo, K., Villa, F., Galbiati, S., Adduci, A., Poggi, G., ... Strazzer, S. (2013). Psychological and adjustment problems due to acquired brain lesions in preschool-aged patients. *Brain Injury, 27,* 677–684. doi:10.3109/02699052.2013.775482

Poggi, G., Liscio, M., Adduci, A., Galbianti, S., Massimino, M., Sommovigo, M., ... Castelli, E. (2005). Psychological and adjustment problems due to acquired lesions in childhood: A comparison of post-traumatic patients and brain tumour survivors. *Brain Injury, 19,* 777–785. doi:10.1080/0269905500110132

Rantanen, K., Nieminen, P., & Eriksson, K. (2010). Neurocognitive functioning of preschool children with uncomplicated epilepsy. *Journal of Neuropsychology, 4,* 71–87. doi:10.1348/174866409X451465

Reilly, C., Atkinson, P., Chin, R. F., Das, K. B., Gillberg, C., Aylett, S. E., ... Neville, B. G. R. (2015). Symptoms of anxiety and depression in school-aged children with active epilepsy: A population-based study. *Epilepsy & Behavior*, *52*, 174–179. doi:10.1016/ j.yebeh2015.09.004.

Richards, S., Pui, C. H., & Gayon, P. (2013). Systematic review and meta-analysis of randomized trials of central nervous system directed therapy for childhood acute lymphoblastic leukemia. *Pediatric Blood and Cancer*, *60*, 185–195. doi:10.1002/pbc.24228

Robinson, K. E., Gerhardt, C. A., Vannatta, K., & Noll, R. B. (2007). Parent and family factors associated with child adjustment to pediatric cancer. *Journal of Pediatric Psychology*, *32*, 400–410. doi:10.1037/t01210-000

Russ, S. A., Larson, K., & Halfon, N. (2012). A national profile of childhood epilepsy and seizure disorders. *Pediatrics*, *129*, 256–264. doi:10.1542/peds.2010-1371

Sarhan, E. M., Walker, M. C., & Selai, C. (2015). Evidence for efficacy combination antiepileptic drugs in treatment of epilepsy. *Journal of Neurological Research*, *5*, 267–276. doi:10.14740/jnr356w

Schmitt, A. (2011). A commentary on childhood leukemia survivors and their return to school: A literature review, case study, and recommendations. *Journal of Applied School Psychology*, *27*, 276–283. doi:10.1080/15377903.2011.590771.

Shah, S. S., Dellarole, A., Peterson, E. C., Bregy, A., Komotar, R., Harvey, P. D., & Elhammady, M. S. (2015). Long-term psychiatric outcomes in pediatric brain tumor survivors. *Child's Nervous System*, *31*, 653–663. doi:10.1007/s00381-015-2669-7

St. Leger, P., & Campbell, L. (2007). Evaluation of a school-linked program for children with cancer. *Health Education*, *108*, 117–129. doi: 10.1108/09654280810855577

Titus, J. B., & Thio, L. L. (2009). The effects of antiepileptic drugs on classroom performance. *Psychology in the Schools*, *49*, 885–891. doi:10.1002/pits.20428

Vance, Y. H., Eiser, C., & Horne, B. (2004). Parents' views of the impact of childhood brain tumours and treatment on young people's social and family functioning. *Clinical Child Psychology and Psychiatry*, *9*, 271–288. doi:10.1177/1359104504041923

Vannatta, K., Gartstein, M. A., Short, A., & Noll, R. B. (1998). A controlled study of peer relationships of children surviving brain tumors: Teacher, peer, and self-ratings. *Journal of Pediatric Psychology*, *23*, 279–287.

Williams, N. A., Davis, G., Hancock, M., & Phipps, S. (2010). Optimism and pessimism in children with cancer in healthy children: Confirmatory factor analysis on the Youth of Life Orientation Test and relations with health-related quality of life. *Journal of Pediatric Psychology*, *35*, 672–682. doi:10.1093/jpepsy/jsop84

Wodrich, D. L. (in press). Impairments related to medical conditions. In F. C. Worrell & T. L. Hughes (Eds.), *Cambridge handbook of applied school psychology*. Cambridge, UK: Cambridge University Press.

Wodrich, D. L. (2005). Disclosing information about epilepsy and type 1 diabetes mellitus: The effect on teachers' understanding of classroom behavior. *School Psychology Quarterly*, *20*, 288–303.

Wodrich, D. L. (2014). *A comprehensive model for understanding pediatric illnesses at school.* Poster presented at the annual meeting of the National Association of School Psychologists, Washington, DC.

Wodrich, D. L., & Cunningham, M. M. (2008). School-based tertiary and targeted interventions: The examples of epilepsy and type 1 diabetes mellitus. *Psychology in the Schools*, *45*, 52–62. doi:10.1002/pits.20278

Wodrich, D. L. Jarrar, R., Buchhalter, J., Levy, R., & Gay, C. (2011). Knowledge about epilepsy and confidence in instructing students with epilepsy: Teachers' responses to a new scale. *Epilepsy & Behavior, 20*, 360–365. doi:10.1015/j.yebeh.2010.12.002

Wodrich, D. L., Kaplan, A. M., & Deering, W. M. (2006). Children with epilepsy in school: Special service usage and assessment practices. *Psychology in the Schools, 43*, 169–181. doi:10.1022/pits.20123

Zyrianova, Y., Alexander, L., & Faruqui, R. (2016). Neuropsychiatric presentations and outcomes in children and adolescents with primary brain tumors: Systematic review. *Brain Injury, 30*, 1–9. doi:10.3109/02699052.2015.1075590.

17

Cardiovascular Disorders

Congenital Heart Disease and Pediatric Acquired Cardiovascular Disease

LYLA E. HAMPTON, ABIGAIL C. DEMIANCZYK, AND CASEY HOFFMAN ■

Congenital heart disease (CHD) is one of the most common birth defects in the United States, affecting 1% of births (i.e., 40,000 newborns) per year (Hoffman & Kaplan, 2002; Reller, Strickland, Riehle-Colarusso, Mahle, & Correa, 2005). Approximately one fourth of cases involve a severe form of CHD that requires medical intervention within the first year of life (Oster et al., 2013). Medical treatment and interventions have vastly improved within the past 50 years, and available surgical techniques (palliation, catheterization) and preoperative advances (e.g., genetic screening, fetal echocardiogram) have led to increased survival (Boneva et al., 2001). As a result, approximately 75% of babies with severe CHD survive to 1 year of age, and 69% survive to 18 years of age (Oster et al., 2013). Furthermore, 90% of individuals with CHD live to adulthood, and currently over 2.4 million Americans are living with a form of CHD (Cassidy et al., 2017). Despite improved survival, individuals with CHD remain at high risk for neurological, cognitive, and psychosocial challenges that affect quality of life across the lifespan (Marino et al., 2012).

HEART DEVELOPMENT

The heart is the first functional organ in the human body (Moorman, Webb, Brown, Lamers, & Anderson, 2003). A primitive heart tube is developed by approximately 21 days of life, and it begins to beat spontaneously by 4 weeks gestation (Moorman et al., 2003). By 8 weeks gestation, the heart has developed into four chambers separated by muscle lining (i.e., septum) to differentiate left and right sides and upper (atria) and lower (ventricles) chambers. Blood flows in one direction through valves in the septum between chambers, with deoxygenated blood entering the heart and leaving through the pulmonary (lung) system, where it is oxygenated and returned to the heart. The oxygenated blood then exits the heart through the circulatory (body) system to provide oxygen and nutrition to the developing organ systems. The rapid fetal brain growth that occurs in the third trimester, including increased size, organization, and brain metabolism, demands increased oxygen and nutrients provided by the heart (Glanzman, Licht, & Wernovsky, 2011). Malformations at the anatomic (valves, chamber size) or hemodynamic level can affect both the rate and quality (e.g., level of oxygenation) of blood flow (Chessa & Plucchinotta, 2015) to the brain as well as other organ systems.

CHD can occur throughout gestational development, both spontaneously and as a result of genetic or environmental influences (Brosig, Sood, & Butcher, 2017). Common genetic diagnoses that are associated with CHD include Down syndrome, 22q.11.2 deletion syndrome (i.e., DiGeorge syndrome), Williams syndrome, and Turner's syndrome. CHD can be detected prenatally by genetic testing, obstetric ultrasound, or fetal echocardiogram (Cassidy et al., 2017). Early detection is encouraged to allow for genetic and family counseling as well as management of high-risk pregnancies.

TYPES OF HEART CONDITIONS

Congenital Heart Defects

The term CHD encompasses a heterogeneous group of diagnoses that range in severity and outcome. The American Heart Association (AHA) currently identifies more than 18 distinct types of CHD, with variations in lesion presentation. There has been an attempt to classify the diagnoses based on severity level (Marino et al., 2012). CHD of increased severity warrants immediate surgery (e.g., transposition of the great arteries, total anomalous pulmonary venous return, single ventricle defects), results in a cyanotic (i.e., blue) presentation due to decreased oxygenated blood flow, has genetic or medical comorbidities, or requires mechanical support devices—e.g., extracorporeal membrane oxygenation (ECMO), ventricular assist device (VAD)—within the first year of life (Marino et al., 2012).

Among the most high-risk diagnoses are single-ventricle defects (SVD). As a group, SVD are the most severe presentations of CHD and result in cyanosis at birth. Hypoplastic left heart syndrome (HLHS) is a SVD characterized by a smaller (hypoplastic) left ventricle and absence of the left atrium. This diagnosis is associated with genetic syndromes (Turner's, Jacobsen's) and requires complex treatment and management. Tricuspid atresia is another SVD characterized by the absence of, or a reduced, tricuspid valve and underdeveloped right ventricle. Pulmonary atresia is characterized by absence of a pulmonary valve and underdeveloped right ventricle and tricuspid valve. Individuals with SVD may require heart transplant, but more often benefit from three-stage surgical palliation. The initial surgery (Norwood procedure) occurs shortly after birth, and the second procedure (bidirectional Glenn procedure) is completed within the year following initial surgery. The third (Fontan) procedure is completed by 3 to 4 years of age. SVD can be detected as early as the second trimester, with associated neurological comorbidities (including delayed brain growth and organization) noted by the third trimester (Licht et al., 2009). Individuals with SVD will require ongoing monitoring and management of their cardiac status, including catheterizations, because they are at risk for infection of the heart (endocarditis) and can be immunocompromised (i.e., at increased risk for viruses and other infections).

The most common and generally one of the least severe of the CHD diagnoses is ventricular septal defect (VSD). VSD is associated with several genetic syndromes (T21, DiGeorge, and Noonan) and occurs when the wall between ventricles fails to close during gestation. Atrial septal defect (ASD) is a similar defect in the walls between the left and right atria, and it is also common in genetic syndromes (T21, VACTERL) or fetal alcohol syndrome. Often VSD and ASD can be monitored or successfully treated with medication, although surgical closure is also completed with more severe or complicated presentations.

Acquired Heart Defects

Acquired heart defects are less prevalent in the pediatric population. Abnormal heart rhythms (i.e., arrhythmias) or cardiac muscle fiber abnormalities (i.e., cardiomyopathy) can occur in both typically developing children and those with CHD. These diagnoses also range in severity, with the most severe requiring pacemakers or heart transplantation. In addition, children who develop rheumatic fever or Kawasaki disease may acquire heart disease due to infection. Kawasaki disease can be associated with inflammation of the coronary arteries or heart muscle (myocarditis). It is most common in children less than 5 years old, and, if it is treated early, lasting impairment is most often avoided.

CASE EXAMPLE

Charlotte is a 7-year-old female who was prenatally diagnosed with HLHS. Charlotte underwent three staged palliative surgeries in her first years of life. Since that time, Charlotte has engaged in routine follow-up and has been admitted to the hospital multiple times for diagnostic cardiac catheterizations, viral illnesses, and other complications related to CHD. During one admission when she was 5 years old, Charlotte required care in the cardiac intensive care unit and was intubated and sedated and received a neuromuscular blocker to paralyze her. Both Charlotte and her parents described it as a traumatic admission. In a more recent admission for a procedure, Charlotte had multiple needle sticks due to difficulties obtaining intravenous access. Afterward, Charlotte experienced temporary vocal cord paresis (muscular weakness) related to being intubated, which resulted in a hoarse voice and difficulty swallowing thin liquids safely.

Charlotte's parents pursued outpatient psychotherapy for her due to her anxiety in the home and medical settings. Charlotte's mother described her as "terrified" during her recent hospitalization and said that she was unable to sleep at night and remained vigilant when any hospital staff entered the room. Charlotte expressed a specific phobia of needle sticks out of worry that they would be painful, and she attempted to refuse these procedures. Charlotte also experienced anxiety in other domains, such as separating from her mother at times. She went to school easily, but she did not like staying at home or being dropped off at new places (e.g., a birthday party) if her mother planned to leave. Charlotte also displayed sleep difficulties, including nightmares after surgeries or lengthy hospitalizations, refusal to go to sleep on her own, and insistence on sleeping with her parents. Her parents tried to encourage her to sleep more independently, but they gave in because they did not want to send her to school exhausted. Socially, Charlotte did well in school and made friends easily. She was generally well behaved at home, and she was involved in many activities in the community.

Weekly individual and family-based health and behavior interventions using an evidence-based cognitive behavioral therapy approach was recommended. Sessions included psychoeducation about feelings, recognizing physical symptoms of anxiety, basic relaxation skills, and how to identify and respond to anxious thoughts. A fear ladder related to Charlotte's needle phobia was established, and gradual exposures were utilized to allow her to practice relaxation skills and coping strategies in anxiety-provoking situations. Charlotte responded well to therapy and was able to identify her existing anxious thoughts (e.g., "I could never handle getting stitches, it would hurt too much and be scary"), to question the validity of her anxious thoughts (e.g., "Is it true that I could never handle stitches? Have I had them before or have I handled other difficult things?"), and to identify more realistic coping thoughts (e.g., "I don't need stitches right now, but I've had them before and been okay. I know deep breathing helps me calm down and that my doctors give me medicine for things that may hurt."). Through gradual exposure and use of techniques like guided imagery, Charlotte had less anxiety during blood work. She also became less fearful during outpatient appointments. Charlotte applied these skills at home to become more independent with sleep.

SCHOOL-RELATED CONCERNS

Children with moderate to severe forms of CHD are at risk for neurobehavioral and school-related deficits (Marino et al., 2012). The deficits can be prevalent but subtle across early childhood to adolescence. Indeed, children with CHD access special education supports from infancy through adolescence at a higher rate than typically developing peers (Bellinger et al., 2003, 2011).

Early Childhood (Birth to Age Five)

Early development can be affected by prolonged hospitalizations and surgical intervention, as well as the adjustment to returning home. Families may focus on primary medical needs without detecting or addressing developmental delays. In infancy, gross motor delays and feeding difficulties are prevalent, and higher rates of cognitive, motor, and language delays have also been found in infants with more complex CHD (Brosig et al., 2017; Gaynor et al., 2015; Mussatto et al., 2014). Mussatto and colleagues (2014) found that over 50% of children (ages 6 months to 3 years) with CHD and without genetic comorbidity demonstrated delays in at least one developmental area. Typically developing infants with CHD remain at risk for developmental concerns up to 3 years of age (Mussatto et al., 2014). Further, motor and language delays in infancy can place a child at risk for later difficulties with social language skills and more complex visuomotor functioning in preschool (Brosig et al., 2017).

In comparison to typically developing peers, preschool-age children with complex CHD are at higher risk for delays in expressive language, visuomotor skills, and early executive function (e.g., organization, motor planning), and overall intelligence performance can range from low-average to average across heterogeneous CHD diagnoses (Karsdorp, Everaerd, Kindt, & Mulder, 2007).

Early childhood assessment is important; ideally, multidisciplinary assessment, including pediatrics, psychology, and developmental specialists (occupational, speech-language, physical therapists), is the best for early detection of delays. The psychological assessment should include standardized developmental assessment, as well as parent behavioral rating questionnaires and clinical interview with families.

School-Age Children

Outcomes for school-age children with severe CHD include slightly lower intelligence (low-average to average) performance in comparison to typically developing peers, as well as increased risk of deficits in pragmatic or social language, visuomotor and fine motor skills, and attention and executive functioning (Karsdorp et al., 2007; Marino et al., 2012; Wernovsky, 2006). Deficits across domains can be subtle but cumulative over time, particularly as demands on independence and academic reasoning (e.g., reading comprehension, mathematical problem-solving) skills increase. In late childhood and adolescence, difficulties in the areas of peer relations and social cognition also begin to emerge (Marino et al., 2012).

Greater risk (15%–25%) of internalizing behaviors (e.g., anxiety, withdrawal, depression, somatic complaints) and externalizing behaviors (e.g., inattention, hyperactivity, aggression) are reported in children with complex CHD, and increased internalizing symptoms are seen as children reach adolescence, regardless of CHD severity (Karsdorp et al., 2007; Marino et al., 2012).

COMORBID NEURODEVELOPMENTAL DIAGNOSES

Social Deficits

Children with complex CHD are at risk for additional developmental delays. Demonstrated deficits in social cognition and language, as well as early language delays, can be consistent with symptoms that comprise the diagnostic criteria for autism spectrum disorder in the *Diagnostic and Statistical Manual of Mental Disorders*, Fifth Edition (DSM-5; American Psychiatric Association, 2013). Specifically, difficulties with social cognition and language are prevalent across both preschool and school-age children, as demonstrated through standardized testing of facial affect recognition and theory of mind, as well as through parent and teacher rating on behavioral questionnaires (Bellinger, 2008; Hövels-Gürich et al., 2002). The addition of language delays, intellectual disability, and genetic comorbidities (e.g., Turner's, 22q11.2) may complicate diagnoses, and it is recommended that diagnostic-specific assessment (e.g., Autism Diagnostic Observation Schedule, Second Edition, Autism Diagnostic Interview, Revised) be completed. Survey research indicates children with CHD have between a two- and fivefold increase of autism diagnosis depending on severity and genetic comorbidity (Cassidy et al., 2017; Marino et al., 2012). Given their higher prevalence of autism, the AHA recommends autism-specific screening for children with CHD at 18 to 24 months of age (Marino et al., 2012).

Attention Deficit Hyperactivity Disorder

Deficits seen in attention, behavior (e.g., impulsivity, hyperactivity), and executive function (e.g., working memory) are prevalent in school-age children and adolescents with CHD, and these symptoms can be consistent with diagnostic criteria for attention deficit hyperactivity disorder (ADHD). Prevalence rates of ADHD have ranged between 25% and 53% in children with varying CHD severity (Cassidy et al., 2017). Families often turn to their pediatrician or primary care physician for help with the behavioral symptoms, but they may also present to a psychologist or school-based clinician for assessment or behavioral management of symptoms. Although a combination of stimulant medication and behavioral management is effective, stimulant medications can be the most immediately effective in addressing symptoms. Use of the medications in children with CHD was initially concerning given reports of adverse cardiac events and unexplained sudden death (Vetter et al., 2008). However, the AHA released a statement in 2008 stating that a diagnosis of CHD is not necessarily a contraindication to stimulant medications, and they advocate for a comprehensive assessment (e.g., ECG, approval from cardiologist), particularly in high-risk patients (Vetter et al., 2008).

CONSIDERATIONS FOR ASSESSMENT OF COGNITIVE AND NEURODEVELOPMENTAL CONDITIONS

Evaluation of school-age children and adolescents with CHD requires a comprehensive battery of measures, given the variety of neurobehavioral complications that may arise as they enter school and are increasingly expected to be independent. A comprehensive battery should include measures of intelligence, academic achievement, attention, executive function, visual and fine motor skills, and social, emotional and behavioral functioning (as rated by parents, teachers, and the child, as applicable). Given the increased rates of both autism and ADHD within the CHD population, the battery should include several behavioral rating questionnaires for parents, teachers, and the child or adolescent when appropriate, as well as measures of social cognition and language (e.g., theory of mind, affect recognition). A clinical interview with the family can identify specific concerns across environments that may guide treatment and intervention options. The reader is encouraged to review Marino et al. (2012) and Cassidy et al. (2017) for a summary of standardized measures commonly used within the CHD population.

PSYCHOLOGICAL ADJUSTMENT AND HEALTH-RELATED QUALITY OF LIFE OUTCOMES

Children with CHD appear to be at greater risk for psychological maladjustment when compared to normative samples. Rates of emotional and behavioral problems reported by parents vary across study, but they can be as high as 41% and are almost always significantly higher than rates of problems reported for the normative sample or control groups (Latal, Helfricht, Fischer, Bauersfeld, & Landolt, 2009). Health-related quality of life (HRQOL), which is defined as the perceived impact of an illness or medical treatment on a patient's ability to function and feel satisfied across a variety of domains, is also rated lower in children with CHD than in controls (Cohen, Mansoor, Langut, & Lorber, 2007; Mellion et al., 2014; Mussatto et al., 2014). Whereas rates of psychological maladjustment do not appear to be dependent on disease severity (Latal et al., 2009), HRQOL for those with the most severe forms of CHD appears to be more affected than HRQOL for those with mild forms of CHD (Mellion et al., 2014).

Medical Treatments and Adjustment

As technologies have advanced, children with congenital and acquired heart disease have begun receiving medical support devices, including implantable cardioverter defibrillators (ICDs), which are used to manage lethal arrhythmias, and VADs, which are implantable devices that pump blood for the heart. ICD placement has been associated with high rates of complications (e.g., inappropriate shocks, lead failure) and lifestyle changes (e.g., avoidance of contact sports), which in turn have been associated with higher rates of anxiety disorders and lower physical quality of life in ICD recipients than in children with pacemakers alone (Sears et al., 2011; Webster et al., 2014). The use of VADs has been associated with depression and anxiety in both patients and their parents (Ozbaran et al., 2012a, 2012b), perhaps due to the prolonged hospitalization and extensive caregiver education prior to hospital discharge, both of which can be very stressful and negatively affect family coping. Of note, many studies investigating psychological adjustment in children with CHD rely only on parent report of child and adolescent functioning. Obtaining self- and teacher reports of a child's functioning is important, as some studies have demonstrated that children with CHD and teachers tend to report fewer adjustment and behavioral difficulties than parents report (Latal et al., 2009; Salzer-Muhar et al., 2002).

Developmental Course of Adjustment Difficulties

The psychological support needs of children with heart disease varies based on how recently they were diagnosed and the level of medical care they currently require. Upon initial diagnosis, children and their families may benefit from additional support to promote emotional adjustment and to assess and treat symptoms of medical traumatic stress associated with initial hospitalization (Kazak et al., 2006). Before and during hospitalizations, children often receive support to promote effective coping and to foster developmentally appropriate discussions about future procedures. Children who experience prolonged illnesses and hospitalizations and thus extended absences from school are at increased risk for poor adjustment, depression, and behavioral problems due to fewer peer interactions and limited physical activities (Roberts & MacMath, 2006). Transitions home from the hospital can also be difficult for children, who have to readjust to home routines and behavioral limits if they were not maintained in the hospital setting (LeRoy et al., 2003). In addition, school-age children may worry about returning to school, due to fears that they will attract attention and face questions about their absence, that they won't fit in with their peers anymore, or that they may have fallen behind academically (Roberts & MacMath, 2006). Long term, children with cardiac conditions often benefit from ongoing support related to adjustment to chronic illness, coping with medically related anxiety, and adherence to the recommendations regarding the appropriate level of physical activity. Researchers have found that parents of children with cardiac conditions often restrict their child's physical activity more than recommended by their child's cardiologist due to their own anxiety and uncertainty about physical activity (Longmuir & McCrindle, 2009).

Family Factors and Adjustment

Special consideration should also be given to the effect that a child with CHD can have on the family system. Years after diagnosis, surgery, and hospitalization, parents of children with CHD continue to endorse higher rates of psychological maladjustment (Woolf-King, Anger, Arnold, Weiss, & Teitel, 2017), parenting stress (Uzark & Jones, 2003), and medical traumatic stress (Franich-Ray et al., 2013; Helfricht, Latal, Fischer, Tomaske, & Landolt, 2008). Siblings of children with CHD may experience adjustment difficulties, particularly during their sibling's hospitalizations, when they may experience prolonged separation from primary caregivers. Adjustment difficulties include worrying about the health and prognosis of the child with CHD, emotional and behavioral challenges related to parental separation and changes in routine, and jealousy about attention given to the child with CHD (Janus & Goldberg, 1997).

RISK AND RESILIENCY FACTORS

Neurodevelopmental Outcomes

Considerable research has focused on identifying biological, medical, and environmental risk and resiliency factors associated with neurodevelopmental outcomes in children with CHD. Biologically, neurodevelopmental differences in children with CHD have been demonstrated in utero. Infants with CHD have been found to have lower brain volumes at birth and increased incidence of white matter hypoxic injuries (Licht et al., 2009). The risk for developmental deficits is also increased in children with cyanotic heart disease, due to their chronic hypoxemia, and in children with suspected or confirmed comorbid genetic abnormality, which occurs in up to 30% of children with CHD (Marino et al., 2012).

Research has explored whether specific aspects of the medical care that children with CHD require have an impact on future neurodevelopment (Bellinger et al., 2011), with results indicating that the causes of neurodevelopmental deficits are multifactorial and cumulative (Marino et al., 2012). Specific medical and surgical factors that have been identified as risk factors include premature birth (gestational age < 37 weeks), mechanical support (ECMO and VAD), heart transplantation, cardiopulmonary arrest and resuscitation, perioperative seizures, abnormalities on neuroimaging, and prolonged hospitalization (Marino et al., 2012).

Environmental factors also have a significant effect on neurodevelopment. Higher socioeconomic status (SES) has been associated with better neurodevelopmental outcomes (Marino et al., 2012). However, parental overprotectiveness, which can limit a child's exposure to developmentally appropriate activities (McCusker et al., 2007), has been hypothesized to explain lower adaptive skills and achievement in children with CHD.

Psychological Maladjustment

Research exploring the risk and resiliency factors associated with psychological adjustment among children with CHD is growing. Overall, the type and severity of CHD have not been linked with behavioral and social-emotional outcomes (Karsdorp et al., 2007), but a number of other factors have been, including neurodevelopmental deficits, long-term complications, the home environment, and the children's own perceptions of themselves and their health status. Neurodevelopmental deficits and long-term complications (e.g., arrhythmias) appear to increase risk for maladjustment (Latal et al., 2009). Specifically, research has demonstrated that parent report of child functioning is lower for children who experience complications or require long-term medication management (Latal et al., 2009). Similarly, parent report of child psychological maladjustment was greater for children with language difficulties or cognitive delays (Latal et al., 2009).

High rates of parental stress are also associated with more emotional and behavioral concerns in children (Latal et al., 2009) and adolescents (DeMaso et al., 2014). Research with older children and adolescents has demonstrated the importance of a youth's self-perceptions in behavioral and HRQOL outcomes. Self-perceptions regarding health, self-worth, and competence accounted for more variance in behavioral problems than sociodemographic and medical factors (Mussatto et al., 2014). Similarly, perceived disease severity was a stronger predictor of HRQOL than actual disease severity (Cohen et al., 2007).

EVIDENCE-BASED INTERVENTIONS

Because the integration of pediatric psychology into cardiology is relatively new, there are only a few studies examining the effectiveness of psychological interventions for children with CHD. McCusker et al. (2010, 2012) have developed interventions for children with CHD that target developmental and school functioning. Their first intervention focused on parental functioning, with six sessions focused on adjustment to diagnosis, feeding interactions, and coping with anxiety (McCusker et al., 2010). Developmental testing at 6-month follow-up revealed that infants from the intervention group performed better on a scale of cognitive development (McCusker et al., 2010). Additionally, mothers from the intervention group breastfed more and had lower levels of maternal anxiety and health-related worry than controls.

McCusker and colleagues (2012) also tested an intervention for children with CHD prior to the transition to school. The intervention consisted of a 1-day parent workshop focused on problem-solving skills, education, and parenting strategies, which was followed up by a single individual session to discuss specific recommendations for each family. At 10-month follow-up, there were no significant results for measures of child behavior at home or school, but children in the intervention group missed fewer days of school and were perceived as "sick" less often by their mothers when compared to the control group (McCusker et al., 2012). Mothers in the intervention group also reported improved mental health and reduced strain associated with parenting a child with a chronic illness compared to control mothers (McCusker et al., 2010).

CULTURAL CONSIDERATIONS

Among children with CHD, health disparities related to race, ethnicity, SES, and type of insurance have been documented. Although rates are improving, pre-natal detection of CHD, which can reduce morbidity and mortality by allowing for planned delivery in a specialized center, is still lowest among mothers living in impoverished or rural communities (Hill, Block, Tanem, & Frommelt, 2015). After birth, infants who are uninsured or underinsured, or who are from ethnic minority or impoverished families, are at increased risk for mortality, hospital readmission, repeat surgery, and neurodevelopmental impairment (Collins, Soskolne, Rankin, Ibrahim, & Matoba, 2017; Ghanayem et al., 2012; Kucik et al., 2014; Lasa, Cohen, Wernovsky, & Pinto, 2013; Marino et al., 2012). Disparities in morbidity and mortality become more apparent over time, as infants transition home and parents or caregivers take over primary responsibility for managing medically complex infants (Collins et al., 2017; Ghanayem et al., 2012; Lasa et al., 2013). Additionally, ethnic minority and impoverished families disproportion-ately face risk factors for poor health outcomes (Berry, Bloom, Foley, & Palfrey, 2010), including lower parental education level, poor social support, more fre-quent housing and transportation challenges, and lower-quality general pediatric care, all of which can affect postdischarge care.

Health disparities have also been documented among parents of children with CHD related to higher rates of parenting stress, medical traumatic stress, and poorer quality of life reported by parents with limited financial and educational means (Davis, Brown, Bakeman, & Campbell, 1998; Lawoko & Soares, 2003). The parental disparities can in turn negatively impact the household environment, which is a risk factor for neurodevelopmental deficits and psychological malad-justment among children with CHD, placing already vulnerable children at even higher risk (DeMaso et al., 2014). Unfortunately, this field is understudied, and additional research is needed to identify the psychosocial needs of high-risk families and to evaluate specific psychosocial interventions that could begin to address these disparities.

LEGAL AND POLICY ISSUES

Some children with heart disease will qualify for accommodations under Section 504 of the Rehabilitation Act of 1973 (a 504 plan). Specific concerns will vary by child, but 504 plans for children with heart conditions typically address issues related to diminished physical stamina, inability to participate in contact sports, need for temperature regulation, access to a water bottle for proper hydration, unlimited access to restrooms (especially when the child is on diuretic medication), use of supplemental oxygen, access to the school nurse, and allowance for extra time on homework and in-class assignments missed due to absence for medical appointments and hospitalizations (see Handout 17.1 for sample accommodations). Teachers are encouraged to ask parents or guardians about the nature of the child's heart condition and any effects on learning or school activities it may have. Most children and teens with CHD can fully participate in the majority of physical and extracurricular activities, but having a thorough understanding of any limitations put in place by the cardiologist is important. Many children will have been followed closely by a team of developmental specialists and may qualify for specific learning accommodations, which would be most appropriately addressed by an individualized education plan (IEP). Handout 17.2 includes resources for working with children with CHD.

For the majority of children and teens with simple heart defects, no special care will be needed at school, but for those with more complicated cardiac conditions, teachers and other school personnel should be aware of signs that may require medical attention, including rapid breathing or shortness of breath, bluish coloring of the skin (cyanosis), and chest discomfort. Schools are encouraged to have a health plan in place (even without a 504 plan) that includes what should be done if the child experiences any concerning symptoms (dizziness, feeling faint, palpitations, and chest pain, as well as bleeding/severe bruising in individuals on anticoagulants). Plans of action may include appropriate interventions, methods for contacting parents, and when to call emergency services. While an automated external defibrillator (AED) is not universally required in the school setting by state law, schools are encouraged to have an AED readily accessible and staff who are trained in both cardiopulmonary resuscitation (CPR) and AED use. On field trips, children with heart disease should be paired with the teacher or another adult who is aware of their diagnosis and familiar with the health plan should any symptoms arise.

REFERENCES

American Psychiatric Association. (2013). *Diagnostic and statistical manual of mental disorders* (5th ed.). Arlington, VA: Author.

Bellinger, D. C. (2008). Are children with congenital cardiac malformations at increased risk of deficits in social cognition? *Cardiology in the Young, 18*(1), 3–9.

Bellinger, D. C., Wypij, D., DuPlessis, A. J., Rappaport, L. A., Jonas, R. A., Wernovsky, G., & Newburger, J. W. (2003). Neurodevelopmental status at eight years in children with dextrotransposition of the great arteries: The Boston Circulatory Arrest Trial. *The Journal of Thoracic and Cardiovascular Surgery, 126*(5), 1385–1396.

Bellinger, D. C., Wypij, D., Rivkin, M. J., DeMaso, D. R., Robertson, R. L., Dunbar-Masterson, C., & Newburger, J. W. (2011). Adolescents with d-transposition of the great arteries corrected with the arterial switch procedure. *Circulation, 124*(12), 1361–1369.

Berry, J. G., Bloom, S., Foley, S., & Palfrey, J. S. (2010). Health inequity in children and youth with chronic health conditions. *Pediatrics, 126*(Suppl. 3), S111–S119.

Boneva, R. S., Botto, L. D., Moore, C. A., Yang, Q., Correa, A., & Erickson, J. D. (2001). Mortality associated with congenital heart defects in the United States: Trends and disparities, 1979–1997. *Circulation 103*, 2376–2381. doi:10.1161/01.CIR.103.19.2376

Brosig, C., Sood, E., & Butcher, J. (2017). Cardiovascular disease. In M. Roberts & R. G. Steele (Eds.), *Handbook of pediatric psychology* (5th ed.). New York, NY: Guilford Press.

Cassidy, A. R., Ilardi, D., Bowen, S. R., Hampton, L. E., Heinrich, K. P., Loman, M. M., Sanz, J. H., & Wolfe, K. R. (2017): Congenital heart disease: A primer for the pediatric neuropsychologist, *Child Neuropsychology, 24*(7), 859–902. doi:10.1080/09297049.2017.1373758

Chessa, M., & Plucchinotta, F. R. (2015). Congenital heart disease: A medical overview. In E. Callus & E. Quadri (Eds.), *Clinical psychology and congenital heart disease* (pp. 3–20). Milan, Italy: Springer.

Cohen, M., Mansoor, D., Langut, H., & Lorber, A. (2007). Quality of life, depressed mood, and self-esteem in adolescents with heart disease. *Psychosomatic Medicine, 69*(4), 313–318.

Collins, J. W., Soskolne, G., Rankin, K. M., Ibrahim, A., & Matoba, N. (2017). African-American: White disparity in infant mortality due to congenital heart disease. *Journal of Pediatrics, 181*, 131–136.

Davis, C. C., Brown, R. T., Bakeman, R., & Campbell, R. (1998). Psychological adaptation and adjustment of mothers of children with congenital heart disease: Stress, coping, and family functioning. *Journal of Pediatric Psychology, 23*(4), 219–228.

DeMaso, D. R., Labella, M., Taylor, G. A., Forbes, P. W., Stopp, C., Bellinger, D. C., & Newburger, J. W. (2014). Psychiatric disorders and function in adolescents with d-transposition of the great arteries. *Journal of Pediatrics, 165*(4), 760–766.

Franich-Ray, C., Bright, M. A., Anderson, V., Northam, E., Cochrane, A., Menahem, S., & Jordan, B. (2013). Trauma reactions in mothers and fathers after their infant's cardiac surgery. *Journal of Pediatric Psychology, 38*(5), 494–505.

Gaynor, J. W., Stopp, C., Wypij, D., Andropoulos, D. B., Atallah, J., Atz, A. M., & Newburger, J. W. (2015). Neurodevelopmental outcomes after cardiac surgery in infancy. *Pediatrics, 135*(5), 816–825.

Ghanayem, N. S., Allen, K. R., Tabbutt, S., Atz, A. M., Clabby, M. L., Cooper, D. S., & Kaltman, J. R. (2012). Interstage mortality after the Norwood procedure: Results of the multicenter Single Ventricle Reconstruction trial. *The Journal of Thoracic and Cardiovascular Surgery, 144*(4), 896–906.

Glanzman, M., Licht, D., & Wernovsky, G. (2011). Neurodevelopment in children with complex congenital heart disease. In M. M. Gleason, J. Rychick, & R. E. Shaddy (Eds.), *Pediatric practice: Cardiology* (pp. 215–230). China: McGraw-Hill.

Helfricht, S., Latal, B., Fischer, J. E., Tomaske, M., & Landolt, M. A. (2008). Surgery-related posttraumatic stress disorder in parents of children undergoing cardiopulmonary bypass surgery: A prospective cohort study. *Pediatric Critical Care Medicine, 9*(2), 217–223.

Hill, G. D., Block, J. R., Tanem, J. B., & Frommelt, M. A. (2015). Disparities in the prenatal detection of critical congenital heart disease. *Prenatal Diagnosis, 35*(9), 859–863.

Hoffman, J. I. E., & Kaplan, S. (2002). The incidence of congenital heart disease. *Journal of the American College of Cardiology, 39*(12), 1890–1900.

Hövels-Gürich, H. H., Konrad, K., Wiesner, M., Minkenberg, R., Herpertz-Dahlmann, B., Messmer, B. J., & von Bernuth, G. (2002). Long term behavioural outcome after neonatal arterial switch operation for transposition of the great arteries. *Archives of Disease in Childhood, 87*, 506–510.

Janus, M., & Goldberg, S. (1997). Treatment characteristics of congenital heart disease and behaviour problems of patients and healthy siblings. *Journal of Paediatrics and Child Health, 33*(3), 219–225.

Karsdorp, P. A., Everaerd, W., Kindt, M., & Mulder, B. J. (2007). Psychological and cognitive functioning in children and adolescents with congenital heart disease: A meta-analysis. *Journal of Pediatric Psychology, 32*(5), 527–541.

Kazak, A. E., Kassam-Adams, N., Schneider, S., Zelikovsky, N., Alderfer, M. A., & Rourke, M. (2006). An integrative model of pediatric medical traumatic stress. *Journal of Pediatric Psychology, 31*(4), 343–355.

Kucik, J. E., Nembhard, W. N., Donohue, P., Devine, O., Wang, Y., Minkovitz, C. S., & Burke, T. (2014). Community socioeconomic disadvantage and the survival of infants with congenital heart defects. *American Journal of Public Health, 104*(11), e150–e157.

Lasa, J. J., Cohen, M. S., Wernovsky, G., & Pinto, N. M. (2013). Is race associated with morbidity and mortality after hospital discharge among neonates undergoing heart surgery? *Pediatric Cardiology, 34*(2), 415–423.

Latal, B., Helfricht, S., Fischer, J. E., Bauersfeld, U., & Landolt, M. A. (2009). Psychological adjustment and quality of life in children and adolescents following open-heart surgery for congenital heart disease: A systematic review. *BMC Pediatrics, 9*(1), 6.

Lawoko, S., & Soares, J. J. (2003). Quality of life among parents of children with congenital heart disease, parents of children with other diseases and parents of healthy children. *Quality of Life Research, 12*(6), 655–666.

LeRoy, S., Elixson, E. M., O'Brien, P., Tong, E., Turpin, S., & Uzark, K. (2003). Recommendations for preparing children and adolescents for invasive cardiac procedures. *Circulation, 108*(20), 2550–2564.

Licht, D. J., Shera, D. M., Clancy, R. R., Wernovsky, G., Montenegro, L. M., Nicolson, S. C., & Vossough, A. (2009). Brain maturation is delayed in infants with complex congenital heart defects. *The Journal of Thoracic and Cardiovascular Surgery, 137*(3), 529–537.

Longmuir, P. E., & McCrindle, B. W. (2009). Physical activity restrictions for children after the Fontan operation: Disagreement between parent, cardiologist, and medical record reports. *American Heart Journal, 157*(5), 853–859.

Marino, B. S., Lipkin, P. H., Newburger, J. W., Peacock, G., Gerdes, M., Gaynor, J. W., . . . Li, J. (2012). Neurodevelopmental outcomes in children with congenital heart disease: Evaluation and management. *Circulation, 126*(9), 1143–1172.

McCusker, C. G., Doherty, N. N., Molloy, B., Casey, F., Rooney, N., Mulholland, C., & Stewart, M. (2007). Determinants of neuropsychological and behavioural outcomes in early childhood survivors of congenital heart disease. *Archives of Disease in Childhood, 92*(2), 137–141.

McCusker, C. G., Doherty, N. N., Molloy, B., Rooney, N., Mulholland, C., Sands, A., & Casey, F. (2010). A controlled trial of early interventions to promote maternal adjustment and development in infants born with severe congenital heart disease. *Child: Care, Health and Development, 36*(1), 110–117.

McCusker, C. G., Doherty, N. N., Molloy, B., Rooney, N., Mulholland, C., Sands, A., & Casey, F. (2012). A randomized controlled trial of interventions to promote adjustment in children with congenital heart disease entering school and their families. *Journal of Pediatric Psychology, 37*(10), 1089–1103.

Mellion, K., Uzark, K., Cassedy, A., Drotar, D., Wernovsky, G., Newburger, J. W., & Marino, B. S. (2014). Health-related quality of life outcomes in children and adolescents with congenital heart disease. *Journal of Pediatrics, 164*(4), 781–788.

Moorman, A., Webb, S., Brown, N. A., Lamers, W., & Anderson, R. H. (2003). Development of the heart: (1) Formation of the cardiac chambers and arterial trunks. *Heart, 89*(7), 806–814.

Mussatto, K. A., Sawin, K. J., Schiffman, R., Leske, J., Simpson, P., & Marino, B. S. (2014). The importance of self-perceptions to psychosocial adjustment in adolescents with heart disease. *Journal of Pediatric Health Care, 28*(3), 251–261.

Oster M. E., Lee K. A., Honein, M. A., Riehle-Colarusso, T., Shin, M., & Correa, A. (2013). Temporal trends in survival among infants with critical congenital heart defects. *Pediatrics, 131*(5), e1502–1508.

Ozbaran, B., Kose, S., Yagdi, T., Engin, C., Erermis, S., Uysal, T., & Ozbaran, M. (2012a). Psychiatric evaluation of children and adolescents with left ventricular assist devices. *Psychosomatic Medicine, 74*(5), 554–558.

Ozbaran, B., Kose, S., Yagdi, T., Engin, C., Erermis, S., Yazici, K. U., & Ozbaran, M. (2012b). Depression and anxiety levels of the mothers of children and adolescents with left ventricular assist devices. *Pediatric Transplantation, 16*(7), 766–770.

Reller, M. D., Strickland, M. J., Riehle-Colarusso, T., Mahle, W. T., & Correa, A. (2008). Prevalence of congenital heart defects in metropolitan Atlanta, 1998–2005. *Journal of Pediatrics, 153*(6), 807–813.

Roberts, J., & MacMath, S. (2006). *Starting a conversation: School children congenital heart disease.* Calgary, Canada: Detselig Enterprises.

Salzer-Muhar, U., Herle, M., Floquet, P., Freilinger, M., Greber-Platzer, S., Haller, A., & Schlemmer, M. (2002). Self-concept in male and female adolescents with congenital heart disease. *Clinical Pediatrics, 41*(1), 17–24.

Sears, S. F., Hazelton, A. G., Amant, J. S., Matchett, M., Kovacs, A., Vazquez, L. D., & Cannon, B. C. (2011). Quality of life in pediatric patients with implantable cardioverter defibrillators. *The American Journal of Cardiology, 107*(7), 1023–1027.

Uzark, K., & Jones, K. (2003). Parenting stress and children with heart disease. *Journal of Pediatric Health Care, 17*(4), 163–168.

Vetter, V. L., Elia, J., Erickson, C., Berger, S., Blum, N., Uzark, K., & Webb, C. L. (2008). Cardiovascular monitoring of children and adolescents with heart disease receiving medications for attention deficit/hyperactivity disorder. *Circulation, 117*, 2407–2423.

Webster, G., Panek, K. A., Labella, M., Taylor, G. A., Gauvreau, K., Cecchin, F., & DeMaso, D. R. (2014). Psychiatric functioning and quality of life in young patients with cardiac rhythm devices. *Pediatrics, 133*(4), e964–e972.

Wernovsky, G. (2006). Current insights regarding neurological and developmental abnormalities in children and young adults with complex congenital cardiac disease. *Cardiology in the Young, 16*(S1), 92–104.

Woolf-King, S. E., Anger, A., Arnold, E. A., Weiss, S. J., & Teitel, D. (2017). Mental health among parents of children with critical congenital heart defects: A systematic review. *Journal of the American Heart Association, 6*(2), e004862.

Handout 17.1.

Education Plans for Children with CHD

Age/Grade	Type(s) Available	Locale/Provider
Birth–Preschool	Individual family service plan (IFSP)	At home/Early intervention
Preschool–Kindergarten	Individualized education plan (IEP)	At home or outside location/Public school
Kindergarten–High School	Individualized education plan (IEP): For educational support Individual healthcare plan (IHP) 504 Plan: For accommodations	At school/Public school

Sample Accommodations

- Physical (504, IHP, IEP)
  - Reduce contact sports or strenuous physical activity
  - Shortened school day (depending on disease severity)
  - Schedule more difficult classes when the child is most alert
  - Monitor fatigue levels
  - Monitor temperature in extreme heat or cold
  - Allow breaks to visit nurse
  - Allow extra set of books for home so that the child does not have to carry them
  - Access to water at all times to stay hydrated
  - Unrestricted use of bathroom if on diuretics
- Medical (504, IHP, IEP)
  - Access to automatic external defibrillator (AED) and staff who are familiar with its use
  - Availability of CPR-trained staff
  - Development of a Cardiac Emergency Response Plan (http://cpr.heart.org/AHAECC/CPRAndECC/Programs/CPRInSchools/UCM_477994_Cardiac-Emergency-Response-Plan.jsp)
  - If child is absent due to medical concerns, in-home tutoring should be provided
  - Modifications related to medication and eating requirements

- Cognitive/Behavioral (504, IEP)
  - Extended time for assignments
  - Preferential seating
  - Small group
  - Restate and repeat instructions
  - Social skills instruction/access to peer mentor
  - Reduced workload

HANDOUT 17.2.

HELPFUL RESOURCES FOR WORKING WITH CHILDREN WITH CHD

- General information regarding CHD and acquired heart conditions:
  - The American Heart Association (http://www.heart.org/HEARTORG/)
  - The Centers for Disease Control and Prevention (https://www.cdc.gov/ncbddd/heartdefects/index.html)
  - National Institutes of Health (https://www.nih.gov/)
- For information about specific state laws, see the American Heart Association's website: http://cpr.heart.org/AHAECC/CPRAndECC/Programs/UCM_473193_Programs.jsp
- Nonprofit organizations that provide information and resources for families and providers:
  - Children's Heart Foundation (http://www.childrensheartfoundation.org/)
  - Mended Little Hearts (http://www.mendedlittlehearts.org)
  - Kids with Heart (https://kidswithheart.org)
  - Little Hearts (https://www.littlehearts.org)
  - Congenital Heart Information Network (http://www.tchin.org/)
  - The Adult Congenital Heart Association (https://www.achaheart.org) offers support and information for adolescents transitioning into early adulthood
- Diagnosis-specific resources
  - Children's Cardiomyopathy Foundation (http://www.childrenscardiomyopathy.org/)
  - Sisters By Heart (http://www.Sistersbyheart.org) and Brothers By Heart (http://sistersbyheart.org/content/brothers-heart) are groups dedicated to single-ventricle (HLHS) diagnoses.
  - Pulmonary Hypertension Association (https://phassociation.org/patients/aboutph/)
  - Kawasaki Disease Foundation (http://www.kdfoundation.org/)
  - 22Q Family Foundation (http://22qfamilyfoundation.org/what-22q/22q-overview)
  - National Association for Down Syndrome (http://www.nads.org/)
- Government and educational resources
  - Early Headstart and Head Start (https://eclkc.ohs.acf.hhs.gov/)
  - National Headstart Association (http://www.nhsa.org/)
  - U.S. Department of Education (https://www.ed.gov/)
  - Supplementary Security Income (www.ssa.gov)

18

Pulmonary Disorders

Cystic Fibrosis and Asthma

DESIREÉ N. WILLIFORD, LISA HYNES, KRISTINE DURKIN, AND CHRISTINA L. DUNCAN ∎

This chapter provides an overview of school-related issues for children with two specific pulmonary disorders (disorders that affect the lungs), asthma and cystic fibrosis. For each disorder, the chapter covers medical care and prognosis, associated risk and protective factors, sociocultural and environmental considerations, legal and policy-related concerns, and the role that school-based professionals play in supporting youth with the disorder.

MEDICAL CARE AND PROGNOSIS

Asthma

Asthma, the most common chronic illness among U.S. children, is an inflammatory disease characterized by wheezing, chest tightness, shortness of breath, and coughing (Centers for Disease Control and Prevention [CDC], 2017a). There is no identified cause of asthma, nor is there a cure, but most children can manage their symptoms with medication and by avoiding individual triggers for an asthma attack, such as pet dander, dust mites, and smoke (CDC, 2017b). Two classes of medications are used in pediatric asthma: rescue medications and controller medications (National Heart, Lung, and Blood Institute [NHLBI], 2014a). Whereas a rescue medication (such as albuterol) is used for quick symptom relief or as a preventive measure before exercise, controller medications (such as inhaled corticosteroids) are used long term and are taken on a daily basis to control airway inflammation. Oral medications, such as prednisone or a leukotriene inhibitor, may be prescribed depending on disease severity and asthma control. Healthcare providers are encouraged to give families an asthma action plan (AAP), which is a written description of the child's care regimen. Achieving and maintaining asthma control often require understanding this plan, addressing environmental triggers, helping children develop skills in self-management, and monitoring symptoms. Still, the typical asthma course involves waxing and waning of symptoms over time. When poorly managed, asthma can increase risk for morbidity (e.g., school absences) and mortality.

Asthma can limit a child's ability to play, to learn, and to sleep, which highlights the importance of school-based health professionals in supporting asthma management (Keeher Engelke, Swanson, & Guttu, 2014; Newacheck & Halfon, 2000). Children who do not respond to signs of asthma symptoms in a timely manner or who do not have or do not regularly use preventive medication are at greater risk of experiencing serious health problems (Akinbami, Moorman, Garbe, & Sondik, 2009). Awareness of risk factors among school personnel is vital to preventing serious problems from developing in the school setting. Developmental risk factors also need to be considered, such as adolescents' potentially being at risk for poor asthma management due to growing independence and decreased parental involvement (Kintner et al., 2015). School-based health professionals can develop different strategies to support younger and older children with asthma. For example, older children may benefit from receiving encouragement and praise for engaging in independent self-management, such as using a rescue inhaler before gym class, whereas younger children may require direct assistance from school-based personnel in recognizing and appropriately responding to asthma symptoms. Moreover, a child's race, ethnicity, or gender may affect the support they receive in managing asthma (Bloom, Jones, & Freeman, 2013). Indeed, minority racial/ethnic status has been linked to using the emergency department for asthma care, to not receiving appropriate asthma medicine prescriptions, to not taking asthma medicines as prescribed, and even to death (Akinbami et al., 2009; Lieu et al., 2002). Overall, school personnel need to consider the individual child's background and developmental needs to effectively support asthma management within the school setting.

Cystic Fibrosis

Cystic fibrosis (CF), which is often diagnosed in infancy and early childhood, is a progressive, inherited disease characterized by abnormal movement of salt and water through body cells (Cystic Fibrosis Foundation [CFF], n.d.; MacKenzie et al., 2014). CF involves thousands of known gene mutations, and it is a complex disease in which symptoms and severity varies across individuals and over time. Common symptoms include mucus buildup in the lungs, pancreas, and other bodily organs; salty-tasting skin; coughing; wheezing or shortness of breath; lung infections; limited growth and weight gain; difficulty with food absorption and elimination; and male infertility (CFF, n.d.; FitzSimmons, 1994). Due to its progressive nature, CF limits life expectancy—the current median survival age is

40 years (Dodge et al., 2007; MacKenzie et al., 2014). Many advancements continue to be made in CF research and it is hoped that new treatments will drastically improve the survival age in the future.

A CF patient's medical regimen involves a series of daily therapies, including airway clearance, inhaled and oral medications, and pancreatic enzyme supplements (CFF, n.d.; Sawicki, Sellers, & Robinson, 2009). Airway clearance (using, for example, an oscillating vest) reduces mucus buildup, whereas medications are used to open airways (bronchodilators), thin mucus (mucolytics), and protect against infection (antibiotics). Finally, children take oral pancreatic enzyme supplements before meals and snacks to facilitate nutrient absorption (CFF, n.d.; Stallings et al., 2008). Overall, the treatment regimen for children with CF is complicated and time-consuming (usually involving $\geq$ 2 hours per day) and may require assistance from individuals in the child's support system, including schools.

CF treatment focuses on good nutrition, preventing and treating breathing problems resulting from infections, encouraging physical activity, and supporting mental health (Beers & Berkow, 1999). School-based health professionals may play a significant role in identifying and reducing risk for CF-related problems and other health and emotional problems among children with CF (MacKenzie et al., 2014; Tapper Strawhacker & Wellendorf, 2004). As is true in asthma, in CF, developmental factors play a role in risk for poorer outcomes (e.g., quality of life, school functioning). Adolescents are at higher risk for serious health problems related to CF, as are females (MacKenzie et al., 2014). Also, given the negative impact of CF on a child's growth, children who do not follow their CF care regimen may be smaller in height and weight and may experience more CF-related problems than children who have achieved better growth. Examples may include increased difficulties with fighting and recovering from infections and compensating for poor digestion (CFF, n.d.; MacKenzie et al., 2014). Youth with CF are also at risk for other serious complications of infection, such as cross-infection, or cross contamination of bacteria, between multiple people with CF (CFF, n.d.; Tapper Strawhacker & Wellendorf, 2004). Additionally, patients from lower socioeconomic backgrounds tend to experience more CF-related problems, which may be related to poor nutrition, exposure to air pollution, exposure to cigarette smoke, respiratory infections, and higher levels of stress (Khan et al., 1995). In sum, identifiable factors like height and weight, signs of illness or infection (e.g., coughing), age, and socioeconomic background play a role in determining risk for CF-related problems among children and adolescents. Mechanisms for identifying and responding to these factors are important when school-based professionals work with these students and their families.

SCHOOL-BASED MANAGEMENT OF ASTHMA AND CF

Children spend a significant portion of their days in school settings; therefore, school-based health professionals are well positioned to support children and young people in achieving academic success through improved health and regular school attendance, whatever health or social obstacles they face (Tapper Strawhacker & Wellendorf, 2004). In 2014, the NHLBI released *Managing Asthma: A Guide for Schools,* which provides detailed strategies for school staff, including school-based health professionals, to improve recognition of symptoms and assistance with management of asthma in academic settings (NHLBI, 2014b). The guide recommends that school-based health professionals take the lead in conducting in-service programs for educators and other staff on the management of asthma and in keeping detailed records of students' AAPs, their use of health resources, and school absences, and in ensuring that children have easy and quick access to their prescribed medications. A number of evidence-based interventions involving school-based professionals in the role of asthma case manager have shown mixed results for positive outcomes related to the child's knowledge of asthma, self-management, self-efficacy, school attendance, and utilization of healthcare services (Moricca et al., 2012; Taras, Wright, Brennan, Campana, & Lofgren, 2004). Case management includes identifying children who might be under-achieving in an academic setting due to asthma, applying direct care to the child for prevention and during symptom exacerbations, and coordinating among parents, educators, and physicians to promote illness management (Bonaiuto, 2007; Keeher Engelke et al., 2014).

To date, evidence-based interventions that focus on the role of school-based health professionals in CF management in children are limited. However, school clinicians play a crucial role in disease management and in boosting school attendance and full participation in school activities. Interventions targeting other pediatric chronic illnesses may be used as a model for potential roles. For example, school clinicians may provide assessment of the student's daily symptom management and may suggest adaptations required in the educational plan for the student to achieve success in the school setting (Holmes et al., 2016). Given the complexity of CF care, in a case-management approach, school-based health professionals can aid students in becoming more knowledgeable and self-sufficient in their CF care, and school-based professionals are well placed to coordinate a team approach among parents, educators, and CF care team providers (Keeher Engelke et al., 2014).

SCHOOL-RELATED CONCERNS AND PSYCHOLOGICAL COMORBIDITIES

As school-based professionals provide support for these children, it is important for them to be aware of the implications that living with asthma and CF have for students. Although children with these conditions may not have a visible disability or cognitive deficit as a result of their illness, students may experience a host of psychosocial stressors. In particular, youth can have difficulty managing their condition, have concerns about regimen nonadherence, experience frequent school absences, require special accommodations or changes to their physical environment, or have concerns about being different or isolated from their peers.

They may also experience mental health concerns, such as anxiety and depression. Therefore, school-based professionals have an important role in normalizing and addressing these experiences, improving youth confidence, and ensuring an optimal environment to promote overall health and academic achievement.

Adherence and Self-Management

Although children are diagnosed with pulmonary disorders by a physician, school personnel serve an important role in identifying changes in severity of the illness, symptom frequency and/or duration, and medication adherence. To investigate nonadherence in a manner that promotes accurate reports by youth, questions should be stated in a nonjudgmental way that normalizes nonadherence (e.g., "Most kids forget to take their medications sometimes. How often do you forget to use your inhaler?"), rather than phrased in a manner that implies expectations of adherence (e.g., "How often do you use your inhaler?"). Additionally, to reduce Yes/No or other less informative or evasive responses, forced-choice answers can be provided for the child (e.g., "once a week," "a few times a week," "most days").

School-based personnel can also play an important role in helping children and families to recognize signs of uncontrolled or worsening asthma and CF. For example, if a school professional notices changes in activity level, increased use of medication during the day, or other potential changes to the student's health, the observations can be communicated to the family. This process can shed light on symptoms occurring in the school setting or during the school day that a parent may not otherwise know about (National Asthma Education and Prevention Program [NAEPP], U.S. Department of Health and Human Services [DHHS], & U.S. Department of Education, 2014). Finally, it is also important for school professionals to be aware of, and to understand, individual student's triggers and symptoms, particularly those that may be present in the school environment (NAEPP et al., 2014).

School-based professionals should ensure that each child has his or her AAP or recommended treatment plan for CF on file and should provide copies to teachers and staff who regularly interact with the child. Furthermore, health professionals should watch for and assess for signs of poorly controlled symptoms, which could include coughing, wheezing, shortness of breath, or chest tightness for asthma and CF. Health-office visits for both routine and acute asthma needs should be consistently documented, as should be urgent calls to parents or guardians for medication, school absences, and hospitalizations.

School Absences and Hospital Stays

Research has shown that an asthma diagnosis and a child's level of asthma control affect school attendance (i.e., absenteeism), economic costs, and perhaps academic performance (NAEPP et al., 2014). Many studies have shown that asthma is the leading cause of chronic-illness-related absences for children (CDC, 2017c), leading to many days missed from school and a large absenteeism cost (e.g., parent's missing work; Nurmagambetov, Khavjou, Murphy, & Orenstein, 2017). The absences are the result of a variety of factors, ranging from routine clinic visits to asthma exacerbations/attacks and poor asthma control (CDC, 2017c; NAEPP et al., 2014). Research has also suggested that absenteeism may be a clinically significant health status indicator for children with asthma, as more frequent absences were found to be related to poorer asthma control and greater asthma severity (Hsu, Qin, Beavers, & Mirabelli, 2016). Additionally, asthma-related absenteeism may affect school success, particularly if a large number of days are missed. Research findings are mixed in this area, however, particularly given that an asthma diagnosis is often confounded by other sociodemographic factors that could affect school attendance (Bloom et al., 2013; Kintner et al., 2015).

Similar to asthma, and given the nature of the illness, CF means that many children have 504 plans that accommodate extensive absences due to exacerbations, hospitalizations, and routine clinic appointments (CFF, n.d.). Research has shown that many absences can lead students to fall behind in school or even to drop out of school due to their not meeting educational milestones. Therefore, without proper supports, youth can feel marginalized or grow to dislike school due to frustration (Jamieson et al., 2014).

Accommodations, Policies, and Legal Considerations

In supporting students with chronic health concerns, school-based health professionals often act as care coordinators between the school and clinical teams and families, and guide school-based decision-making and actions (Keeher Engelke et al., 2014). According to the most recent version of *Managing Asthma: A Guide for Schools*, partnership among the family, physician, and school is vital to success for youth with asthma (NAEPP et al., 2014). Supportive school personnel and policies can help youth to feel a sense of normalcy and not to be limited in the school environment due to their condition (that is, they can participate in physical and extracurricular activities). There has also been some evidence to show that school-based health professionals can improve outcomes like academic success and self-management behaviors among children with asthma (Keeher Engelke et al., 2014). However, it can be difficult for staff members to choose the most suitable course of action for each child living with asthma or CF. School systems may need to develop new policies to be responsive to trends in care for these youth, for example.

Safety is an important area of concern in the school environment, particularly regarding lowering the risk for triggering an asthma attack or transmitting infection among students with CF. Specifically, for many youth with asthma, it is important to minimize exposure to dust, smoke, fumes, and strong smells, because these exposures can trigger a symptom flare. For schools with more than one student diagnosed with CF, it is extremely important that the children remain a safe distance (6 or more feet) from one another to decrease the likelihood of cross-infection (CFF, n.d.; Tapper Strawhacker & Wellendorf, 2004). For youth with CF, school-based professionals can promote a healthier school environment by taking a series of four actions. The first action is to reduce the time that children with CF are in close proximity (less than 6 feet from one another). Overlap in class and activity schedules and gathering locations (e.g., classrooms, bathrooms, drinking fountains) also should be minimized (CFF, n.d.). The remaining three tasks apply more globally to the entire school environment and focus on encouraging students, teachers, and staff to engage in health-promoting behaviors: (1) washing hands frequently, (2) avoiding coming to school ill and covering coughs and sneezes appropriately, and (3) staying up to date on vaccinations (Tapper Strawhacker & Wellendorf, 2004). These efforts can significantly decrease the likelihood of serious infections among children with CF, which lead to school absences, worsened disease severity, and even death (CFF, n.d.).

Regardless of potential barriers and challenges, the needs of the individual student with asthma or CF should be assessed so that appropriate accommodations, or 504 plans, can be devised and implemented. The accommodations might include posting assignments online, seating that enables easy access to snacks and fluids or supplies and medications, unrestricted bathroom access, and the ability to modify accommodations in response to changing health status. Additional accommodations for students with CF and asthma might include making time during the day to take medication (such as use an inhaler or take pancreatic enzyme supplements) and to complete required therapies (e.g., airway clearance), facilitating access to the nurse, and setting up a school-based medical emergency plan (CFF, n.d.; Tapper Strawhacker & Wellendorf, 2004). Physical activity-related accommodations also promote the health and well-being of young people with asthma and CF; therefore, procedures should support children's opportunities to take part in these activities. For instance, clinic teams can create AAPs (or other plans in the case of CF) that include taking medication before exercise and then share the plans with relevant school personnel. It is preferred that school professionals normalize the need for accommodations and work with families to ensure the accommodations do not draw a great deal of attention to the student, to prevent school or activity avoidance and social embarrassment.

Awareness of state laws regarding the provision of educational resources (e.g., home tutoring if a child experiences frequent or prolonged absences) will help schools inform and advocate for families. If a school plans to serve a role in care coordination, however, special mechanisms must be in place to carefully establish and maintain communication among the school, clinic-based teams, and families. School policy should account for issues related to permission to have contact with clinic teams, to monitor and act on children's symptoms and needs, and to discuss clinical decisions with families (Tapper Strawhacker & Wellendorf, 2004). School personnel need to be mindful of these policies as well as family preferences about privacy and care coordination. For example, the family of a child with CF may not want a school-based health professional to share their child's diagnosis with students or school staff. Overall, consideration of legal issues related to privacy and creating a nonjudgmental, child-centered school ethos should be the focus of school policies.

Social Environment and Peers

School is a social environment; thus, peer interactions are an important consideration for chronically ill students. When observing children with asthma and CF, it is important for school professionals to note if the students appear to be isolated or are experiencing peer-based discrimination related to their health. Youth with CF can become dissatisfied with their bodies, particularly given the disease's impact on growth and puberty, and they may feel different from their peers. They also may be embarrassed by the attention drawn to their symptoms (e.g., coughing, gastrointestinal concerns). Students with CF may also feel that peers perceive them negatively when they engage in care-related activities, such as airway clearance (Pinquart, 2013). Similarly, youth with asthma may avoid activities (e.g., participating on a school sports team) due to concerns about performance limitations caused by symptoms; consequently, these children may have fewer opportunities to experience positive peer interactions. Youth also can feel socially isolated due to frequent absences from school and its outings, which can make it difficult for them to establish and maintain friendships and romantic relationships (Jamieson et al., 2014). Indeed, social embarrassment is a significant barrier for many youth with CF, sometimes leading to avoidance of school and other social activities (Teicher, 1969; Withers, 2012). This is also true for youth with severe asthma. Finally, another notable area is career and education options for the future, as some students may feel a sense of limited independence due to their condition, particularly youth with CF (Jamieson et al., 2014). Transition IEPs (individualized educational plans) can be helpful in targeting a balance between future goals and CF care (CFF, n.d.; Tapper Strawhacker & Wellendorf, 2004).

Psychological Comorbidities with Asthma and CF

Not surprisingly, youth with chronic illness, including CF and asthma, are at risk for psychological distress, including high rates of both anxiety and depression (Ferro & Boyle, 2015; Goodwin, Fergusson, & Horwood, 2004). In fact, the CF Foundation guidelines recommend that CF care centers conduct routine psychological screening, with a particular focus on anxiety and depression, in patients with CF and their caregivers (Quittner et al., 2016). In addition, psychological distress has been linked to worsened health outcomes and decreased medication adherence (Hilliard, Eakin, Borrelli, Green, & Riekert, 2015; Smith, Modi, Quittner, & Wood, 2010). Accordingly, school-based providers can serve an important role in detecting potential signs of psychological distress in students with asthma or CF, such as changes in mood, demeanor, or activity level, restlessness, fatigue, irritability, suicidal ideation/self-harm behaviors, decreased socializing/increased isolation, or decreasing academic performance. Any signs of potential psychological distress should be discussed with the student and communicated to the family and other members of the care team, as appropriate. Referrals to therapeutic services and other resources for managing psychological distress can also be provided to students and their caregivers. It is important to note that, when having these conversations with youth and caregivers, school-based personnel should normalize the stress and demands associated with managing a chronic illness, emphasize the potential benefits of resources and therapeutic services, and use language and a tone that communicate empathy.

CASE EXAMPLES TO ILLUSTRATE KEY CONCEPTS

Asthma

Mario is a 6-year-old male of Mexican and African American descent, who lives with his mother, stepfather, and two younger siblings (ages 2 and 5 years) in an apartment in an urban community. Mario was diagnosed with moderate persistent asthma and allergies at age 5 after several episodes of bronchitis and "infantile wheezing." Despite prescriptions for an inhaled corticosteroid (ICS) and rescue bronchodilator (albuterol), Mario continues to experience asthma exacerbations approximately 1 to 2 times a week during the school year, and about once a month during the summer. His triggers for asthma flares are physical activity or exertion (e.g., physical education class), cigarette smoke, and seasonal allergies. Since experiencing a severe and frightening asthma attack during recess in kindergarten, Mario avoids most physical activity at school. He frequently complains of difficulty breathing and dizziness prior to recess or gym class. Mario's fear escalates until his teacher sends him to the school nurse for evaluation and rescue medication. Mario's mother also reports that a few times a month, he wakes up with wheezing and chest tightness and these symptoms quickly intensify, resulting in Mario's becoming panicky and difficult to console. Thus, he misses an excessive number of school days and the absences have led to his mother's missing too much work at a local bakery, putting her employment at risk. When Mario's mother was questioned about his asthma care, she appeared confused about the importance of daily preventive medication use and instead said that Mario's asthma seemed to be best controlled with his rescue medication (albuterol). She also stated that Mario has tantrums when taking any asthma medication because he says that he is "choking" from the spacer mask on his face. She admitted that it is easier to just give Mario albuterol when he needs it rather than fight Mario to give him preventive medication each day. In support of his mother's report, the medical team's review of Mario's prescription refills showed sporadic replacement of preventive medication, but frequent refills for albuterol.

Cystic Fibrosis

Rachel is a 16-year-old Caucasian female who was diagnosed with CF soon after birth. She resides primarily with her single mother, a 16-year-old fraternal twin brother (who is free of the diagnosis), and a 12-year-old brother who also has CF. Rachel's parents divorced when she was 8 years old and neither has remarried. Rachel's father has a history of alcoholism, but reportedly has been sober the past year. The children stay with their father every other weekend and many holidays. Rachel's mother works as a nursing assistant, while her father is employed as a car mechanic. Rachel's CF has deteriorated significantly over the past couple of years, resulting in frequent school absences due to hospitalizations and clinic visits to treat exacerbations. Although Rachel was involved in school sports and organizations in junior high, her participation has declined dramatically in high school. She reported that she was embarrassed because her peers were afraid they could catch something infectious from her because she was always coughing, particularly in physical activities. Because she does not participate in these activities anymore, Rachel said that she has become increasingly disconnected from her friends. When she gets home from school, she tends to go to her room and watch television, away from her brothers, who "annoy" her. Rachel rarely helps with chores around the house because she is "too tired." In fact, she sleeps a lot and her school grades have dropped from A's and B's to largely C's and D's due to absence-related poor homework and classwork completion. Rachel reports that being at school is very stressful now because she feels behind in her schoolwork and "just can't catch up." It has become so challenging that she says she may just drop out and try to get her GED. Rachel's mother expressed additional concern that Rachel does not eat well (e.g., she prefers to eat in her room), has lost weight over the past several months, and refuses to let her mother help with or monitor her CF treatments. Rachel's mother reported that any discussion of CF care leads to a screaming argument with her daughter. Moreover, Rachel's father reportedly lets Rachel skip treatments when she is staying with him, because he feels that she is old enough to make her own decisions.

CONCLUSION AND FUTURE DIRECTIONS

As described throughout this chapter and as is highlighted in the case examples, there are several considerations for school-based personnel to apply when presented with a child with asthma or CF. First, knowledge of the condition, its medical care and prognosis, and associated risk, preventive, and sociocultural factors may be helpful in terms of identifying, understanding, and supporting the child. Knowledge can also assist in identifying potential barriers for youth and families, as well as aid in coming up with ways to circumvent some of the barriers. Furthermore, there are specific strategies for identifying and managing asthma and CF in the school setting, as well as school-related concerns and psychological comorbidities. Topics of particular relevance include school absences and hospital stays, the physical environment, school-based accommodations, other legal and policy-related concerns, social environment and peers, and psychological distress, including anxiety and depression. Although there are common issues and patterns seen in youth with asthma and CF, each student is unique in his or her background, struggles, and support needs in disease management and school functioning. It is beyond the scope of this chapter to provide a comprehensive summary of potential difficulties in the school environment and evidence-based guidance to address these challenging situations; however, information regarding important considerations (Handout 18.1) and potential resources for school personnel, students, and their families (Handout 18.2) is included at the end of this chapter.

REFERENCES

Akinbami, L. J., Moorman, J. E., Garbe, P. L., & Sondik, E. J. (2009). Status of childhood asthma in the United States, 1980–2007. *Pediatrics, 123*(3), S131–S145. doi:10.1542/peds.2008-2233C

Beers, M. H., & Berkow, R. (Eds.). (1999). *The Merck manual* (17th ed., pp. 2366–2371). Whitehouse Station, NJ: Merck Research Laboratories.

Bloom, B., Jones, L. I., & Freeman, G. (2013). Summary health statistics for U.S. children: National Health Interview Survey, 2012. National Center for Health Statistics. Retrieved from http://www.cdc.gov/nchs/data/series/sr_10/sr10_258. pdf

Bonaiuto, M. (2007). School nurse case management: Achieving health and educational outcomes. *Journal of School Nursing, 23*, 202–208.

Centers for Disease Control and Prevention. (2017a). *Asthma.* Retrieved from https://www.cdc.gov/asthma/default.htm

Centers for Disease Control and Prevention. (2017b). *Learn how to control asthma.* Retrieved from https://www.cdc.gov/asthma/faqs.htm

Centers for Disease Control and Prevention. (2017c). *Asthma's impact on the nation.* Retrieved from https://www.cdc.gov/asthma/impacts_nation/default.htm

Cystic Fibrosis Foundation. (n.d.). *About cystic fibrosis.* Retrieved from https://www.cff.org/What-is-CF/About-Cystic-Fibrosis/

Dodge, J. A., Lewis, P. A., Stanton, M., & Wilsher, J. (2007). Cystic fibrosis mortality and survival in the UK: 1947–2003. *European Respiratory Journal, 29*(3), 522–526. doi: 10.1183/09031936.00099506

Ferro, M. A., & Boyle, M. H. (2015). The impact of chronic physical illness, maternal depressive symptoms, family functioning, and self-esteem on symptoms of anxiety and depression in children. *Journal of Abnormal Child Psychology, 43*(1), 177–187. doi:10.1007/s10802-014-9893-6

FitzSimmons, S. C. (1994). The changing epidemiology of cystic fibrosis. *Current Problems in Pediatrics, 24*(5), 171–179. doi:10.1016/0045-9380(94)90034-5

Goodwin, R. D., Fergusson, D. M., & Horwood, L. J. (2004). Asthma and depressive and anxiety disorders among young persons in the community. *Psychological Medicine, 34*(8), 1465–1474. doi:10.1017/S0033291704002739

Hilliard, M. E., Eakin, M. N., Borrelli, B., Green, A., & Riekert, K. A. (2015). Medication beliefs mediate between depressive symptoms and medication adherence in cystic fibrosis. *Health Psychology, 34*(5), 496–504. doi:10.1037/hea0000136

Holmes, B. W., Sheetz, A., Allison, M., Ancona, R., Attisha, E., Beers, N., . . . Weiss-Harrison, A. (2016). Role of the school nurse in providing school health services. *Pediatrics*, e20160852. doi:10.1542/peds.2016-0852

Hsu, J., Qin, X., Beavers, S. F., & Mirabelli, M. C. (2016). Asthma-related school absenteeism, morbidity, and modifiable factors. *American Journal of Preventive Medicine*, *51*(1), 23–32. doi:10.1016/j.amepre.2015.12.012

Jamieson, N., Fitzgerald, D., Singh-Grewal, D., Hanson, C. S., Craig, J. C., & Tong, A. (2014). Children's experiences of cystic fibrosis: A systematic review of qualitative studies. *Pediatrics*, *133*(6), e1683–e1697. doi:10.1542/peds.2014-0009

Keeher Engelke, M., Swanson, M., & Guttu, M. (2014). Process and outcomes of school nurse case management for students with asthma. *Journal of School Nursing*, *30*(3), 196–205. doi:10.1177/105984051350708.

Khan, T. Z., Wagener, J. S., Bost, T., Martinez, J., Accurso, F. J., & Riches, D. W. (1995). Early pulmonary inflammation in infants with cystic fibrosis. *American Journal of Respiratory Critical Care Medicine*, *151*(4), 1075–1082. doi:10.1164/ajrccm.151.4.7697234

Kintner, E. K., Cook, G., Marti, N., Allen, A., Stoddard, D., Harmon, P., . . . Van Egeren L.A. (2015). Effectiveness of a school and community-based academic asthma health education program on use of effective asthma self-care behaviors in older school-age students. *Pediatric Nursing*, *20*, 62–75. doi:10.1111/jspn.12099.

Lieu, T. A., Lozano, P., Finkelstein, J. A., Chi, F. W., Jensvold, N. G., Capra, A. M., . . . Farber, H. J. (2002). Racial/ethnic variation in asthma status and management practices among children in managed Medicaid. *Pediatrics*, *109*(5), 857–865. doi:10.1542/peds.109.5.857

MacKenzie, T., Gifford, A. H., Sabadosa, K. A., Quinton, H. B., Knapp, E. A., Goss, C. H., & Marshall, B. C. (2014). Longevity of patients with cystic fibrosis in 2000 to 2010 and beyond: Survival analysis of the Cystic Fibrosis Foundation Patient Registry. *Annals of Internal Medicine*, *161*, 233–241. doi:10.7326/M13-0636

Moricca, M. L., Grasska, M. A., BMarthaler, M., Morphew, T., Weismuller, P. C., & Galant, S. P. (2012). School asthma screening and case management: Attendance and learning outcomes. *The Journal of School Nursing*, *29*(2), 104–112. doi:10.1177/1059840512452668

National Asthma Education and Prevention Program [NAEEP], National Heart, Lung, and Blood Institute [NHLBI], U.S. Department of Health and Human Services [DHHS], & U.S. Department of Education. (2014). *Managing asthma: A guide for schools*. Retrieved from https://www.nhlbi.nih.gov/files/docs/resources/lung/asth_sch.pdf

National Heart, Lung, and Blood Institute. (2014a). *What is asthma?* Retrieved from https://www.nhlbi.nih.gov/health/health-topics/topics/asthma/

National Heart, Lung, and Blood Institute. (2014b). *Managing asthma: A guide for schools* (NIH 14-2650). Retrieved from https://www.nhlbi.nih.gov/files/docs/resources/lung/NACI_ManagingAsthma-508%20FINAL.pdf.

Newacheck, P. W., & Halfon, N. (2000). Prevalence, impact, and trends in childhood disability due to asthma. *Archives of Pediatric and Adolescent Medicine*, *154*(3), 287–293. doi:10.1001/archpedi.154.3.287

Nurmagambetov, T., Khavjou, O., Murphy, L., & Orenstein, D. (2017). State-level medical and absenteeism cost of asthma in the United States. *Journal of Asthma*, *54*(4), 357–370. doi:10.1080/02770903.2016.1218013

Pinquart, M. (2013). Do the parent–child relationship and parenting behaviors differ between families with a child with and without chronic illness? A meta-analysis. *Journal of Pediatric Psychology, 38*(7), 708–721. doi:10.1093/jpepsy/jst020

Quittner, A. L., Abbott, J., Georgiopoulos, A. M., Goldbeck, L., Smith, B., Hempstead, S. E., . . . Elborn, S. (2016). International Committee on Mental Health in Cystic Fibrosis: Cystic Fibrosis Foundation and European Cystic Fibrosis Society consensus statements for screening and treating depression and anxiety. *Thorax, 71*(1), 26–34. doi:10.1136/thoraxjnl-2015-207488

Sawicki, G. S., Sellers, D. E., & Robinson, W. M. (2009). High treatment burden in adults with cystic fibrosis: Challenges to disease self-management. *Journal of Cystic Fibrosis, 8*(2), 91–96. doi:10.1016/j.jcf.2008.09.007

Smith, B. A., Modi, A. C., Quittner, A. L., & Wood, B. L. (2010). Depressive symptoms in children with cystic fibrosis and parents and its effects on adherence to airway clearance. *Pediatric Pulmonology, 45*(8), 756–763. doi:10.1002/ppul.21238

Stallings, V. A., Stark, L. J., Robinson, K. A., Feranchak, A. P., Quinton, H., Clinical Practice Guidelines on Growth and Nutrition Subcommittee, & Ad Hoc Working Group. (2008). Evidence-based practice recommendations for nutrition-related management of children and adults with cystic fibrosis and pancreatic insufficiency: Results of a systematic review. *Journal of the American Dietetic Association, 108*(5), 832–839. doi:10.1016/j.jcf.2008.09.007

Tapper Strawhacker, M. A., & Wellendorf, J. (2004). Caring for children with cystic fibrosis: A collaborative clinical and school approach. *The Journal of School Nursing, 20*(1), 5–11. doi:10.1177/10598405040200010301

Taras, H., Wright, S., Brennan, J., Campana, J., & Lofgren, R. (2004). Impact of school nurse case management on students with asthma. *Journal of School Health, 74*, 213–219.

Teicher, J. D. (1969). Psychological aspects of cystic fibrosis in children and adolescents. *California Medicine, 110*(5), 371–374.

Withers, A. L. (2012). Management issues for adolescents with cystic fibrosis. *Pulmonary Medicine, 2012*, 134132. doi:10.1155/2012/134132

HANDOUT 18.1

IMPORTANT CONSIDERATIONS FOR SCHOOL PERSONNEL

Learn

1. Learn about the child's condition, including a basic level of understanding of, and appreciation for, the medical care, prognosis, and level of treatment involvement.
2. Learn about risk and protective factors for the illness, as well as relevant sociocultural considerations.
3. Learn the legal and policy-related issues involved with supporting the child's success, including school-based accommodations and related accommodation plans.

Identify, Manage, and Intervene

1. Become an active observer and notice changes in the student's behavior, mood, or demeanor.
2. Ask nonjudgmental questions about symptoms, psychological distress, and medication adherence.
3. Help youth learn to recognize symptoms and signs of their condition, and provide direction, as needed, to help them understand their care regimen and learn better disease self-management.
4. Develop a checklist of potential barriers to school engagement and structure the environment to reduce barriers to participation.
5. Inform parent/guardian and the care team, as applicable and appropriate, about behavior observed in the school setting as well as conversations with youth.
6. Provide resources and information to families to help them best advocate for their child (e.g., referrals for therapeutic services, self-help resources, information on 504 plans)

Disseminate and Implement

1. Spread awareness about laws, regulations, and guidelines and the importance of supporting children with chronic illnesses and improving their likelihood of success.
2. Work with other school-based professionals to implement a coordinated school health program.

Handout 18.2

Additional Resources for Families and Educators

Coordinated School Health Program/Collaborative Model of School Health
- Whole School, Whole Community, Whole Child (WSCC)
  https://www.cdc.gov/healthyschools/wscc/wsccmodel_update_508tagged.pdf
  https://www.cdc.gov/healthyschools/wscc/index.htm

Asthma Care in the School Setting
- https://www.cdc.gov/healthyschools/asthma/strategies.htm
- https://www.jmcsh.org/content/jmcsh/documents/asthma_mgmt_schl.pdf

American Lung Association—*Open Airways for Schools*
- http://www.lung.org/assets/documents/asthma/open-airways-for-schools.pdf
- http://www.lung.org/openairways

Allergy and Asthma Foundation of America (http://www.aafa.org/page/asthma.aspx)
- Asthma Care Training (ACT) for Kids Initative (https://www.cdc.gov/asthma/interventions/act_researchbase.htm)
- Parent and healthcare professional materials and tool, including free downloads

American Academy of Allergy, Asthma, and Immunology (https://www.aaaai.org/)

Allergy and Asthma Network (http://www.allergyasthmanetwork.org)
- Allergy & Asthma Network Mothers of Asthmatics (AANMA): http://www.asthmacommunitynetwork.org/node/2547

American Thoracic Society (http://www.thoracic.org/)

Cystic Fibrosis Foundation (https://www.cff.org/)

National Heart, Lung, & Blood Institute (https://www.nhlbi.nih.gov/)
- *Managing Asthma: A Guide for Schools*: https://www.nhlbi.nih.gov/health-pro/resources/lung/asthma-management-school-guide
- https://www.nhlbi.nih.gov/health/resources/lung

19

Type 1 and Type 2 Diabetes

KATHERINE A. S. GALLAGHER AND MARISA E. HILLIARD ∎

OVERVIEW

Type 1 Diabetes

Type 1 diabetes (T1D) is an autoimmune condition in which the pancreas stops producing insulin, a hormone that converts sugar (glucose) into energy for cells (American Diabetes Association, 2017). This results in elevated blood glucose levels (i.e., hyperglycemia), which must be treated with exogenous insulin to return them to normative levels. Low blood glucose levels (i.e., hypoglycemia) also occur and must be treated with exogenous glucose to return them to target levels. Both severe hypoglycemia and hyperglycemia carry significant risk for short- and long-term health complications, including disorientation, diabetic ketoacidosis, nerve damage, cardiac problems, blindness, stroke, and death. T1D onset is typically acute and requires urgent medical care to manage extreme hyperglycemia. Although the exact cause of T1D is unknown, researchers suspect that a combination of a genetic predisposition with an environmental stressor (e.g., viral illness) triggers the onset of the condition (Skyler et al., 2016).

T1D management involves tasks that occur throughout the day and night, primarily frequent monitoring of blood glucose levels and responding to the levels by taking insulin or glucose, with the goal of returning levels to a specified range. Common causes of hyperglycemia include carbohydrate intake, sedentary behavior, stress, illness, dehydration, and hormonal activity; common causes of hypoglycemia include administration of insulin, physical activity, and skipping or postponing meals or snacks. However, in people with diabetes, glucose levels often fluctuate without an identifiable cause, necessitating frequent monitoring. Blood glucose is typically monitored using a blood glucose meter, which measures glucose in a blood droplet obtained via fingerprick. Typical recommendations include at least 4 to 5 blood glucose checks per day, including before meals, upon waking, and before sleep, as well as in other situations (e.g., if feeling unwell, and before and after physical activity). Some youth use a continuous glucose monitor, comprised of a sensor worn under the child's skin that measures glucose every 5 minutes and sends data to a handheld receiver or a mobile device or smartphone. Continuous glucose monitors require less frequent fingerprick checks and can also send glucose values to other devices (e.g., parents' smartphones, teachers' or nurses' tablets). Students with T1D should be permitted to check and treat their glucose levels frequently throughout the school day.

Exogenous (e.g., injected) insulin is required to return rising blood glucose levels to a safe range and sustain life. Calculations to determine the necessary dose of insulin are based on current blood glucose level, number of carbohydrates consumed or planned to be eaten, and awareness of impending physical activity or other circumstances that might affect glucose levels. Each person with T1D has a unique regimen of insulin needs, determined by the treating medical provider. For many youth, insulin is dosed according to individualized ratios of insulin to carbohydrates, and children often take a basal amount of insulin at specified times per day and then require a bolus of insulin before meals and snacks. Insulin is administered via a syringe, which requires the insulin to be drawn up from refrigerated vials, via small portable "pen" that contains insulin and a needle; or via a pump attached to the body that infuses insulin throughout the day at adjustable levels based on need.

Type 2 Diabetes

Type 2 diabetes (T2D) is a metabolic condition in which the body stops producing enough insulin or becomes less effective at using insulin to convert glucose into energy. This results in elevated glucose levels, and there is less risk for hypoglycemia. T2D onset is typically slower, often without acute medical problems or diagnosis. Risk factors for T2D include genetic predisposition, low physical activity, and central adiposity. Although prevalence of pediatric T1D in the United States is higher than pediatric T2D, T2D prevalence is increasing quickly, particularly among racial and ethnic minority groups (Mayer-Davis et al., 2017).

For many youth with T2D, the primary treatment is careful attention to nutritional intake and physical activity as recommended by their treating medical providers. Youth with T2D may be prescribed insulin injections, oral medications, both, or neither, depending upon medical recommendations. Recommendations for blood glucose monitoring vary, and most youth with T2D are not required to check their glucose levels as frequently as youth with T1D.

Related Conditions

Other, less common forms of diabetes include other genetic variants of diabetes, diabetes during pregnancy (gestational diabetes), and diabetes in the context of another medical condition or treatment (e.g., steroid-induced diabetes). These topics are beyond the scope of this chapter, which focuses on T1D and T2D in children and adolescents.

DIABETES AT SCHOOL

Educating Staff and Students

It is important to inform the faculty, administrators, and support staff (e.g., recess monitors, food service staff) who regularly interact with the student about the child's diagnosis and treatment needs, and that there are circumstances during which it is necessary for staff to provide additional supports or allowances. For instance, there will be times when the child with diabetes must leave class to visit the nurse, either at scheduled (e.g., before lunch) or at unscheduled times (e.g., to check or treat an out-of-range glucose level). The child may need to carry a bag, snacks, water, medications, and a smartphone or other device to monitor blood glucose or to administer insulin. Youth with diabetes can eat most foods and may need to take insulin or medication prior to eating, so it is often helpful to coordinate with the classroom teacher, family, and school nurse ahead of time to ensure the student can participate in food-related events. Youth with diabetes should be allowed to make choices about where to complete diabetes-care tasks (e.g., in classroom, nursing office), and questions about care tasks should be addressed with the child or family individually. Staff should be trained to respond in case of emergency, such as administering glucose orally or via a glucagon injection for a severe hypoglycemic event. Table 19.1 supplies a list of additional resources about diabetes management at school.

It is also important to help peers understand basic facts about diabetes: diabetes is not "contagious," the child is not at fault for having diabetes, and it is not necessary for peers to monitor or to correct the child's food choices. Peers can be informed that children with diabetes check their blood glucose and take medicine using special tools, some of which may make noise or remain attached to the child's body, and care tasks might occur in the classroom or in the nurse's office. Peers can also be informed that children with diabetes may need to eat snacks at certain times. Importantly, peers should be instructed that children with diabetes can do all the same activities as children without diabetes. When possible, provide developmentally appropriate diabetes education materials to students, such as reading a book to the class to increase knowledge of, and to normalize, diabetes. To the degree they are interested, the child and parents may wish to be involved in shaping the education plan and to participate in this education.

Symptom Response and Management

Diabetes typically requires completion of many care tasks throughout the day, and collaboration among school staff and families is helpful to ensure tasks are

Table 19.1. WEBSITES AND RESOURCES FOR PROFESSIONALS

Resource	Target Populations	What is Offered
American Diabetes Association www.diabetes.org/living-with-diabetes/parents-and-kids/	All ages, caregivers	Educational resources about diabetes, handouts for families and providers about a range of topics
American Diabetes Association: Safe at School www.diabetes.org/living-with-diabetes/parents-and-kids/diabetes-care-at-school/	Providers and caregivers for school-age youth	Legal protections for children with diabetes, position statements and resources for care at school, sample written care plans
American Association of Diabetes Educators: Position Statement on Management of Children with Diabetes in the School Setting https://www.diabeteseducator.org/docs/default-source/practice/practice-resources/position-statements/diabetes-in-the-school-setting-position-statement_final.pdf)	School-based providers	Legal framework for diabetes care at school, specific recommendations and tasks for which diabetes educators can provide support to school staff
American Diabetes Association: Position Statement on Diabetes Care in the School Setting http://care.diabetesjournals.org/content/38/10/1958	School-based providers, caregivers	Guidelines for diabetes medical management plans at school, responsibilities of the various stakeholders (e.g., caregivers, school staff, youth)
Lilly Glucagon www.lillyglucagon.com	Providers and caregivers	Step-by-step instructions about how to use glucagon to treat severe hypoglycemia, as well as a free smartphone app
Beyond Type 1 www.beyondtype1.org	Adolescents and young adults, caregivers	Educational resources about diabetes and mental health concerns, reading and sharing stories about people with diabetes
College Diabetes Network www.collegediabetesnetwork.org	Adolescents and young adults transitioning to college and employment	Resources about diabetes management away from home and at work, connecting with college-age peers with diabetes, scholarships
T1EverydayMagic www.t1everydaymagic.com/	Younger children and preteens, newer-onset diabetes	Free e-books, recipes, diabetes-themed activities to support healthy adjustment to diabetes

completed appropriately and at the correct times, to ensure the child's health and safety. Given the nature and frequency of required diabetes care tasks during the school day, this is particularly relevant for youth with T1D and students with T2D who take insulin. Staff and families should develop a plan for maintenance care, including when and where the child is expected to check blood glucose and take insulin or medications (e.g., nurse's office, classroom), who assists in task completion, and in what situations parents will be involved or contacted (e.g., in event of high or low blood glucose). A plan should also be developed to respond when a child does not present to the predetermined location for diabetes care tasks, such as a staff member's fetching the child.

Staff and families are also advised to develop a plan for response care, such as in the event of an out-of-range blood glucose or of illness. In addition to contacting caregivers, the plan may include more frequent blood glucose monitoring, testing for ketones, administration of additional insulin or sugar-free fluids, administration of fast-acting glucose orally or via intramuscular injection, and determinations about when a child should leave school or receive urgent medical care. In children with T1D, hypoglycemia and hyperglycemia require urgent attention. Children may have rapid behavioral and emotional changes when experiencing an out-of-range blood glucose. Children experiencing hypoglycemia may feel nervous, shaky, dizzy, hungry, irritable, or tearful, and they may appear pale. Children experiencing hyperglycemia may feel irritable, angry, or thirsty, they may require frequent urination, and they may have headache or abdominal pain. In addition, experiencing high or low blood sugars can be distressing or children may feel unable to control themselves. Hypoglycemia and hyperglycemia are both dangerous if left untreated, and out-of-range blood sugars should be monitored and treated with haste. If a child with diabetes demonstrates unusual or disruptive behavior, an adult should prompt or assist the child to check blood glucose immediately. If blood glucose is out of range, staff should follow the child's agreed-upon diabetes care plan. It is often recommended that children be allowed to check their blood glucose or seek adult assistance if they suspect or notice an out-of-range blood glucose.

DIABETES-RELATED PSYCHOLOGICAL AND BEHAVIORAL CONCERNS

People with diabetes have an elevated risk for experiencing depressive symptoms (Lawrence et al., 2006), which makes diabetes management more difficult and increases their risk of poor health outcomes (Hood, Rausch, & Dolan, 2011; McGrady & Hood, 2010). Contributors to the risk for depressed mood include biological factors, such as inflammation (Hood et al., 2012; Moulton, Pickup, & Ismail, 2015), low engagement in self-management behaviors due to low mood or energy (McGrady & Hood, 2010), and the ongoing stress of managing and coping with a chronic medical condition (Van Bastelaar et al., 2010). In addition, many children develop diabetes distress and burnout, which may have some overlap with depressive symptoms but are distinct in their specific link to the stressors of daily diabetes care (Fisher, Gonzalez & Polonsky, 2014). Declines in self-management behaviors may be associated with diabetes distress and burnout, in that children can become fatigued or overwhelmed by the daily burden of diabetes management and may begin avoiding tasks, which can result in suboptimal diabetes health outcomes (Hilliard et al., 2016).

Anxiety symptoms also occur in youth with diabetes, and the anxiety may relate to suboptimal diabetes management behaviors and health outcomes (Herzer & Hood, 2010). Anxiety may be caused by fear of injection pain, needle phobia, worries about parent reactions to out-of-range blood glucose values, or discomfort with completing diabetes tasks in front of peers (Wasserman et al., 2017). Many families report fear of hypoglycemia, particularly when diabetes is newly diagnosed or in a child who has difficulty noticing signs of dropping or low blood glucose (Driscoll, Raymond, Naranjo & Patton, 2016). Although attention to blood glucose fluctuations is a necessary part of diabetes management, extreme fear of hypoglycemia can interfere with other important health behaviors, such as sleep, food choices, engaging in physical activity, and administering insulin as recommended by medical professionals.

At different developmental stages, responsibility for executing diabetes care shifts between parents and youth, which can lead to tension or misunderstandings among family members, inconsistent adherence to the care tasks, and ultimately poorer health outcomes (Anderson, 2004; Markowitz, Garvey, & Laffel, 2015). Understanding the family's perspectives on the child's level of responsibility for self-management tasks, as well as the degree to which the child requires an adult to conduct tasks or to directly supervise task completion, is essential to ensure that expectations at school match those at home. Importantly, some adult monitoring of children's diabetes task completion is recommended at all ages, but the direct involvement of adults in task execution may differ.

Children with diabetes may experience both subtle and overt diabetes-related stigma and bullying (Browne, Ventura, Mosely, & Speight, 2013; Schabert, Browne, Mosely, & Speight, 2013). At school, peers unfamiliar with diabetes may make unhelpful comments or jokes that can be hurtful (e.g., referring to a diabetes care device and asking, "Are you a robot?"). Even well-intentioned peers and staff may ask questions or make comments that can be frustrating to hear on a regular basis (e.g., "You can't eat that!"). Individuals often confuse T1D and T2D and hold inaccurate views about diabetes etiology or treatment recommendations (e.g., "Did you eat too much sugar?"), which children may not know how to respond to or to correct. Misinformation can also lead to overt stigmatization as well (e.g., "I'm not touching you, I might catch diabetes!").

Youth with diabetes have higher rates of disordered eating behaviors, including binge eating, restricting, and covert eating, as well as body image concerns (Young-Hyman & Davis, 2010; Young et al., 2013). Children with diabetes are asked to closely monitor food intake, count carbohydrates, and control their eating in ways that children without diabetes are usually not asked to do, which may evolve into unhealthy levels of dietary restriction. Because insulin can cause weight gain, youth may manipulate insulin doses to lose weight. Some children may eat extra snacks without informing their parents or taking insulin, which may cause high blood sugar levels and contribute to family conflict. Because physical activity is known to reduce insulin resistance and can help treat mild hyperglycemia (Schmitz et al., 2002), exercise is an important component of diabetes management; however, some children may engage in excessive exercise after a binge episode or to control their weight.

Diabetes may also be associated with neurocognitive concerns. Severe hypoglycemic episodes in early childhood can affect motor and visuospatial functioning, memory, and attention. Chronic hyperglycemia in adolescence may impact executive function and information processing (Desrocher & Rovet, 2004; Schwartz, Wasserman, Powell, & Axelrad, 2014).

RISK AND PROTECTIVE FACTORS

Diabetes-related risk and protective factors occur at the individual, family, social, and societal levels. The Pediatric Self-Management Model (Modi et al., 2012) and the Diabetes Resilience Model (Hilliard, Harris, & Weissberg-Benchell, 2012) summarize the research on modifiable and nonmodifiable influences that may affect self-management behaviors and health outcomes. For example, at the individual level, psychological distress (whether related to diabetes or not) is a risk factor for less engagement in diabetes self-management behaviors and suboptimal health outcomes, while feelings of self-confidence and optimism are considered protective factors. On a family level, parental distress and psychological problems, family conflict, and either too much or too little parental involvement in diabetes care are risk factors, while collaborative parental involvement that matches the child's developmental level is one of the strongest predictors of positive diabetes outcomes. Likely due to the correlations with lower socioeconomic status or having fewer parental resources for diabetes-related oversight, living in a single-parent household often predicts poor outcomes. Socially, data are mixed on the impact of peer relationships on diabetes outcomes; some data suggest that negative peer influences and overattention to social cues can be risk factors, while other data suggest that feeling supported by peers in relation to diabetes care can be protective. Recent data from a large survey of adolescents with T1D in Australia indicate that an individual's diabetes-related strengths (e.g., feelings of self-efficacy and support from others related to diabetes) predicted diabetes outcomes even after controlling for symptoms of depression and anxiety and parent–child conflict about diabetes (Hilliard et al., 2017), findings suggesting that identifying and supporting a child's protective factors may be an important step in helping the child to overcome risks and to achieve optimal diabetes outcomes.

CONSIDERATIONS FOR ASSESSMENT AND INTERVENTION

Assessment

A diagnostic interview, conducted by a qualified behavioral health clinician, will help identify the family's needs and potential goals for therapy. In addition to gathering relevant history, obtaining details about current difficulties for which the youth and family are seeking support, and screening for mental health concerns, it may be relevant to discuss diabetes-specific topics that can affect psychological well-being and functioning at school.

Clinicians may choose to inquire about diabetes management and how its demands are shared between the child and caregivers. Diabetes management is most successful when viewed by families as a collaborative effort, and it is important to set this expectation with families. Consider asking "Who helps you with your diabetes tasks?" and be specific about individual responsibilities (e.g., "For blood sugar checks, who pokes the finger?" or "Who helps you remember your pills?"). When asking about engagement in diabetes management behaviors, use language that normalizes imperfection. For instance, rather than asking "Do you ever miss a blood sugar check?" consider asking "When was the last time you checked blood sugar?" This allows an immediate opportunity for praise and exploration ("Great, you checked a couple of days ago—what helped you get the blood sugar check done that day?"). Asking "What time of day is hardest for you to check your blood sugar?" may allow the child to feel more comfortable being honest about the frequency of the behavior. It is also helpful to assess barriers to diabetes self-management tasks, such as "What makes it hard to exercise?" or "What gets in the way of taking insulin before eating?"

To assess diabetes distress, say "Diabetes can be really tough—what are the toughest parts for you about having diabetes?" It may also be helpful to discuss parts of diabetes management that are going well (e.g., consistently taking medications at home, enjoying physical activity) to identify and reinforce the child's strengths.

Given the risks of parent–child conflict about diabetes management, school providers may wish to assess family communication and relationships around diabetes. Speak with the child about diabetes-related communication, such as "What kinds of things do you and your parents argue about related to diabetes?" It may help to be more specific—for example, ask "When you have a high blood sugar, do you tell one of your parents? How does your parent react? What do they say?"

Children with diabetes may have different levels of comfort with telling friends and peers about diabetes. Ask children "Who at school knows you have diabetes?" and "How did they respond when you told them you had diabetes?" The answers to these questions could provide insight into children's social and emotional supports, and possibly allow the clinician to highlight positive experiences and the benefits of talking about feelings or difficult experiences. Also consider asking "What is it like for you when other kids ask questions about your diabetes?" and "How do you respond?" The answers to these questions can help clinicians identify and encourage adaptive interpretation and response to questions from peers, as well as to screen for possible or perceived bullying experiences. Table 19.2 lists validated measures that may offer additional insights for assessment and treatment, as well as aid in tracking targeted outcomes over the course of therapy.

Intervention

Psychosocial interventions for children with diabetes typically involve identifying and addressing psychological, behavioral, and interpersonal difficulties that could negatively affect diabetes management, health outcomes, and quality of life. Evidence-based intervention approaches to promote positive outcomes in children with diabetes target different levels of the child's environment using individual, family-based, and multisystemic approaches (Hilliard, Powell, & Anderson, 2017). There is very limited research on school-based psychosocial interventions for children with diabetes, yet data from other evidence-based interventions can inform school-based clinicians' efforts.

Adherence to recommended diabetes management tasks is a common reason for children with diabetes to be referred for behavioral health services. Multicomponent interventions, such as those that target self-management barriers (e.g., low mood or self-efficacy) and that also strengthen diabetes-related skills (e.g., communication, problem-solving, and coping skills), are more effective at enhancing diabetes management than programs that focus exclusively on a single target, such as diabetes education, or direct behavioral processes, such as reminders and routines (Hood, Rohan, Peterson, & Drotar, 2010).

Using positive reinforcement to promote adaptive diabetes-related behaviors is strongly encouraged. Children can be given positive attention for a wide range of behaviors, such as visiting the nurse at predetermined times, checking blood glucose, taking medication or insulin, engaging in physical activity, choosing nutritious foods in moderate quantities, telling peers about diabetes, remaining calm when managing an out-of-range blood glucose, or asking for help. Positive reinforcement can be provided via specific labeled praise ("Thank you for checking your blood sugar"), positive nonverbal attention (thumbs up, smiling, nodding), or more structured behavioral reinforcement plans (e.g., earning "points" or incentives for completing specific tasks; Handout 19.1).

Out-of-range blood glucose levels can cause behavior changes and must be treated urgently. However, a hypo- or hyperglycemic episode is not a license to engage in disruptive or aggressive behavior, and children can be encouraged to learn to respond and cope adaptively to blood glucose changes. Therefore, consequences for undesired behavior—not for the blood glucose level itself—may

Table 19.2. DIABETES BEHAVIORAL HEALTH CONCERNS AND SCREENING MEASURES

Behavioral Health Concern	Screening Tools	Measure Details
Depressive symptoms (not diabetes-specific)	Patient Health Questionnaire-9 (PHQ-9; Kroenke, Spitzer, & Williams, 2001)	Nine items, ages 13+
	Center for Epidemiological Studies-Depression Scale for Children (CES-DC; Faulstich, Carey, Ruggiero, Enyart, & Gresham, 1986)	20 items, ages 6–17
Diabetes distress and burnout	Problem Areas in Diabetes–Child and Teen versions (PAID-C; Evans, et al., 2019; PAID-T; Shapiro et al., 2018)	PAID-C: 11 items, ages 8-12 PAID-T: 14 items, ages 12-18
Diabetes-related family conflict	Diabetes Family Conflict Scale – Revised (DFCS-R; Hood, Butler, Anderson, & Laffel, 2007)	20 items, ages 8+
Disordered eating	Eating Attitudes Test (EAT-26; Garner, Olmsted, Bohr, & Garfinkel, 1982)	26 items plus five functioning-related questions, adolescent and older
	Children's Eating Attitudes Test (ChEAT; Smolak & Levine, 1994)	26 items, ages 8–13
Anxiety (includes measures that are specific to diabetes and those that are not)	General Anxiety Disorder-7 (GAD-7; Spitzer, Kroenke, Williams, & Lowe, 2006)	Seven items plus one functioning-related question, ages 13+
	Penn State Worry Questionnaire for Children (PSWQ-C; Chorpita, Tracey, Brown, Collica, & Barlow, 1997)	14 items, ages 7–17
	Children's Hypoglycemia Fear Survey (HFS-C; Green, Wysocki, & Reineck, 1990)	25 items, ages 6–18

Note. This is not a comprehensive list of measures. Rather, the authors included brief, well-validated screening tools that are also free and accessible via the original peer-reviewed article referenced for each measure, with permission from the measure's authors, and/or online. Readers may also refer to the American Diabetes Association Psychosocial Position Statement (Young-Hyman et al., 2016) for additional psychosocial screening measures.

be applied after the child's blood glucose is safely back in range, according to the family's usual approach to responding to misbehavior.

Cognitive-behavioral therapy (CBT) is well established as an effective intervention for anxiety and depression in youth (Higa-McMillan, Francis, Rith-Najarian, & Chorpita, 2016; Weersing, Jeffreys, Do, Schwartz, & Bolano, 2017). Although there is little research on CBT for children with diabetes, data from adults with diabetes suggest CBT that addresses diabetes-specific stressors may help to alleviate distress and enhance coping and self-management (Gonzalez, Fisher, & Polonsky, 2011; Wei et al., 2017). Using CBT strategies, clinicians can help children address learned helplessness (e.g. "No matter how hard I try, my blood sugar still goes high; what's the point of trying?") and build self-efficacy around their self-management skills. Clinicians can help youth address unhelpful thoughts that contribute to diabetes distress and to learn adaptive problem-solving and coping skills.

To address feeling self-conscious about diabetes at school, role-playing and learning assertive communication skills may help children build confidence in speaking with peers about diabetes or completing care tasks in front of others. It may be helpful to partner with classroom teachers to support children in addressing questions and to ensure there are acceptable options for youth to complete diabetes care tasks in a manner with which they are most comfortable.

To address academic challenges related to neurocognitive sequelae of diabetes, fluctuating blood glucose levels, leaving class for diabetes management tasks, and the cognitive burden of diabetes management demands, clinicians can work with children individually on strategies to optimize classroom behavior, to enhance study habits and time-management skills, and to optimize diabetes routines to reduce cognitive burden. Teachers are likely to be essential partners in interventions to promote an optimal learning environment and adaptive classroom behavior. It may also be helpful to refer children with diabetes for cognitive testing.

Collaboration with the child's medical team to offer coordinated care may be necessary when addressing specific diabetes-related management or communication concerns. For youth whose behavioral or psychological difficulties appear predominantly related to diabetes, referral to a diabetes-specific mental health provider may be advisable.

Case Example

Juan is a 13-year-old Hispanic male with T1D who was referred to see his school's psychologist due to his being "sick of diabetes" and having management difficulties at school and home. At the time of his assessment, Juan had had T1D for 4 years, and he used syringes for insulin injections.

During his interview, Juan acknowledged that he hated having diabetes and commented "I feel like I'm not normal," when he had to stop during soccer practice to check blood glucose or have a snack. Juan had told only one or two close friends about his diabetes. He avoided going to the nurse's office at school to check his blood glucose because he was embarrassed to leave class early or to arrive late to lunch. Juan also worried that the nurse would call his mother if he had high blood glucose levels, because his mother often became frustrated and asked "Why is it high? What did you eat?" Finally, Juan was also concerned about high academic achievement. For their part, Juan's parents described him as a "good boy" who performed well in school and had many friends, but who was "controlling" and resisted their involvement in his diabetes care. They noted that Juan would not allow them to help with diabetes tasks and he often became argumentative when they asked questions about diabetes.

Treatment emphasized individual CBT-based interventions for diabetes distress and anxiety and family-based interventions to enhance diabetes-related communication and parental involvement in care. Individually, Juan learned to identify unhelpful thinking patterns (e.g., perfectionism and mind-reading) that contributed to distress and parental conflict, and he began practicing a wider range of adaptive coping skills. At school, the nurse was enlisted to fetch Juan when he did not present to her office at lunchtime, which helped increase his attendance in her office. Juan's parents were asked to discontinue questions about causes of high blood glucose, to view blood glucose numbers as data rather than "good" or "bad," and to emphasize praise for adaptive diabetes-related behaviors. The family also learned healthy communication skills, such as "I statements," and shared decision-making, to reduce conflict. Juan's anxiety, diabetes distress, and family conflict decreased significantly.

CULTURAL CONSIDERATIONS

In a large national sample of youth with T1D, white youth were more likely than African American and Hispanic youth to be prescribed an insulin pump; and African American youth had more actue diabetes medical problems and poorer health outcomes overall than white and Hispanic youth (Willi et al., 2015). These concerning disparities suggest that there may be systematic differences in how minority youth are treated by the healthcare system. Research on racial and ethnic differences in psychosocial factors among youth with T1D is limited, largely due to the fact that the majority of youth with T1D are Caucasian. However, there is some research that suggests that minority youth with T1D may believe that diabetes is not very serious or they may discount the risk of long-term complications (Naranjo, Schwartz, & Delamater, 2015).

The prevalence of T2D is rising fastest among youth from racial and ethnic minority groups (Mayer-Davis et al., 2017), and data also show there are disparities in quality of life and parental burden among minority youth with T2D (Butler, 2017). Stress, particularly chronic or toxic stress, may differ across racial and ethnic groups (Naranjo et al., 2015), and stress has been linked with poorer diabetes health outcomes (Hilliard et al., 2016). Lower socioeconomic status is often a correlate of minority status, which means that some youth with T2D may have less access to healthcare resources, live in neighborhoods with low access to fresh healthy foods and safe places to exercise, and have many people in their families or neighborhoods with T2D. Family factors, such as parental literacy and health literacy and family structure or single-caregiver homes, may also play a role in diabetes management and outcomes in youth with diabetes (Naranjo et al., 2015).

LEGAL AND POLICY ISSUES

Although children with diabetes are able to live full, healthy lives and to engage in the same activities as their peers without diabetes, their unique healthcare needs may require accommodations to ensure full access to, and participation, in educational, extracurricular, and occupational opportunities. In the school setting, diabetes is covered under Section 504 of the Rehabilitation Act of 1973, a federal civil rights law that prohibits discrimination due to a disability. Developing a 504 plan for educational accommodations in public schools helps to ensure that children receive necessary resources to fully engage with their educational environment, and prevents censure or disadvantage due to diabetes-related care needs. The American Diabetes Association has created a range of materials to guide schools, healthcare providers, and families in how best to support students with diabetes, including sample 504 plans, which are freely available to the public via the association's website (www.diabetes.org). Sample 504 plan accommodations for a child with diabetes include: multiple staff members are trained to check blood glucose, to administer insulin, and to inject glucagon (a fast-acting intramuscular glucose injection for severe hypoglycemia); the child has permission to eat whenever and wherever necessary; alternate arrangements are available for classroom time missed for medical appointments, because of high or low blood glucose, or illness related to diabetes, without penalty; and many others. Table 19.1 lists resources on legal protections and management recommendations for children with diabetes in the school setting.

CONCLUSIONS

Diabetes is a chronic medical condition that affects many thousands of children in the United States, and school providers play an important role in helping students live well with diabetes. Assistance with, or supervision of, daily self-management tasks, monitoring for urgent medical concerns, and facilitating appropriate accommodations are some of the key roles of school-based professionals in supporting health and well-being in the school setting. If learning or psychological concerns are evident, assessing for possible diabetes-related contributors can help school personnel and medical providers ensure the child's needs are being met. Given the complexity and individualization of diabetes management, all school-based care should be conducted in close collaboration with the child's treating medical team and family.

REFERENCES

American Diabetes Association. (2017). Standards of medical care in diabetes—2017. *Diabetes Care, 40*(1), S1–135.

Anderson, B. J. (2004). Family conflict and diabetes management in youth: Clinical lessons from child development and diabetes research. *Diabetes Spectrum, 17*(1), 22–26.

Browne, J. L., Ventura, A., Mosely, K., & Speight, J. (2013). "I call it the blame and shame disease": A qualitative study about perceptions of social stigma surrounding type 2 diabetes. *BMJ Open, 3*(11), e003384.

Butler, A. M. (2017). Social determinants of health and racial/ethnic disparities in type 2 diabetes in youth. *Current Diabetes Reports, 17*(8), 60.

Chorpita, B. F., Tracey, S. A., Brown, T. A., Collica, T. J., & Barlow, D. H. (1997). Assessment of worry in children and adolescents: An adaptation of the Penn State Worry Questionnaire. *Behavior Therapy Research, 35*(6), 569–581.

Desrocher, M., & Rovet, J. (2004). Neurocognitive correlates of type 1 diabetes mellitus in childhood. *Child Neuropsychology, 10*, 36–52.

Driscoll, K. A., Raymond, J., Naranjo, D., & Patton, S. R. (2016). Fear of hypoglycemia in children and adolescents and their parents with type 1 diabetes. *Current Diabetes Reports, 16*(8), 1–9.

Evans, M. A., Weil, L. E. G., Shapiro, J. B., Anderson, L. M., Vesco, A. T., Rychlik, K., Hilliard, M. E., Antisdel, J., & Weissberg-Benchell, J. (2019). Psychometric properties of the parent and child problem areas in diabetes measures. *Journal of Pediatric Psychology, 44*, 703–713.

Faulstich, M. E., Carey, M. P., Ruggiero, L., Enyart, P., & Gresham, F. (1986). Assessment of depression in childhood and adolescence: An evaluation of the Center for Epidemiological Studies Depression Scale for Children (CES-DC). *American Journal of Psychiatry, 143*(8), 1024–1027.

Fisher, L., Gonzalez, J. S., & Polonsky, W. H. (2014). The confusing tale of depression and distress in patients with diabetes: A call for greater clarity and precision. *Diabetic Medicine, 31*(7), 764–772.

Garner, D. M., Olmsted, M. P., Bohr, Y., & Garfinkel, P. E. (1982). The eating attitudes test: Psychometric feastures and clinical correlates. *Psychological Medicine, 12*(4), 871–878.

Gonzalez, J. S., Fisher, L., & Polonsky, W. H. (2011). Depression in diabetes: Have we been missing something important? *Diabetes Care, 34*(1), 236–239.

Green, L. B., Wysocki, T., & Reineck, B. M. (1990). Fear of hypoglycemia in children and adolescents with diabetes. *Journal of Pediatric Psychology, 15*, 633–641.

Herzer, M., & Hood, K. K. (2010). Anxiety symptoms in adolescents with type 1 diabetes: Association with blood glucose monitoring and glycemic control. *Journal of Pediatric Psychology, 35*(4), 415–425.

Higa-McMillan, C. K., Francis, S. E., Rith-Najarian, L., & Chorpita, B. F. (2016). Evidence base update: 50 years of research on treatment for child and adolescent anxiety. *Journal of Clinical Child & Adolescent Psychology, 45*(2), 91–113.

Hilliard, M. E., Hagger, V., Hendrieckx, C., Anderson, B. J., Trawley, S., Jack, M. M., . . . Speight, J. (2017). Strengths, risk factors, and resilient outcomes in adolescents with type 1 diabetes: Results from Diabetes MILES Youth–Australia. *Diabetes Care, 40*(7), 849–855.

Hilliard, M. E., Harris, M. A., & Weissberg-Benchell, J. (2012). Diabetes resilience: A model of risk and protection in type 1 diabetes. *Current Diabetes Reports, 12*(6), 739–748.

Hilliard, M. E., Yi-Frazier, J. P., Hessler, D., Butler, A. M., Anderson, B. J., & Jaser, S. (2016). Stress and A1c among people with diabetes across the lifespan. *Current Diabetes Reports, 16*(8), 1–10.

Hilliard, M. E., Powell, P. W., & Anderson, B. J. (2016) Evidence-based behavioral interventions to promote diabetes management in children, adolescents, and families. *American Psychologist, 71*, 590–601.

Hood, K. K., Butler, D. A., Anderson, B. J., & Laffel, M. B. (2007). Updated and revised Diabetes Family Conflict Scale. *Diabetes Care, 30*(7), 1764–1768.

Hood, K. K., Rausch, J. R., & Dolan, L. M. (2011). Depressive symptoms predict change in glycemic control in adolescents with type 1 diabetes: Rates, magnitude, and moderators of change. *Pediatric Diabetes, 12*, 718–723.

Hood, K. K., Lawrence, J. M., Anderson, A., Bell, R., Dabalea, D., Daniels, S., . . . Dolan, L. M. (2012). Metabolic and inflammatory links to depression in youth with diabetes. *Diabetes Care, 35*, 2443–2446.

Hood, K. K., Rausch, J. R., & Dolan, L. M. (2011). Depressive symptoms predict change in glycemic control in adolescents with type 1 diabetes: Rates, magnitude, and moderators of change. *Pediatric Diabetes, 12*, 718–723.

Hood, K. K., Rohan, J. M., Peterson, C. M., & Drotar, D. (2010). Interventions with adherence-promoting components in pediatric type 1 diabetes: Meta-analysis of their impact on glycemic control. *Diabetes Care, 33*(7), 1658–1664.

Kroenke, K., Spitzer, R. L., & Williams, J. B. W. (2001). The PHQ-9: Validity of a brief depression severity measure. *Journal of General Internal Medicine, 16*(9), 606–613.

Lawrence, J. M., Standiford, D. A., Loots, B., Klingensmith, G. J., Williams, D. E., Ruggiero, A., . . . McKeown, R. E. (2006). Prevalence and correlates of depressed mood among youth with diabetes: The SEARCH for Diabetes in Youth study. *Pediatrics, 117*(4), 1348–1358.

Markowitz, J. T, Garvey, K. C., & Laffel, L. M. B. (2015). Developmental changes in the roles of patients and families in type 1 diabetes management. *Current Diabetes Reviews, 11*(4), 231–238.

Mayer-Davis, E. J., Lawrence, J. M., Dabelea, D., Divers, J., Isom, S., Dolan, L., . . . Wagenknecht, L. (2017). Incidence trends of type 1 and type 2 diabetes among youths, 2002–2012. *New England Journal of Medicine, 376*(15), 1419–1429.

McGrady, M. E., & Hood, K. K. (2010). Depressive symptoms in adolescents with type 1 diabetes: Associations with longitudinal outcomes. *Diabetes Research and Clinical Practice, 88*(3), e35–e37.

Modi, A. C., Pai, A. L., Hommel, K. A., Hood, K. K., Cortina, S., Hilliard, M. E., . . . Drotar, D. (2012). Pediatric self-management: A framework for research, practice, and policy. *Pediatrics, 129*(2), e473–85.

Moulton, C. D., Pickup, J. C., & Ismail, K. (2015). The link between depression and diabetes: The search for shared mechanisms. *The Lancet Diabetes & Endocrinology, 3*(6), 461–471.

Naranjo, D., Schwartz, D. D., & Delamater A. M. (2015). Diabetes in ethnically diverse youth: Disparate burden and intervention approaches. *Current Diabetes Reviews, 11*, 251–260.

Schabert, J., Browne, J. L., Mosely, K., & Speight, J. (2013). Social stigma in diabetes: A framework to understand a growing problem for an increasing epidemic. *The Patient—Patient-Centered Outcomes Research, 6*(1), 1–10.

Schmitz, K. H., Jacobs, D. R., Jr., Hong, C. P., Steinberger, J., Moran, A., & Sinaiko, A. R. (2002). Association of physical activity with insulin sensitivity in children. *International Journal of Obesity and Related Metabolic Disorders, 26*(10), 1310–1316.

Schwartz, D. D., Wasserman, R., Powell, P. W., & Axelrad, M. E. (2014). Neurocognitive outcomes in pediatric diabetes: A developmental perspective. *Current Diabetes Reports, 14*(10), 533. doi:10.1007/s11892-014-0533-x.

Shapiro, J. B., Vesco, A. T., Weil, L. E. G., Evans, M. A., Hood, K. K., & Weissberg-Benchell, J. (2018). Psychometric properties of the problem areas in diabetes: Teen and parent of teen versions. *Journal of Pediatric Psychology, 43*, 561–571.

Skyler, J. S., Bakris, G. L., Bonifacio, E., Darsow, T., Eckel, R. H., Groop, L., . . . Ratner, R. E. (2016). Differentiation of diabetes by pathophysiology, natural history, and prognosis. *Diabetes, 66*(2), 241–255.

Smolak, L., & Levine, M. P. (1994). Psychometric properties of the Children's Eating Attitudes Test. *International Journal of Eating Disorders, 16*(3), 275–282.

Spitzer, R. L., Kroenke, K., Williams, J. B. W., & Lowe, B. (2006). A brief measure for assessing generalized anxiety disorder. *Archives of Internal Medicine, 166*, 1092–1097.

Van Bastelaar, K. M. P., Pouwer, F., Geelhoed-Duijvestijn, P. H. L. M., Tack, C. J., Bazelmans, E., Beekman, A. T., . . . Snoek, F. J. (2010). Diabetes-specific emotional distress mediates the association between depressive symptoms and glycaemic control in type 1 and type 2 diabetes. *Diabetic Medicine, 27*, 798–803.

Wasserman, R. M., Eshtehardi, S. S., Cao, V. T., Anderson, B. J., Marrero, D. G., McKinney, B. M., & Hilliard, M. E. (2017). Developmental shifts in worries about life with type 1 diabetes (T1D) from childhood through young adulthood. *Diabetes, 66*(Suppl 1), 868–P.

Weersing, V. R., Jeffreys, M., Do, M. C. T., Schwartz, K. T. G., & Bolano, C. (2017). Evidence base update of psychosocial treatments for child and adolescent depression. *Journal of Clinical Child & Adolescent Psychology, 46*(1), 11–43.

Wei, C., Allen, R. J., Tallis, P. M., Ryan, F. J., Hunt, L. P., Shield, J. P. H. & Crowne, E. C. (2017). Cognitive behavioral therapy stabilizes glycaemic control in adolescents with type 1 diabetes—Outcomes from a randomized controlled trial. *Pediatric Diabetes,19*(1), 106–113. doi:10.1111/pedi.12519.

Weissberg-Benchell, J., & Antisdel-Lomaglio, J. (2011). Diabetes-specific emotional distress among adolescents: Feasibility, reliability, and validity of the Problem Areas in Diabetes-Teen version. *Pediatric Diabetes, 12*, 341–344.

Willi, S. M., Miller, K. M., DiMeglio, L. A., Klingensmith, G. J., Simmons, J. H., Tamborlane, W. V., . . . Lipman, T. H. (2015). Racial-ethnic disparities in management and outcomes among children with type 1 diabetes. *Pediatrics, 135*(3), 424–434.

Young, V., Eiser, C., Johnson, B., Brierley, S., Epton, T., Elliott, J., & Heller, S. (2013). Eating problems in adolescents with type 1 diabetes: A systematic review with meta-analysis. *Diabetic Medicine, 30*, 189–198.

Young-Hyman, D., de Groot, M., Hill-Briggs, F., Gonzalez, J. S., Hood, K. K., & Peyrot, M. (2016). Psychosocial care for people with diabetes: A position statement of the American Diabetes Association. *Diabetes Care, 39*(12), 2126–2140.

Young-Hyman, D. L., & Davis, C. L. (2010). Disordered eating behavior in individuals with diabetes. *Diabetes Care, 33*(3), 683–689.

HANDOUT 19.1.

SAMPLE DIABETES SELF-CARE CHART

_____'s Diabetes Self-Care Chart

My points goal for this week is: _____ Points

I will earn: _____ (reward)

	MONDAY	TUESDAY	WEDNESDAY	THURSDAY	FRIDAY
Came to nurse/staff office					
Completed blood sugar check					
Took insulin before meal					
Total					

Diabetes Chart: Provider Instructions

1. Children can earn stickers or points each day when they complete agreed-upon diabetes-related behaviors and tasks. Staff can use the chart above to track task completion as well as data (e.g., blood glucose values, carb counts, insulin units given). Stickers and points for completing self-care behaviors, such as checking blood sugar, should be given independent of diabetes numbers.
2. Each day when the child completes tasks, provide positive attention (e.g., smile) or labeled praise (e.g., "Thanks for coming to take your medicine") to reinforce the behavior. At the end of the week, consider a small token or reward the child may earn if they achieve a certain amount of points.
3. If there are multiple designated times per day when the child is asked to visit the nurse's office for a blood glucose check and/or insulin, providers may consider allowing the child to earn a point for each time he or she visits the nurse at the prescribed time. Consider having a daily point limit to avoid reinforcing excessive nurse visits or time out of class.

Provider Considerations:

1. Reward behaviors, not numbers: It is normal for children and adolescents to experience variations in blood glucose, and they may have a high or low blood glucose even when they have followed all medical instructions. Be sure to reinforce the behaviors that children have control over, such as visiting the nurse's office before meals and completing diabetes tasks as directed. Avoid criticism or excessive questioning about possible causes for out-of-range blood glucose (e.g., "What did you eat?"); instead, focus on problem-solving (e.g., "Okay, let's decide how to get your sugars back in range").

2. Consider adding or substituting additional target behaviors: Three essential school-based diabetes tasks are presented in the chart, but once the child masters them, consider adding or substituting new tasks on the tracking sheet. Behavior goals should be specific, measurable, attainable, realistic, and timely (i.e., SMART goals). For example, if the child forgets to come get a snack before gym class, consider formally tracking and reinforcing this behavior (e.g., "Visited nurse's office at 10:00 AM and ate snack"). Also, highlight the behavior you'd like to increase. For example, if the child tends to argue or complain, emphasize the goal behavior (e.g., "Completed blood glucose check the first time I asked" or "Used an inside voice") or an appropriate substitute behavior (e.g., "Told me something that made her happy today while checking blood glucose"). Avoid nonspecific goals ("Be respectful") or goals that focus on what a child shouldn't do (e.g., "Didn't yell").

20

Hematologic/Oncologic Disorders and HIV

JENNIFER L. HARMAN, MEGAN L. WILKINS, AND NIKI JURBERGS ■

Schools across the country serve children with a variety of health-related conditions. Some of these conditions are hematologic, meaning they are related to blood or bone marrow (e.g., sickle cell disease, hemophilia), and some conditions are oncologic diagnoses, meaning cancer (e.g., leukemia, neuroblastoma, medulloblastoma, retinoblastoma). Some, but not all, cancers are considered blood cancers (e.g., leukemia). Similarly, not all blood-related diseases are primarily conceptualized as hematologic disorders. For example, diseases involving blood-borne pathogens (e.g., human immunodeficiency virus [HIV], hepatitis B, hepatitis C) are commonly characterized as infectious diseases.

This chapter briefly reviews pediatric cancer, sickle cell disease, and HIV, while focusing on factors of particular relevance to school-based clinicians and teachers. Each condition's description includes a case example to emphasize practical applications of the material presented. Subsequently, pertinent considerations for assessment and intervention work in the school setting are highlighted for the three conditions concurrently.

PEDIATRIC CANCER

Brief Overview of Pediatric Cancer

Over 15,000 children and adolescents are diagnosed with cancer in the United States each year (National Cancer Institute, 2017). The most common diagnoses include acute lymphoblastic leukemia (ALL) and other blood cancers, medulloblastoma and other brain tumors, and neuroblastoma and other solid tumors. Prevalence rates for different cancer diagnoses vary across sex and ethnicity. Treatment for pediatric cancer takes many forms and might include surgery, chemotherapy, radiation therapy, immunotherapy, stem cell transplant, and other targeted therapies, depending on the diagnosis. Although there is still significant variability in outcomes, advances in treatment over the past four decades have pushed overall survival rates to nearly 80% (National Cancer Institute, 2017; U.S. Cancer Statistics Working Group, 2017). This means more and more children are entering classrooms as cancer survivors. Some treatment protocols, such as treatment for ALL, take as long as 2 years or more and allow for children to attend school during portions of their treatment. Because of the long-term effects and health risks (e.g., cognitive and physical side effects, increased risk of second cancers, etc.), health providers now conceptualize pediatric cancer and survivorship as a chronic illness (Armstrong et al., 2014; Hudson et al., 2013; Robison & Hudson, 2014). The disease itself and its invasive treatments often produce a variety of acute and long-term side effects that affect how students function in the classroom both during and after treatment.

Case Example

Lucy was 7 years old and had just entered second grade when she was diagnosed with ALL. The first few months of her more than 2 years of treatment were very intense. She received oral, intravenous, and intrathecal (injected directly into the cerebral spinal fluid via the spine) chemotherapy and steroids, and she endured frequent, invasive medical procedures, such as lumbar punctures and bone marrow biopsies. Side effects of her treatment included nausea, vomiting, fatigue, pain, peripheral neuropathy (numbness or weakness of the extremities), and hair loss. Lucy was given a number of medications to manage some of her symptoms (e.g., pain, nausea), but these medications also produced side effects (e.g., drowsiness, constipation). Lucy's treatment also affected her immune system and made it difficult for her to fight off infections. She spent most of her time at the hospital, either in clinic or admitted to the inpatient unit. Once Lucy was in remission and transitioned to the longer maintenance phase of her treatment, Lucy's oncologist cleared her to return to school. Her parents were worried that she would struggle academically, knowing she had missed much of the first semester of instruction and would continue to miss school frequently for medical appointments for the next 2 years. Although they wanted Lucy to attend school as much as possible, they had to prioritize her physical health, which might mean keeping her home during flu season or other times when she would be at higher risk of getting sick. Lucy was understandably nervous about seeing her classmates. Her appearance had changed since she last saw her friends. Chemotherapy caused her hair to fall out and steroids had led to weight gain, particularly in her face. Lucy also knew she had missed out on a great deal socially, such as time together on the playground, play dates, and birthday parties.

Common School-Related Concerns and Mental Health Comorbidities of Childhood Cancer

Being diagnosed with and treated for cancer can be a very difficult experience for a child. In addition to the obvious medical challenges, children are faced with disruption to their normal routines and, potentially, their overall social, emotional, and academic development (Fuemmeler, Elkin, & Mullins, 2002; Gerhardt et al., 2007; Mancini et al., 1989; Noll, LeRoy, Bukowski, Rogosch, & Kulkarni, 1991; Sanger, Copeland, & Davidson, 1991; Willard et al., 2017). Children with cancer are at risk for a variety of difficulties that might require support in the school setting (Table 20.1).

PHYSICAL CONCERNS

Pain and fatigue are among the most common short- and long-term side effects of cancer therapy (Collins et al., 2000; Gibson et al., 2005; Hedén, Pöder, von Essen, & Ljungman, 2013; Olson & Amari, 2015; Varni, Burwinkle, & Katz, 2004). These and other somatic symptoms may make it difficult for a student to attend school, remain focused and on-task throughout the day, and function at his or her best. Students may experience treatment-related problems with fine motor functioning that make writing, including taking notes in class and completing assignments and tests, difficult, particularly when given a time limit. Physical appearance may be altered, which might be distressing to the student, as it was for Lucy, and might put the child at risk for bullying. Children with cancer may lose their hair and, in some cases (e.g., patients with brain tumors who receive cranial-spinal radiation therapy), it might not grow back evenly or at all. When the immune system is suppressed, students must wear masks at school to protect them from infection. In addition to making students look different from their peers, masks can be uncomfortable and can impact social functioning by restricting communication. Children with cancer may experience significant weight loss or weight gain secondary to either medication side effects or damage to endocrine functioning (Hudson et al., 2013). Some patients with solid tumors are treated with limb-sparing surgery or amputation, which typically alters both functional mobility and appearance.

SOCIAL, EMOTIONAL, AND BEHAVIORAL CONCERNS

Research has consistently shown that children with cancer do not exhibit greater rates of depression or anxiety than their healthy peers (Canning, Canning, & Boyce, 1992; Noll et al., 1991; Phipps, Jurbergs, & Long, 2009). Of course, this does not mean these children do not experience emotional distress during treatment. Lucy, for example, was very fearful of needles and had a difficult time adjusting to frequent "sticks." In fact, procedural distress is common (Dahlquist & Shroff Pendley, 2005). Other sources of emotional distress include coping with loss of function, fear of relapse or recurrence, survivor's guilt, and difficulties socially reintegrating with peers. During treatment, children often have access to support and intervention from psychologists or other mental health professionals. Once

Table 20.1. INTERVENTIONS AND ACCOMMODATIONS FOR COMMON
SYMPTOMS OR PROBLEMS

Symptom/ Problem	Interventions/Accommodations	Applicable Diseases
MEDICAL, PHYSICAL, AND PHYSICAL FUNCTIONING		
Medication side effects	• Be aware of student's medications and possible side effects • Monitor student for side effects • Keep school nurse informed and involved • See interventions for pain, nausea, fatigue, etc.	Cancer HIV SCD
Compromised immune function (e.g., low white blood cell counts)	• Allow student to wear a mask, as needed • Increase hand-washing of all within the classroom and school setting • Seat student away from peers with symptoms of illness • Encourage enforcement of school policies related to keeping sick students out of the classroom	Cancer HIV SCD
Nausea and/ or frequent restroom use	• Provide free pass to the restroom	Cancer SCD
Fatigue	• Allow partial school day • Decrease workload • Allow naps/rest breaks; rest in a quiet place	Cancer
Pain	• Allow student to rest in a quiet place • Encourage student to utilize relaxation strategies* • Offer nurse-led school-based pain group* • Provide cognitive-behavioral therapy for pain*	Cancer SCD
Peripheral neuropathy and/ or fine motor deficits	• Reduce paper and pencil task demands • Avoid having student copy from the board or from a book • Provide copies of classroom notes, study guides, assignments, etc. • Shorten assignments that require handwriting • Allow typed assignments in lieu of handwritten ones • Allow use of dictation or voice transcription software • Allow extended time • Provide occupational therapy	Cancer HIV SCD

Table 20.1. CONTINUED

Symptom/ Problem	Interventions/Accommodations	Applicable Diseases
Crutches, wheelchair (e.g., post amputation)	• Assign a peer helper to carry books • Provide second set of books for home • Ensure safety when traveling halls of school (e.g., early dismissal from class, provision of a peer escort) • Provide physical therapy	Cancer
General weakness and/ or decreased physical stamina	• Modify physical education (PE) curriculum requirements • Provide second set of books for home • Assign locker close to classes • Allow partial school day • Provide scheduled rest periods • Provide physical therapy • Provide occupational therapy	Cancer SCD
Need for continual hydration	• Allow water at desk • Provide free pass to the restroom	SCD
Increased sensitivity to extreme temperatures	• Allow student to stay inside during recess in extreme heat or cold • Allow jacket/uniform deviation	SCD
Hearing loss	• Ensure student is wearing hearing aids • Provide FM trainer • Have student sit at front of classroom.	Cancer
Vision loss Vision impairment	• Provide low-vision interventions • Provide preferential seating at front of classroom	Cancer SCD
Hair loss	• Allow student to wear a hat	Cancer
COGNITIVE AND ACADEMIC		
Executive dysfunction	• Teach use of outlines and organizers • Break long assignments into individual steps • Give explicit directions; give only one instruction at a time • Provide copies of classroom notes, study guides, assignments, etc. • Teach student to "stop and think" before beginning an assignment • Use modeling to teach planning skills • Have the student verbalize plans for completing an assignment or task • Encourage the student to review work after completion • Emphasize accuracy over speed • Provide computer-based cognitive remediation*	Cancer HIV SCD

(*continued*)

Table 20.1. CONTINUED

Symptom/ Problem	Interventions/Accommodations	Applicable Diseases
Attention deficits	• Provide preferential seating • Provide a structured and organized environment • Provide clear rules and expectations • Provide frequent reinforcement and praise for on task behavior • Have the student privately repeat directions to teacher • Highlight important directions • Require the student to utilize an assignment book • Allow frequent breaks within the classroom • Provide computer-based cognitive remediation*	Cancer HIV SCD
Processing speed deficits	• Encourage accuracy over speed • Provide the student with handouts of class material ahead of time • Provide extended time to complete tasks and assignments • Allow student to audiotape important lessons and review sessions • Refrain from calling on the student to quickly respond to questions in class • Provide the student with advanced warning of questions/specific topics if required to speak in class • Provide the student with early notification of upcoming projects and assignments	Cancer HIV SCD
Working memory deficits	• Slow the presentation of new information • Provide the student with handouts of class material ahead of time • Refrain from calling on the student to quickly respond to questions in class • Provide the student with advanced warning of questions/specific topics if required to speak in class • Teach the student to underline important points while reading and then review them at the end of each page • Teach the student to write down the steps used to solve a problem • Encourage the student to take frequent breaks while studying • Encourage the student to use assignment notebooks and to-do lists • Teach the student to use verbal mediation to assist with completing steps of a task • Provide computer-based cognitive remediation*	Cancer HIV SCD

Table 20.1. CONTINUED

Symptom/ Problem	Interventions/Accommodations	Applicable Diseases
SOCIAL, EMOTIONAL, AND BEHAVIORAL		
Social skills deficits	• Engage the student in social skills groups* • Provide direct social skills instruction*	Cancer SCD
Anxiety, depression, and/ or adjustment difficulties	• Encourage student to engage in behavioral activation • Avoid providing excess attention to anxiety-related discussions • Provide cognitive-behavioral therapy*	Cancer HIV SCD
Emotional lability, outbursts, or easily upset	• Implement individualized behavior plans • Assist student in developing and implementing a plan for reaction to frustrations • Provide labeled praise for use of appropriate behavioral responses to frustrations • Serve as a role model for the student	Cancer HIV SCD
School avoidance and/ or refusal	• Expect student to attend school if physically able and cleared by medical team • Collaborate with parents and medical team to create cohesive behavioral approach to school refusal behavior • Welcome student to the school and the classroom upon arrival • Avoid allowing student to leave earlier than the predetermined time unless medically necessary • Consider assigning a peer buddy, especially for younger students	Cancer SCD

Note. * Indicates empirically supported intervention strategy.

back at school, students may benefit from additional professional support in the school environment.

COGNITIVE AND ACADEMIC CONCERNS

When a child is first diagnosed with cancer, school is not likely to be the first thing on the parents' minds. However, it is in the best interest of the child to make a plan for education as soon as possible. In many cases, students may continue school at home (e.g., via homebound instruction) or they may receive instruction through hospital-based school services. Educators should expect to be flexible, both with expectations and with scheduling, when working with children with cancer, as their physical functioning and needs often change rapidly.

SCHOOL REINTEGRATION

Integrating or reintegrating into the classroom after completion of therapy, or in some cases during therapy, can be a challenge for students, parents, and educators. There are many factors to consider, such as the student's medical status and any ongoing medical needs, academic readiness, instructional needs, and social and emotional needs. Students may require medication administration at school. They may have physical limitations or activity restrictions that require modified physical education, wheelchair-accessible classrooms, or the provision of ongoing rehabilitation services (e.g., physical, occupational, or speech and language therapies).

Social aspects of re-entry may be facilitated by communicating with peers before, and at the time of, classroom re-entry. Children with cancer often enjoy making a presentation to their classmates to educate them on the cancer experience. This gives the student control over what information is shared and provides a structured, supervised setting for asking and answering questions.

Educators are encouraged to work closely with families and medical teams to understand a student's individual needs at the time of re-entry and to continue monitoring needs as the student progresses, particularly at times of significant educational transitions (e.g., to a new school, to high school), which is often done best via a formal educational plan. Although individual educational needs vary across students, all cancer survivors will need a plan for managing absences, both planned and unplanned, and including accommodations and expectations for missed assignments and tests. Lucy, for example, continued to miss a full day of school every month for appointments, even after her cancer treatment was complete.

COGNITIVE LATE EFFECTS

Children who are treated with chemotherapy and/or radiation therapy to the central nervous system (CNS; i.e., brain and spine), such as children with brain tumors or ALL, are at risk of decreased attention and working memory and slowed processing speed (Jacola et al., 2016; Knight et al., 2014; Winter et al., 2014). These weaknesses typically emerge after the completion of treatment, which can be confusing to educators who perceive the child to be healthy. In fact, cognitive deficits typically worsen over time. Underlying deficits in attention, working memory, and processing speed can lead to secondary deficits in overall IQ and academic skills.

When Lucy was able to return to school for third grade, she was at grade level in all subjects thanks to her homebound instruction. Lucy was a hard worker and had always been a strong student. By the middle of her fifth grade year, however, her parents and teachers noticed that she was having trouble paying attention, seemed forgetful, made frequent careless mistakes, and worked slower than her classmates. Formal assessment of her neurocognitive and psychoeducational functioning revealed that Lucy had begun to develop weaknesses in attention, working memory, and processing speed secondary to her cancer treatment. These weaknesses made it difficult for Lucy to keep up in class and, as a result, her grades began to drop. It was initially difficult for her teachers to understand how her history of cancer, which had long been in remission, could be causing these changes. Lucy was even accused of being "lazy" and "not trying." This was not the case. In fact, Lucy was trying harder than ever, and she was very frustrated by her new-found academic difficulties.

Risk Factors and Protective Factors

Premorbid functioning is often a good predictor of how a child will function after cancer treatment. This means that well-adjusted, successful students who are treated for cancer are likely to be successful in the school environment after treatment. Conversely, students with cognitive, academic, or psychosocial weaknesses before their cancer diagnosis are more likely to struggle in these areas following treatment (Kazak, 2006). Additionally, and as explained above, patients with CNS disease or CNS-directed therapy, such as patients with brain tumors and ALL, are at the highest risk for developing cognitive, academic, and psychosocial problems. Young age at diagnosis is associated with poorer cognitive outcomes, as are greater treatment intensity and neurological complications, such as stroke and hydrocephalus (Mulhern, Merchant, Gajjar, Reddick, & Kun, 2004; Reddick et al., 2014).

Educators have very little control over many of the factors that put students going through cancer treatment at risk of difficulties in the school setting. Fortunately, educators can have a positive effect by contributing to school-related protective factors. As is true for any school population, school–home communication is linked to improved academic and behavioral outcomes in the classroom (Christenson & Conoley, 1992). The provision of individualized accommodations and interventions, as discussed in detail below, can also facilitate a student's best performance. Lucy benefitted from ongoing communication and collaboration among her family, educational team, and medical team. An individualized education plan (IEP) under the other health impairment (OHI) designation was created for her and was updated annually, with input from her parents and teachers, which provided ongoing support for Lucy and her changing needs. Although things would never be the same for Lucy after being treated for ALL, adjusting expectations and offering flexible support allowed her to be successful throughout her formal education.

SICKLE CELL DISEASE

Brief Overview of Sickle Cell Disease (SCD)

SCD is a group of chronic, inherited conditions that affect red blood cells. Red blood cells contain a protein called hemoglobin, and hemoglobin carries oxygen throughout the body. In individuals with SCD, the body produces an altered form of hemoglobin that causes red blood cells to become hard, sticky, and crescent-shaped. As a result, red blood cells have difficulty passing through blood vessels. Instead, the sickled red blood cells form clumps and obstruct blood flow. This leads to the episodes of extreme pain known as vaso-occlusive pain crises. Obstructed blood flow also can cause severe tissue damage and significantly harm vital organs (National Heart Lung and Blood Institute [NHLBI], 2014).

Many SCD treatment plans involve prophylactic (i.e., preventative) penicillin use, because infections can become fatal when they progress quickly in individuals with SCD (NHLBI, 2014). Chronic blood transfusions, which necessitate absences from school, also are often required for children with SCD who have suffered a cerebral infarction (i.e., stroke). Yet, transfusions themseleves are associated with various risks, including, but not limited to, increased viscosity of the blood and associated neurological complications (Yawn et al., 2014). Individuals with SCD who are not treated with chronic blood transfusions may be treated with oral hydroxyurea (Lemaneck & Ranalli, 2009). In very severe cases of SCD, a bone marrow stem cell transplant may be considered. Stem cell transplantstion is currently the only potentially curative treatment available for SCD; however, stem cell transplants come with a host of risks and not all patients who undergo a transplant remain disease-free (Fitzhugh, Abraham, Tisdale, & Hsieh, 2014).

Approximately one out of every 1,940 infants born in the United States is diagnosed with SCD through newborn screening (Therrell, Lloyd-Puryear, Eckman, & Mann, 2015). An overwhelming majority of these infants are of African descent or have parents who self-identify as black; a minority of the infants are of Latin American, Middle Eastern, or Asian Indian descent (Yawn et al., 2014). Various forms of SCD exist (e.g., HbSS, HbSC, HbSβ°thalassemia, HbSβ+thalassemia, etc.). HbSS is the most common type of SCD. This type of SCD and HbSβ°thalassemia are frequently referred to as sickle cell anemia. Sickle cell anemia is typically associated with the most severe clinical manifestations of SCD. Conversely, sickle cell trait occurs when an individual has inherited only one sickle cell gene from one parent, rather than inheriting two sickle cell genes— one from each parent. Individuals with sickle cell trait do not have SCD and often do not have any of the symptoms or complications associated with SCD; however, in rare instances, individuals with sickle cell trait experience complications associated with SCD (NHLBI, 2014).

Case Example

Sammy was a 13-year-old male in the sixth grade who had been diagnosed with SCD as a newborn. He was seen in the hematology clinic a minimum of once per month. Sammy had no history of strokes; however, he continued to be monitored for signs of stroke given his increased risk. Although Sammy had been prescribed oral hydroxyurea, he experienced a number of SCD-related complications. He was previously hospitalized on two occasions for acute chest syndrome, a known pulmonary complication of SCD; he was hospitalized for vaso-occlusive pain crises five times over the previous 2 years. During each hospitalization, Sammy missed several days of school. Sammy had a history of academic delays and was retained in the first grade due to the number of absences he accumulated, but he had no history of special education programming. Throughout much of his sixth grade year, he received Tier 3 intervention services; however, he continued to perform poorly. He recently completed a hospital-based psychological assessment, for which he had been referred due to poor school performance and known neurocognitive weaknesses associated with SCD. Results of his evaluation revealed difficulties with executive function and below-average broad cognitive and academic functioning. Although Sammy did not yet have special education services or an IEP, he had a Section 504 plan in place for medically indicated accommodations (e.g., reduced physical activity, protection from extreme heat or cold, access to water at all times, frequent restroom breaks, and a plan for pain management). Accommodations related to pain management were particularly important for Sammy because he suffered debilitating chronic pain related to complications of SCD. Luckily, the staff at Sammy's school were able to facilitate his independent implementation of nonpharmacological pain interventions in the school setting through utilization of his "Pain Passport" (see Handout 20.1).

Common School-Related Concerns and Mental Health Comorbidities of SCD

SCD is a chronic condition with the potential to affect cognitive, academic, social, emotional, and behavioral functioning (Smith & Baker, 2011). Similarly, physical symptoms and sequelae associated with SCD can affect a student's performance (Lemanek & Ranalli, 2009). Indeed, as with cancer, a variety of school-related concerns exist for students with SCD (see Table 20.1).

PHYSICAL CONCERNS
As is true with cancer, pain and fatigue are common among students with SCD (Yawn et al., 2014). These difficulties may contribute to problems with sustained attention and focus, and they also may make it hard for students to demonstrate optimal school-related potential (Lemanek & Ranalli, 2009; Smith & Baker, 2011). Sammy experienced chronic, debilitating pain; he commonly stated that it was hard for him to pay attention and do his best at school because of his pain. Tools like a Pain Passport may be utilized to help students maximize pain management in the school setting. Similarly, allowing frequent breaks as needed for students with SCD can help with fatigue. Students with SCD also must remain hydrated throughout the day and need to actively work to avoid dehydration and becoming overheated (Wang, 2008). Because of this, students like Sammy benefit from being allowed to have water with them at all times and from being allowed to use the restroom whenever needed throughout the school day. Similarly, these students need to avoid extreme temperatures (Wang 2008). Therefore, students like Sammy benefit from being allowed to stay inside when it is very hot or very cold outside. Some male students with SCD experience involuntary, painful erections (Lemanek

& Ranalli, 2009). The teacher may assist students with SCD avoid their embarrassment by using a nonverbal communication system if one of these occurs during class. Additionally, many students with SCD have visual impairments (Yawn et al., 2014) and benefit from individualized accommodations and modifications (e.g., larger print, seats close to the front of the room) to address these impairments. Finally, schools serving students with SCD should be aware that a fever constitutes a medical emergency for these students. It is essential to have a plan in place to ensure prompt medical attention to students with SCD if a fever occurs at school (Yawn et al., 2014).

Social, Emotional, and Behavioral Concerns

Students with SCD often have a history of frequent school absences due to pain, illnesses, medical appointments, and hospitalizations; however, school avoidance, school refusal, peer-related concerns, and anxiety also may occur in students with chronic conditions like SCD (Barakat, Lash, Lutz & Nicolaow, 2006). Indeed, students with SCD are at increased risk for peer victimization (Smith & Baker, 2011). School personnel are encouraged to remain vigilant for peer-related interactions that occur in the school setting. Teachers, guidance counselors, school psychologists, and administrators may need to intervene to address bullying and individual cases of peer victimization. Similarly, school personnel may need to facilitate plans to address school avoidance and school refusal, and home–school–medical clinic communication and collaboration are imperative for successful interventions with such behaviors among these students. Indeed, students with SCD who also have a history of school avoidance and school refusal can be successfully treated with a behavioral intervention akin to those indicated for use with school refusal and school avoidance in general. Essentially, students with SCD should not be allowed to miss school unless there is a need for medical attention or they are attending necessary medical appointments.

Students with SCD who report increased stress and negative mood report same-day increased pain and decreased participation in school and social activity (Gil et al., 2003). Teachers, guidance counselors, and school psychologists can reinforce use of stress-reduction strategies in the school setting. In Sammy's case, use of a Pain Passport (see Handout 20.1) helped him function in spite of his chronic pain.

Some students with SCD also struggle with pica, or persistent ingestion of nonnutritive, nonfood substances (Ivascu et al., 2001). Teachers and school personnel may be informed of a student's pica if it is thought to transcend settings. When this occurs, collaboration among school personnel, medical providers, treating psychologists, and the family is imperative to ensure fidelity of targeted behavioral interventions across settings.

Cognitive and Academic Concerns

Even in the absence of a history of strokes, SCD commonly affects the central nervous system (Schatz & McClellan, 2006; Smith & Baker, 2011). Therefore, SCD is conceptualized as a neurodevelopmental disorder in addition to a chronic medical condition (Smith & Baker, 2011). Sammy's cognitive profile and history of poor academic achievement are consistent with known neurodevelopmental weaknesses among this population. Indeed, students with SCD often have weaknesses in overall cognitive abilities, executive function, processing speed, working memory, attention, short- and long-term memory, visuospatial abilities, and language, as well as difficulties in reading, writing, and math (Daly, Kral, & Tarazi, 2011; Smith & Baker, 2011). These cognitive and academic weaknesses can deleteriously affect learning and performance in the school setting. Therefore, some students with SCD benefit from consideration for special education services that allow for the provision of an IEP.

Risk Factors and Protective Factors

Like Sammy, students with SCD may experience frequent absences from school due to medical appointments or sequelae of SCD. Similarly, as noted above, pain and fatigue also may negatively impact attention and concentration, particularly on days when these symptoms are bothersome. Students with SCD also may experience more difficulty in the school setting than many of their peers due to known neurocognitive correlates of SCD. Furthermore, delayed puberty, which is common among individuals with SCD, is one of many factors thought to increase risk for peer victimization among this population (Smith & Baker, 2011).

Family functioning significantly impacts the emotional coping and physical functioning of students with SCD (Lemanek & Ranalli, 2009). As with cancer and HIV, home–school–medical clinic communication and collaboration can help promote success for these students across settings. Adherence to medical treatment (e.g., taking hydroxyurea as directed), adequate hydration, and avoidance of extreme temperatures are also examples of actionable protective factors for students with SCD, and allowing a free hall pass for restroom breaks can help these students protect their kidney function (Yawn et al., 2014).

HIV

Brief Overview of HIV

Another chronic condition that teachers, school-based clinicians, and education staff should be knowledgeable about is HIV infection. HIV is a blood-borne virus that attacks white blood cells in the immune system. It can be transmitted sexually, through needles, from mother to child in utero or during birth, and through breast milk. HIV cannot be transmitted through saliva, sweat, or casual contact (e.g., hugging, sharing utensils, toilet seats). Once considered an acute illness with high morbidity and mortality, HIV infection is now considered a chronic and manageable illness, with patients' life expectancies similar to those for individuals with other chronic illnesses (Samji et al., 2013). Children in schools may have perinatally acquired HIV, although this type of transmission is increasingly rare, or new infections. At present, nonperinatal transmission of HIV is the most prevalent route of infection and disproportionately affects adolescents and young adults, as well as ethnic minorities and young men who have sex with men. Adolescents and young adults are overrepresented in new infections; in 2015, youth age 13 to 24 accounted for 20% of all new infections (Centers for Disease Control and Prevention [CDC], 2016). Although there has been a drop in HIV acquisition over time (CDC, 2017), certain geographic regions of the United States continue to exhibit higher than expected rates of infection. These include large urban areas and large sections of the Southern United States. HIV infection is also overrepresented among people in poverty, highlighting the relationship between poverty and poor access to preventive healthcare. Prevention efforts aim toward reducing rates of infection in these overrepresented groups.

Case Example

Jamal is an 18-year-old African American man with HIV, diagnosed during his senior year in high school. He has a history of learning challenges and was diagnosed with a learning disability in early elementary school. Since then, he received academic support in a co-teaching environment and earned average grades. Since learning about his diagnosis, which was made after he donated blood, Jamal has exhibited social isolation at home and at school. He is preoccupied with thoughts about not having HIV and feels "normal" when he is not taking his medication. Thus, he takes his medication inconsistently, and his immune functioning has been variable but has declined in the last several months. Jamal has disclosed his HIV status only to his mother and older brother, and not to anyone at his school. As a result, he experiences feelings of isolation while at school and has been more distractible in class than is typical for him. His mother has also noted a decrease in his academic functioning. She is concerned about Jamal's ability to graduate from high school and to continue to a nearby university as planned.

Jamal may now be at risk for further school- and learning-related difficulties due to executive function weaknesses associated with HIV. These weaknesses are above and beyond those that were previously present and accounted for by Jamal's learning disability. If Jamal chooses to disclose his HIV status to school personnel, he should be offered school-based counseling services to provide support regarding the perceived stigma in the community, to improve symptoms of social isolation, and to mitigate any related social issues. Furthermore, school personnel also may wish to update his psychological evaluation to see if changes to his current support services may be indicated based on possible newly identified executive function deficits.

PHYSICAL CONCERNS
With adherence to medications prescribed, HIV can be controlled and individuals with HIV infection can live normal lives. Those living with HIV are typically

monitored regularly by an infectious diseases medical specialist, who gathers labs (e.g., immune system functioning and levels of virus in blood) and monitors and manages symptoms and side effects of medication treatment or HIV. Treatment guidelines now recommend all youth infected with HIV begin medication treatment as soon as possible, regardless of immune functioning. Thus, youth with HIV are often started on medications during the first few weeks of diagnosis. Medication advancements have allowed most youth to start treatment with a combination medication, often one pill, once daily. Despite this, youth with HIV often have difficulties with compliance; low family support and poverty increase the risk for noncompliance. This is in addition to the typical adolescent struggle with identity and social acceptance, which is compounded by the social stigma of HIV. Efficacious interventions to improve medication adherence are varied but include use of motivational interviewing techniques and cognitive-behavioral therapy (Simoni, Pearson, Pantalone, Marks, & Crepaz, 2006).

SOCIAL, EMOTIONAL, AND BEHAVIORAL CONCERNS

Despite efforts to reduce stigma through policy change and social programs to educate the public with factual information about HIV and to improve tolerance of individuals with HIV, HIV-related stigma continues to be pervasive in many communities. The stigma may be compounded by other social stress, particularly for gay youth, who are more likely to face peer bullying and reduced family support. Thus, youth with HIV are often faced with the stigma daily and experience shame regarding their diagnosis. This may lead to decreased peer relationships or increased experience of social anxiety in the school setting. Relatedly, youth may struggle with disclosing their diagnosis to others. This further complicates medication adherence, as research has demonstrated the benefit of social support in improving medication adherence (Edwards, 2006; Simoni, Frick & Huang, 2006). Thus, stigma is one of the primary barriers to successful treatment of HIV. Youth are often concerned about disclosure to others and so avoid medical treatment. Stigma also causes increased incidence of anxiety and depressive disorders in youth with HIV, and both depression and anxiety are overrepresented in people with HIV. For example, rates of depressive disorders among youth with HIV have been estimated to be 20% to 40% (Ferrando, 2009; Walsh et al., 2017). Recommended treatment includes both cognitive-behavioral therapy and psychiatric consultation.

LEGAL AND ETHICAL ISSUES

School mental health providers for youth with HIV could be faced with ethical issues regarding disclosure of HIV status to the youth's sexual partners. Some states have criminal exposure laws that hold knowingly exposing a sexual partner to HIV as a felony offense. Thus, during the course of treatment, youth should be educated on their obligation to disclose to sexual partners; however, due to stigma, this does not always occur. It is unclear if this constitutes mandated reporting in accord with the Tarasoff precedent and duty to warn. Clinicians must balance patient confidentiality with legal and ethical responsibilities to protect others.

Disclosure of HIV status in schools is not required in any state (Todd, 2015). In 2013, an Illinois state law that required families to disclose HIV status to school administration was repealed. This was the last known legislation mandating reporting of a student's HIV status to schools. Disclosure of HIV status to schools is considered an individual family decision. Given widespread adoption of universal precautions with blood products and other bodily fluids, there is no identified risk to others with nondisclosure of HIV status in schools. Given this and the prevalence of HIV-related stigma, youth with HIV in schools are probably not identified. They may have accommodations through an IEP or Section 504 plan for other identified disabilities, such as learning disorders or attention deficit hyperactivity disorder. However, it is unlikely a student with HIV will receive school accommodations for his or her primary illness (e.g., other health impairment).

COGNITIVE AND ACADEMIC CONCERNS

The impact of HIV infection on cognitive functioning in youth is not completely known. Early in the epidemic, profound cognitive impairment was observed in children with untreated HIV (Smith & Wilkins, 2014), and it is thought to have been related to the presence of encephalopathy, a brain disease related to viral infection without treatment. Recent evidence suggests youth with HIV experience more subtle executive function deficits, regardless of treatment patterns and medication adherence (Nichols et al., 2013, 2016). A pattern of slower processing speed and working memory deficits has been reported (Phillips et al., 2016). On academic measures, youth with HIV have not been found to perform lower than their noninfected counterparts on most measures, with the exception of youth with a history of encephalopathy and related cognitive impact, who perform significantly below the expected range for their age (Garvie et al., 2014). Among those with non-perinatal HIV infection, cognitive impact has been reported, but treatment has not been shown to improve functioning over time (Nichols et al., 2016). Despite living with HIV for shorter periods of time, over two thirds of youth with HIV diagnosed in adolescence and young adulthood showed deficits in episodic memory and fine-motor skills when compared to normative samples (Nichols et al., 2013).

CONSIDERATIONS FOR ASSESSMENT
AND INTERVENTION

Assessment

Students like Jamal, Sammy, and Lucy may experience school-related difficulties due to disease- and treatment-related neurocognitive weaknesses. Traditional psychological or neuropsychological assessment, which may be conducted within the medical or school setting, often is useful for students with cancer (particularly those who received CNS-directed therapy), HIV, or SCD. In fact, although these students may attend schools that superbly implement response to intervention or multitiered systems of support, schools would be remiss to discount the utility of traditional assessment results in informing appropriate intervention services and accommodations for students with cancer, HIV, or SCD. When psychological and neuropsychological assessments are conducted in the medical setting, and appropriate parental consent is obtained, schools can adopt the findings of the reports and/or collaborate with the clinicians doing the testing in the medical setting to provide information about school-based behaviors and to identify and coordinate needed interventions. The usefulness of assessment in the medical setting also may be enhanced when combined with other school-based methods of assessment. For example, at the time of school re-entry, and in light of missed instruction, academic achievement assessment can provide useful information about a student's current skills to help inform instructional programming; however, the utility of assessment is also bolstered when curriculum-based assessment is done at the school and results are used in concert with traditional assessment results.

Although curriculum-based measurement could be used to further elucidate information regarding academic skills, some information is best provided by traditional psychological or neuropsychological assessment. In fact, with regard to pediatric cancer, serial monitoring of cognitive functioning is standard of care for those who received CNS-directed therapy, because it often leads to cognitive late effects that emerge long after therapy is completed (Annett, Patel, & Phipps, 2015).

Executive function deficits are associated with cancer, SCD, and HIV, and, as discussed elsewhere in this chapter, visuospatial processing difficulties may emerge and negatively impact functioning in the classroom setting. Similarly, SCD and various pediatric cancers are associated with neurocognitive declines (Annett et al., 2015; Daly et al., 2011; Smith & Baker, 2011). Therefore, school-based monitoring of functioning is essential, and teachers should closely observe the classroom performance of any student with a current or previous cancer diagnosis or with SCD or HIV. Identifying and intervening before neurocognitive weaknesses lead to additional learning-related declines are imperative.

Accommodations and Interventions

As discussed, students with cancer, HIV, or SCD may experience a variety of symptoms or difficulties associated with their disease and treatment. The experience of each student is unique. Table 20.1 lists a number of common problems that these students may encounter and accommodations and individualized interventions to address them. Psychological or neuropsychological assessment results often help inform which accommodations and interventions best meet the needs of individual students with HIV, SCD, or cancer. For example, cognitive remediation and computer-based working memory trainings, such as Cogmed®, which could be done in the school setting, have demonstrated efficacy among students with SCD (Hardy, Hardy, Schatz, Thompson, & Meier, 2016) and among student survivors of ALL and pediatric brain tumors (Cox et al., 2015; Hardy,

Willard, Allen, & Bonner, 2013). Empirical evidence further supports the use of direct instruction in appropriate social interactions and use of social skills groups to address social problem-solving deficits that may occur among students with cancer (Schulte, Vannatta, & Barrera, 2014).

Regardless of the interventions and accommodations a student with HIV, SCD, or cancer receives, these students frequently benefit from a 504 plan or an IEP. Specifically, a student with SCD, HIV, or cancer may qualify for a 504 plan as outlined in Section 504 of the Rehabilitation Act of 1973 if the student's diagnosis results in a physical or mental impairment that limits the student's ability to engage in one or more major life activities (e.g., engagement in self-care, performance of manual tasks, walking, seeing, hearing, speaking, breathing, learning, working; U.S. Department of Education, 2000). A student with SCD, cancer, or HIV also may qualify for an IEP, as delineated in the Individuals with Disabilities Education Improvement Act (Federal Register, 2006). Because students with SCD, HIV, or cancer often experience neurocognitive weaknesses associated with their medical diagnosis and treatments that impair learning, these students frequently benefit from special education services and the provision of an IEP. Indeed, students with SCD or with cancer commonly qualify for special education services under the OHI eligibility category.

In spite of the many challenges faced by students with cancer, SCD, or HIV, these students can be successful in the classroom with the support of the educational team. Teachers, academic interventionists, school psychologists, guidance counselors, occupational therapists, physical therapists, speech–language pathologists, and administrators are each uniquely qualified to ensure these students obtain indicated individualized support services. In turn, the educational team has the great responsibility and honor of setting the stage for the success of students with cancer, SCD, or HIV.

RESOURCES

- *Educating the Child with Cancer: A Guide for Parents and Teachers.* Keane, N. (Ed.). 2013. Bethesda, MD: Candlelighters Childhood Cancer Foundation.
- *Together* website powered by St. Jude Children's Research Hospital: www.together.stjude.org
- Disease Fact Sheets for pediatric cancers, SCD, and HIV: www.stjude.org/disease.
- National Cancer Institute: www.cancer.gov; www.cancer.gov/types/childhood-cancers; https://www.cancer.gov/types/aya
- National Heart, Lung, and Blood Institute: www.nhlbi.nih.gov/health/health-topics/topics/sca/
- Sickle Cell Disease Association of America: www.sicklecelldisease.org
- Sickle Cell Information Center: https://scinfo.org

- National Resource Center for HIV/AIDS Prevention among Adolescents: https://whatworksinyouthhiv.org/
- The Body, The Complete HIV/AIDS Resource: www.thebody.com

REFERENCES

Annett, R. D., Patel, S. K., & Phipps, S. (2015). Monitoring and assessment of neuropsychological outcomes as standard of care in pediatric oncology. *Pediatric Blood and Cancer, 62*(S5), S460–S513. doi:10.1002/pbc.25749

Armstrong, G. T., Kawashima, T., Leisenring, W., Stratton, K., Stovall, M., Hudson, M. M., . . . Oeffinger, K. C. (2014). Aging and risk of severe, disabling, life-threatening, and fatal events in the Childhood Cancer Survivor Study. *Journal of Clinical Oncology, 32*, 1218–1227.

Barakat, L. P., Lash, M., Lutz, L. M., & Nicolaow, D. C. (2006). Psychosocial adaptation of children and adolescents with sickle cell disease. In R. T. Brown (Ed.), *Comprehensive handbook of childhood cancer and sickle cell disease: A biopsychosocial approach* (pp. 471–495). New York, NY: Oxford University Press.

Canning, E. H., Canning, R. D., & Boyce, W. T. (1992). Depressive symptoms and adaptive style in children with cancer. *Journal of the American Academy of Child & Adolescent Psychiatry, 31*, 1120–1124.

Centers for Disease Control and Prevention. (2017). CROI HIV Incidence Press Release. Retrieved from https://www.cdc.gov/nchhstp/newsroom/2017/croi-hiv-incidence-press-release.html

Centers for Disease Control and Prevention. (2016). HIV Surveillance Report, 27. Retrieved from http://www.cdc.gov/hiv/library/reports/hiv-surveillance.html

Christenson, S. L. & Conoley, J. C. (Eds.). (1992). *Home–school collaboration: Enhancing children's academic and social competence.* Silver Spring, MD: National Association of School Psychologists.

Collins, J. J., Byrnes, M. E., Dunkel, I. J., Lapin, J., Nadel, T., Thaler, H. T., . . . Portenoy, R. K. (2000) The measurement of symptoms in children with cancer. *Journal of Pain and Symptom Management, 19*, 363–377.

Cox, L. E., Ashford, J. M., Clark, K. N., Martin-Elbahesh, K., Hardy, K. K., Merchant, T. E., . . . Conklin, H. M. (2015). Feasibility and acceptability of a remotely administered computerized intervention to address cognitive late effects among childhood cancer survivors. *Neuro-oncology Practice, 2*, 78–87.

Dahlquist, L. M., & Shroff Pendley, J. (2005). When distraction fails: Parental anxiety and children's responses to distraction during cancer procedures. *Journal of Pediatric Psychology, 30*, 623–628.

Daly, B., Kral, M. C., & Tarazi, R. M. (2011). The role of neuropsychological evaluation in pediatric sickle cell disease. *The Clinical Neuropsychologist, 25*(6), 903–925. doi:10.1080/13854046.2011.560590

Edwards, L. V. (2006). Perceived social support and HIV/AIDS medication adherence among African American women. *Qualitative Health Research, 16*, 679–691.

Federal Register. (2006). Assistance to States for the Education of Children with Disabilities and Preschool Grants for Children with Disabilities; Final Rule, 34 C. F. R. § 300. Retrieved from https://www.federalregister.gov/documents/2016/12/19/

2016-30190/assistance-to-states-for-the-education-of-children-with-disabilities-preschool-grants-for-children

Ferrando, S. J. (2009). Psychopharmacologic treatment of patients with HIV/AIDS. *Current Psychiatry Reports, 11*(3), 235–242.

Fitzhugh, C. D., Abraham, A. A., Tisdale, J. F., & Hsieh, M. M. (2014). Hematopoietic stem cell transplant for patients with sickle cell disease: Progress and future directions. *Hematology/Oncology Clinics of North America, 28*(6), 1171–1185. doi:10.1016/j.hoc.2014.08.014

Fuemmeler, B. F., Elkin, T. D., & Mullins, L. L. (2002). Survivors of childhood brain tumors: Behavioral, emotional, and social adjustment. *Clinical Psychology Review, 22*, 547–585.

Garvie, P. A., Zeldow, B., Malee, K., Nichols, S. L., Smith, R. A., Wilkins, M. L., & Williams, P. (2014). Discordance of cognitive and academic achievement outcomes in youth with perinatal HIV exposure. *Pediatric Infectious Diseases Journal, 33*, 232–238. doi:10.1097/INF.0000000000000314

Gerhardt, C. A., Dixon, M., Miller, K., Vannatta, K., Valerius, K. S., Correll, J., & Noll, R. B. (2007). Educational and occupational outcomes among survivors or childhood cancer during the transition to emerging adulthood. *Journal of Developmental Behavioral Pediatrics, 28*, 448–455.

Gibson, F., Mulhall, A. B., Richardson, A., Edwards, J. L., Ream, E., & Sepion, B. J. (2005). A phenomenologic study of fatigue in adolescents receiving treatment for cancer. *Oncology Nursing Forum, 32*, 651–660.

Gil, K. M., Carson, J. W., Porter, L. S., Ready, J., Valrie, C., Redding-Lallinger, R., & Daeschner, C. (2003). Daily stress and mood and their association with pain, health-care use, and school activity in adolescents with sickle cell disease. *Journal of Pediatric Psychology, 28*(5), 363–373. doi:10.1093/jpepsy/jsg026

Hardy, K. K., Willard, V. W., Allen, T. M., & Bonner, M. J. (2013). Working memory training in survivors of pediatric cancer: A randomized pilot study. *Psycho-Oncology: Journal of the Psychological, Social, and Behavioral Dimensions of Cancer, 22*, 1856–1865.

Hardy, S. J., Hardy, K. K., Schatz, J. C., Thompson, A. L., & Meier, E. R. (2016). Feasibility of home-based computerized working memory training with children and adolescnets with sickle cell disease. *Pediatric Blood and Cancer, 63*, 1578–1585.

Hedén, L., Pöder, U., von Essen, L., & Ljungman, G. (2013). Parents' perceptions of their child's symptom burden during and after cancer treatment. *Journal of Pain and Symptom Management, 46*, 366–375.

Hudson, M. M., Ness, K. K., Gurney, J. G., Mulrooney, D. A., Chemaitilly, W., Krull, K. R., . . . Robison, L. L. (2013). Clinical ascertainment of health outcomes among adults treated for childhood cancer. *Journal of the American Medical Association, 309*, 2371–2381.

Ivascu, N. S., Sarnaik, S., McCrae, J., Whitten-Shirney, W., Thomas, R., & Bond, S. (2001). Characterization of pica prevalence among patients with sickle cell disease. *Archives of Pediatrics and Adolescent Medicine, 155*(11), 1243–1247. doi:10.1001/archpedi.155.11.1243

Jacola, L. M., Edelstein, K., Liu, W., Pui, C. H., Hayashi, R., Kadan-Lottick, N. S., . . . Krull, K. R. (2016). Cognitive, behavior, and academic functioning in adolescent and young adult survivors of childhood acute lymphoblastic leukaemia: A report from the Childhood Cancer Study. *Lancet Psychiatry, 3*, 965–972. doi: 10.1016/S2215-0366(16)30283-8

Kazak, A. (2006). Pediatric Psychosocial Preventative Health Model (PPPHM): Research, practice and collaboration in pediatric family systems medicine. *Families, Systems, and Health, 24*, 381–395. doi:10.1037/1091-7527.24.4.381

Knight, S. J., Conklin, H. M., Palmer, S., Schreiber, J., Armstrong, C. L., Wallace, D., . . . Gajjar, A. (2014). Working memory abilities among children treated for medulloblastoma: A longitudinal study of parent report and performance. *Journal of Pediatric Psychology, 39*, 501–511. doi:10.1093/jpepsy/jsu009

Lemanek, K. L., & Ranalli, M. (2009). Sickle cell disease. In M. C. Roberts & R. G. Steele (Eds.), *Handbook of pediatric psychology* (4th ed., pp. 303–318). New York, NY: Guilford Press.

Mancini, A. F., Rosito, P., Canino, R., Calzetti, G., Di Caro, A., Salmi, S., . . . Missiroli, G. (1989). School-related behavior in children with cancer. *Pediatric Hematology and Oncology, 6*, 145–154.

Mulhern, R. K., Merchant, T. E., Gajjar, A., Reddick, W. E., & Kun, L. E. (2004). Late neurocognitive sequelae in survivors of brain tumors in childhood. *Lancet, 5*, 399–408.

National Cancer Institute (2017). *Childhood cancers*. Retrieved from https://www.cancer.gov/types/childhood-cancers

National Heart, Lung, and Blood Institute. (2014). Evidence-based management of sickle cell disease: Expert panel report. Retrieved from http://www.nhlbi.nih.gov/health/dci/Diseases/Sca/

Nichols, S. L., Bethel, J., Garvie, P. A., Patton, D. E., Thornton, S., Kapogiannis, B. G., . . . Woods, S. P. (2013). Neurocognitive functioning in antiretroviral therapy-naïve youth with behaviorally acquired HIV. *Journal of Adolescent Health, 53*, 763–771. doi:10.1016/j.jadohealth.2013.07.006

Nichols, S. L., Bethel, J., Kapogiannis, B. G., Li, T., Woods, S. P., Patton, E. D., . . . Garvie, P. A. (2016). Antiretroviral treatment initiation does not differentially alter neurocognitive functioning over time in youth with behaviorally acquired HIV. *Journal of Neurovirology, 22*, 218–230. doi:10.1007/s13365-015-0389-0

Noll, R. B., LeRoy, S., Bukowski, W. M., Rogosch, F. A., & Kulkarni, R. (1991). Peer relationships and adjustment in children with cancer. *Journal of Pediatric Psychology, 16*, 307–326.

Olson, K., & Amari, A. (2015). Self-reported pain in adolescents with leukemia or a brain tumor. *Cancer Nursing, 38*, E43–E53.

Phillips, N., Amos, T., Kuo, C., Hoare, J., Ipser, J., Thomas, K. G. F., & Stein, D. J. (2016). HIV- associated cognitive impairment in perinatally infected children: A meta-analysis. Pediatrics, *138*(5). doi:10.1542/peds.2016-0893

Phipps, S., Jurbergs, N., & Long, A. (2009). Symptoms of post-traumatic stress in children with cancer: Does personality trump health status? *Psycho-Oncology, 18*, 992–1002.

Reddick, W. E., Taghipour, D. J., Glass, J. O., Ashford, J. M., Xiong, X., Wu, S., . . . Conklin, H. M. (2014). Prognostic factors that increase the risk for reduced white matter volumes and deficits in attention and learning for survivors of childhood cancers. *Pediatric Blood and Cancer, 61*, 1074–1079.

Robison, L. L., & Hudson, M. M. (2014). Survivors of childhood and adolescent cancer: Life-long risks and responsibilities. *National Review of Cancer, 14*, 61–70.

Samji, H., Cescon, A., Hogg, R., Modur, S., Althoff, K., Buchacz, K., . . . Gange S. J., for the North American AIDS Cohort Collaboration on Research and Design (NA-ACCORD) of IeDEA. (2013). Closing the gap: Increases in life expectancy among treated HIV-positive individuals in the United States and Canada. *PLoS One, 8*(12) e81355. doi:10.1371/journal.pone.0081355.

Sanger, M. S., Copeland, D. R., & Davidson, E. R. (1991). Psychosocial adjustment among pediatric cancer patients: A multidimensional assessment. *Journal of Pediatric Psychology, 16,* 463–474.

Schatz, J., & McClellan, C. B. (2006). Sickle cell disease as a neurodevelopmental disorder. *Mental Retardation and Developmental Disabilities Research Reviews, 12,* 200–207.

Shulte, F., Vannatta, K., & Barrera, M. (2014). Social problem solving and social performance after a group social skills intervention for childhood brain tumor survivors. *Psychooncology, 23,* 183–189.

Simoni, J. M., Frick, P. A., & Huang, B. (2006). A longitudinal evaluation of a social support model of medication adherence among HIV-positive men and women on antiretroviral therapy. *Health Psychology, 25*(1) 74–81. doi:10.1037/0278-6133.25.1.74

Simoni, J. M., Pearson, C. R., Pantalone, D. W., Marks, G., & Crepaz, N. (2006). Efficacy of interventions in improving highly active antiretroviral therapy adherence in HIV-1 RNA viral load: A meta analytic review of randomized controlled trials. *Journal of Acquired Immune Deficiency Syndrome, 43,* S23–25.

Smith, J. T., & Baker, D. A. (2011). Sickle cell disease. In S. Goldstein & C. Reynolds (Eds.), *Handbook of neurodevelopmental and genetic disorders in children* (2nd ed., pp. 338–361). New York, NY: Guilford Press.

Smith, R. A., & Wilkins, M. L. (2014). Perinatally acquired HIV infection: Long-term neuropsychological consequences and challenges ahead. *Child Neuropsychology, 21*(2), 234–268.

Therrell, B. L., Lloyd-Puryear, M. A., Eckmas, J. R., & Mann, M. Y. (2015). Newborn screening for sickle cell disease in the United States: A review of data spanning 2 decades. *Seminars in Perinatology, 39,* 238–251. doi:10.1053/j.semperi.2015.03.008

Todd, A. (2015). Mandatory HIV status disclosure for students in Illinois: A deterrent to testing and a violation of the Americans with Disabilities Act, *Northwestern Journal of Law & Social Policy, 10*(2), 426–460.

U.S. Cancer Statistics Working Group. (2017). *United States cancer statistics: 1999–2014. Incidence and mortality Web-based report.* Available at http://www.cdc.gov/uscs

U.S. Department of Education. (2000). Nondiscrimination on the basis of handicap in programs or activities receiving federal financial assistance, 34 C. F. R. § 104. Retrieved from https://www2.ed.gov/policy/rights/reg/ocr/34cfr104.pdf

Varni, J. W., Burwinkle, T. M., & Katz, E. R. (2004). The PedsQL in pediatric cancer pain: A prospective longitudinal analysis of pain and emotional distress. *Journal of Developmental and Behavioral Pediatrics, 25,* 239–246.

Walsh, A. S. J., Wesley, K. L., Tan, S. Y., Lynn, C., O'Leary, K., Wang, K., . . . Rodriguez, C. (2017). Screening for depression among youth with HIV in an integrated care setting. *AIDS Care, 29,* 851–857. doi:10.1080/09540121.2017.1281878

Wang, W. C. (2008). Sickle cell anemia and other sickling syndromes. In J. P. Greer, J. Foerster, G. M. Rodgers, F. Paraskevas, & B. E. Glader (Eds.), *Wintrobe's clinical hematology* (12th ed., pp. 1038–1082). Philadelphia, PA: Lippincott Williams & Wilkins.

Willard, V. W., Cox, L. E., Russell, K. M., Kenney, A., Jurbergs, N., Molnar, A. E., & Harman, J. (2017). Cognitive and psychosocial functioning of preschool-aged children with cancer. *Journal of Developmental and Behavioral Pediatrics, 38,* 638–645.

Winter, A. L., Conklin, H. M., Tyc, V. L., Stancel, H. H., Hinds, P. S., Hudson, M. M., & Kahalley, L. S. (2014). Executive function late effects in survivors of brain tumors and acute lymphoblastic leukemia. *Journal of Clinical and Experimental Neuropsychology, 36,* 818–830.

Yawn, B. P., Buchanan, G. R., Afenyi-Annan, A. N., Ballas, S. K., Hassell, K. L., James, A. H., . . . John-Sowah, J. (2014). Management of sickle cell disease: Summary of the 2014 evidence-based report by expert panel Members. *JAMA, 312*(10), 1033–1048. doi:10.1001/jama.2014.10517

HANDOUT 20.1.

PAIN PASSPORT

This passport may help you get throughthe school day in spite of not feeling your best at times. Knowing what makes your discomfort or pain worse and planning for use of coping tools ahead of time can make all the difference in the world.

Things that trigger my discomfort are:
Ways I can overcome these include:

Warning signs that I am starting to not feel my best include:
Things I can do when I notice these signs include:

If I start to feel uncomfortable at school I can:
I know I can be successful at school because:

21

Obesity in Children and Adolescents

JANE GRAY, ALISON J. LEE, AND STEPHEN PONT ■

OVERVIEW OF OBESITY, RELATED COMORBIDITIES, AND BEHAVIORAL HEALTH CONCERNS

Obesity is a highly prevalent concern in American schoolchildren, with 17% of children and adolescents in the United States being classified as obese (Ogden, Carroll, Flegal, & Kit, 2014). The risk of obesity increases with age: 8.9% of preschool-age children, 17.5% of 6- to 11-year-olds, and 20.5% of 12- to 19-year-olds meet the criteria for obesity (Ogden, Carroll, Fryar, & Flegal, 2015). In childhood, obesity is defined as having a body mass index (BMI) of ≥ 95th percentile, while overweight is defined as having a body mass index (BMI) of ≥ 85th percentile. When data for overweight are included, 31.8% of youth ages 2-19 are overweight or obese (Ogden et al., 2014). Pediatric obesity is associated with a myriad of chronic health issues, including type 2 diabetes, asthma, obstructive sleep apnea, hypertension, joint problems, polycystic ovarian syndrome, non-alcoholic fatty liver, and premature mortality (Pulgarón, 2013). In addition, obesity has negative psychological effects in youth, including symptoms of depression, disordered eating, low self-esteem, and poor quality of life (Small & Aplasca, 2016). The physical and psychological effects of obesity are exacerbated by the social response to individuals affected by excess weight. Stigmatization can be pervasive and damaging, and it may contribute to adverse weight-related health outcomes, including stress, binge eating, decreased physical activity, increased weight gain over time, social isolation, and avoidance of healthcare services (Hunte & Williams, 2009; Puhl & Suh, 2015). Given the importance of the school environment in a child's ecological context, it is critical that school professionals understand the problem of childhood obesity, as well as effective strategies for addressing the problem and its social impact.

Key Medical Terms and Procedures

Obesity is a medical term referring to the BMI category of the 95th percentile and above. Although the term is used in scientific and medical contexts, research has shown that individuals respond negatively to the use of this term due to the stigma it carries (Puhl, Peterson, & Luedicke, 2011, 2013). It is preferable to use terms related to weight (e.g., *excess weight, overweight, unhealthy weight*). It is also preferable to use person-first language, such as *children with obesity*, or *children with overweight/excess weight*.

Some of the more common medical conditions associated with, or caused by, obesity include the following conditions.

Acanthosis nigricans is a darkening and thickening of the skin associated with insulin resistance and with the development of type 2 diabetes. It is most often apparent on the back of the neck. Some individuals will also develop acanthosis nigricans in their armpits, on the abdominal area, on the inner thighs, and sometimes on the face. It is important that parents understand that acanthosis nigricans is due to increased pigment in the skin and cannot be washed off with soap, bathing, or other chemicals. As children and adolescents move to a healthier weight, acanthosis nigricans will often soften or resolve.

Type 2 diabetes occurs when the body becomes less sensitive to the effects of insulin. Insulin is produced in the pancreas and allows the body to move sugar (or glucose) from the bloodstream into the cells so that the sugar can be used for energy production by the cells. Blood sugar levels increase as the body becomes resistant to insulin. Some children are diagnosed with prediabetes, which refers to blood sugar levels in an at-risk range. Some physicians may prescribe medication for children with prediabetes; however, most often the treatment plan includes lifestyle changes to improve nutrition and physical activity.

Hypertension is high blood pressure. Hypertension, if untreated for long periods of time, can lead to stroke, heart attack, kidney failure, and other medical problems. Occasionally blood pressure can rise to high levels quickly and create a medical emergency. The plan for hypertension in children and adolescents may include monitoring of blood pressure in nonclinical settings, such as at school, because many children and adults experience anxiety and resultant blood pressure elevation when in a clinic or hospital. Treatment plans for children with obesity and hypertension typically include lifestyle changes to manage excess weight and, in some cases, medication to regulate blood pressure.

Abnormal cholesterol can be either due to elevated "bad" cholesterol (i.e., LDL— low density lipoproteins—or triglycerides), or due to low levels of "good" cholesterol (i.e., HDL—high density lipoproteins). Unless levels are very high, initial treatment typically involves lifestyle changes to manage excess weight.

Non-alcoholic fatty liver disease (NAFLD) or non-alcoholic steatohepatitis (NASH) is due to fat deposition in the liver. Over time, this leads to liver inflammation, followed by cirrhosis, or irreversible scarring of the liver, that can ultimately lead to liver failure. A challenge with this condition is its asymptomatic nature; typically, adolescents do not feel symptoms and are unaware of the condition until their physician detects liver inflammation by a blood test. By the time individuals feel the symptoms of liver disease (fatigue, bleeding, jaundice, loss of appetite, nausea, swelling), the damage is irreversible.

Obstructive sleep apnea occurs when a child stops breathing at night due to soft tissue in the throat that obstructs the airway. Loud snoring is a risk factor and is associated with obstructive sleep apnea; however, many adolescents with snoring do not have sleep apnea. Symptoms of apnea include gasping for air while sleeping, nighttime enuresis, and daytime sleepiness despite good sleep hygiene. Treatment includes wearing a sleep apnea mask attached to a bilevel positive airway pressure (BiPAP/BPAP) or continuous positive airway pressure (CPAP) machine. This increases the pressure in the airway, preventing closure of the airway. It typically takes some adjustment for children and adolescents to become comfortable sleeping with the mask and the blowing airflow. Sometimes a tonsillectomy or nasal steroids can also relieve symptoms of mild to moderate obstructive sleep apnea. Left untreated, sleep apnea can lead to heart and lung failure.

The comorbidities above are mainly addressed by changing lifestyle, as opposed to treatment with medical procedures. For children and teens with severe obesity or conditions that are more severe or have been more longstanding, medication to regulate blood sugar or blood pressure, use of CPAP for sleep apnea, or tonsillectomy to address sleep apnea may be necessary.

CASE EXAMPLES

Estevan

Estevan is an 8-year-old Latino boy. He is in third grade at a primarily Latino school, and he lives with his biological mother, father, and siblings (ages 2, 5, and 12). His parents are undocumented immigrants from Mexico and their primary language is Spanish. His father works in construction and his mother stays at home. Their family has very limited financial resources. Estevan is described as a happy boy and has a few friends at school. His pediatrician took blood work and discovered high cholesterol and blood glucose levels; therefore, the pediatrician diagnosed Estevan with obesity and prediabetes. Estevan's parents are concerned about the risk for diabetes because his mother has type 2 diabetes and many extended family members have diabetes and heart disease. They are very open to learning information about how to cook differently at home, but they report little access to healthy foods.

Sarah

Sarah, a 14-year-old Caucasian girl, is a ninth grader at a mostly middle-class suburban high school. Her parents are divorced and she lives primarily with her mother.

She has an older sister who is also in high school and whose weight is within healthy norms, and a younger brother whose weight appears typical, but whose BMI falls within the overweight category. Sarah has obesity. She has no medical comorbidities but is experiencing significant depression and bullying. She played volleyball in middle school but decided not to try out in high school, instead participating in the school newspaper. Her parents have poor communication with one another and the structure is very different in each household. Sarah's mother's household is very "healthy," with few processed foods, and her father's household is described as having lots of snacks and sodas. Sarah's mother has called the school counselor several times because Sarah often cries after school and recently told her mother that she is frequently called names related to her size and that her friends have started avoiding her. She is afraid to talk to any adults at school about her concerns.

OBESITY AND SCHOOL-RELATED CHALLENGES

Academic Achievement

The association between healthy behaviors and academic achievement (e.g., attendance, graduation rates, grades, and standardized test scores) is well documented (Basch, 2011; Bradley & Greene, 2013; Busch et al., 2014; Michael, Merlo, Basch, Wentzel, & Wechsler, 2015; Rasberry et al., 2011, 2017). Middle-school students with overweight scored 11% lower than the national percentile for reading scores compared to peers without overweight/obesity (Shore et al., 2008). Students with overweight have also been found to have poorer school attendance, more disciplinary issues, and less sport participation than their peers (Geier et al., 2007; Shore et al., 2008). Some of these issues may be caused, or exacerbated, by weight-based victimization (Puhl & Luedicke, 2012).

Peer Victimization and Weight Stigma

Research indicates that peer victimization is associated with poor academic outcomes (Schwartz, Gorman, Nakamoto, & Toblin, 2005), and students with obesity are often targets of teasing, bullying, and victimization, particularly in the school setting. Weight bias begins early; preschool-age children ascribe negative attributes to youth with larger bodies (Spiel, Paxton, & Yager, 2012; Su & Aurelia, 2012). Students with overweight or obesity are more socially isolated and are more likely to be bullied than students without overweight or obesity, even after accounting for a variety of demographic, social, and academic factors (Goldfield et al., 2010; Lumeng et al., 2010). Weight-based victimization persists into and throughout the teenage years, with adolescents reporting the main reason peers are bullied or teased at school is due to their weight status (Puhl, Luedicke, & Heuer, 2011).

The experience of weight stigma can result in numerous adverse physical and psychological outcomes for youth. Physical consequences related to weight stigma include decreased physical activity (Losekam, Goetzky, Kraeling, Rief, & Hilbert, 2010) unhealthy eating patterns (Haines, Neumark-Sztainer, Eisenberg, & Hannan, 2006), and increased weight gain over time (Jackson, Beeken, & Wardle, 2014). Generally, being bullied is associated with increased anxiety, feelings of depression, isolation, decreased self-esteem, and behavior problems (Mamun, O'Callaghan, Williams, & Najman, 2013), with body image being an additional challenge for victims of weight-based bullying (Jensen & Steele, 2009; Puhl & Latner, 2007). Peer victimization puts children at risk for suicide (Geoffroy et al., 2016), and a higher rate of suicide attempts is reported among adolescents with obesity (Eaton, Lowry, Brener, Galuska, & Crosby, 2005). Not surprisingly then, the rate of suicidal ideation and attempted suicide among adolescents subjected to weight-based teasing is two to three times higher than the rate for adolescents not subjected to such teasing (Eisenberg, Neumark-Sztainer, & Story, 2003). These findings highlight the importance of addressing weight stigma, particularly in the school setting, due to the documented potential for serious adverse outcomes.

Educators can be susceptible to weight bias. Teachers may expect less from, and have more negative attitudes toward, students with obesity. Longitudinal research looking at students from later elementary school years into middle school found that a higher BMI z-score was significantly associated with worsening teacher perceptions of academic ability for girls and boys, independent of standardized test scores (Kenney, Gortmaker, Davison, & Austin, 2015). This bias can be found in physical education as well, with coaches expecting students with obesity to have poorer physical abilities compared to students without obesity, and female students with obesity experiencing higher levels of bias with respect to physical performance, cooperation, reasoning, and social skills than their male peers (Peterson, Puhl, & Luedicke, 2012). This is particularly concerning because evidence suggests that, in general, females report weight discrimination at significantly higher rates and lower BMI levels than males (Puhl, Andreyeva, & Brownell, 2008).

School professionals have an important opportunity to help protect youth with obesity from the above-mentioned risks. First and foremost, it would be helpful for all professionals to engage in continuing education about weight bias to develop increased awareness, knowledge, and skills related to this issue. The Rudd Center website listed at the end of this chapter has helpful tools for this purpose. Children like Estevan and Sarah are at particular risk for the negative consequences of weight stigma and peer victimization. While Estevan has some social support and is not reporting victimization, he should be monitored for any changes in his peer relationships. A nonjudgmental, supportive relationship with Estevan's family will highlight the family's strengths and motivation in the face of social and economic stressors. Sarah is clearly struggling with peer victimization, which has the potential to worsen her academic, social, and emotional functioning. In her case, a supportive school environment, including empathetic connections with school professionals, can be protective.

CONSIDERATIONS FOR ASSESSMENT AND INTERVENTION IN THE SCHOOL SETTING

Assessment of Obesity

Screening for obesity in schools can have an important role in increasing awareness of students' risk for other health conditions. Some states utilize screening measurements, such as the Cooper Institute's Fitnessgram (http://www.cooperinstitute.org/fitnessgram), or other independently developed fitness assessment and BMI measurement protocols. When the fitness or BMI screening tests are done respectfully, using nonstigmatizing language and thoughtful communication with families, they can play an important role in supporting the health of students. Some states have also implemented screening for acanthosis nigricans, which can be helpful in identifying students at risk for diabetes.

In order to determine if a child is at a healthy weight, the child must be plotted on a growth chart by age and sex for weight, height, and BMI. Recommendations are then made based upon the age of the child and the degree to which the child is above a healthy weight. The American Academy of Pediatrics recommends:

- For children 2 to 5 years old with a BMI in the 95th to 99th percentile, weight maintenance; if the BMI is ≥ 99th percentile, gradual weight loss of no more than 1 pound per month.
- For children 6 to 11 years old with a BMI in the 95th to 99th percentile, weight maintenance or gradual weight loss of no more than 1 pound per month; if the BMI is ≥ 99th percentile, gradual weight loss of no more than 2 pounds per week.
- For adolescents 12 to 18 years old with a BMI in the 95th to 99th percentile and BMI ≥ 99th percentile, gradual weight loss of no more than 2 pounds per week. (Barlow, 2007)

Weight loss and evaluation of healthy changes should all be carried out under the supervision and guidance of a physician.

In addition to screening for excess weight, it is helpful for school professionals to screen for potential mental health concerns, including depressive symptoms and behavioral problems, as these concerns have been shown to be associated with both excess weight and success with treatment (Anderson, He, Schoppe-Sullivan, & Must, 2010; Hommel, Odell, Sander, Baldassano, & Barg, 2011; Zeller et al., 2004). Behavioral health intervention for these issues may assist with overall success with weight management. Additionally, it is helpful for school professionals to screen for maladaptive eating behaviors, including binge eating or secretive eating, and to recommend further assessment and treatment by a medical and behavioral health specialist in the community if those behaviors are present.

Intervention for Obesity

School professionals have an important opportunity to address childhood obesity, given the amount of time children spend in school, the number of meals eaten on the school campus, and the availability of safe space and equipment for physical activity. Experts recommend a comprehensive school-based approach to prevent obesity (Sobol-Goldberg, Rabinowitz, & Gross, 2013; Wang et al., 2015). For ideas on implementing schoolwide health and obesity-prevention programming, the CDC's "Make a Difference at Your School" toolkit can be helpful (CDC, 2013).

The United States Preventive Services Task Force (USPSTF) recommends comprehensive, intensive behavioral interventions in order to achieve meaningful BMI reduction and a benefit for metabolic and cardiovascular risk factors (O'Connor et al., 2017). Initial signs of success may include changes in eating and physical activity behaviors, which promote slowing of the rate of weight gain, stabilization of weight, stabilization of BMI, and eventually a decrease in BMI. These behavioral changes can also improve comorbidities associated with obesity, including high blood pressure (Shi, Krupp, & Remer, 2014). Effective behavioral interventions include a parental component and provide foundational information about physical activity and nutrition. Including a parental component is of particular importance with younger children, because parents and caregivers have more control over the child's nutrition and physical activity. The majority of research on interventions for pediatric obesity is focused on elementary- and middle-school-age children; there is less empirical evidence about interventions with adolescents or very young children (Sobol-Goldberg et al., 2013; Wang et al., 2015). School interventions for obesity vary in terms of format (individual or group), content (nutrition education, physical activity education, actual physical activity, goal planning, parent involvement), and length/intensity of intervention, but generally the research has indicated that addressing health behaviors in the school setting can have an impact on student BMI and associated health indicators (Berry et al., 2014; Coppins et al., 2011; Johnston et al., 2013; Toruner & Savaser, 2010).

It is useful for schools to be aware of specialty clinics and programs available in medical and community settings, particularly for children with severe obesity who may need more intensive intervention and medical oversight. Comprehensive weight-management programs for children with obesity should have an interprofessional team that includes a behavioral health specialist. Typical treatment plans for children with severe obesity and associated medical and psychological comorbidities involve intensive behavioral changes in nutrition and physical activity, in addition to management of the medical comorbidities and mental health concerns (Spear et al., 2007). Collaborative goal setting can provide structure and motivation for children and families as they begin making these behavioral changes (see handout 21.1). Weight-management teams typically try to use a strengths-based approach to assist families in recognizing their strengths and resources, to identify barriers and realistic solutions, and to facilitate connections to additional resources in order to enhance engagement and adherence (American

Academy of Pediatrics, 2013; Flaherty, Stirling, & The Committee on Child Abuse and Neglect, 2010). For Estevan and Sarah, school-based screening and assessment would assist them in getting medical and behavioral health assistance. For Estevan, it would be particularly helpful for the family to have access to an intervention that is delivered in Spanish. A full assessment of the family environment and family's resources would help inform appropriate recommendations. In Sarah's case, an intervention that addresses her weight management, as well as the bullying and depression she is experiencing, would be important.

Risk and Protective Factors

Several risk factors have been identified in the literature, including parental obesity, maternal weight gain during pregnancy, chronic maternal depression, poor sleep, low family income, and behavioral risk factors, such as excess caloric intake, low physical activity, and sedentary behavior (Bammann et al., 2014; Lampard, Franckle, & Davison, 2014; Magee & Hale, 2012; Tamayo, Christian, & Rathmann, 2010). Of these risk factors, behavioral risk factors are most easily addressed in school, by encouraging healthy nutrition and both structured (e.g., physical education and team sports) and unstructured (e.g., recess) physical activity. The literature has not identified many protective factors against obesity beyond breastfeeding during infancy (Wang, Collins, Ratliff, Xie, & Wang, 2017). It may be helpful for school professionals to provide information to families on the benefits of breastfeeding, in order to provide some protection for younger siblings of students.

CULTURAL CONSIDERATIONS

Obesity rates among black and Latino youth are significantly higher than among white or Asian youth, and in some lower socioeconomic status communities, up to two thirds of children have overweight or obesity (Ogden et al., 2014; Skinner, Perrin, & Skelton, 2016). Low socioeconomic status can create a forced choice along a hierarchy of immediate needs that may, understandably, affect a family's ability to implement lifestyle changes, such as improved diet and increased physical activity (Payne, 2005). Furthermore, poverty influences obesity-related risk factors, such as the availability of environments in which to be safely physically active and the cost of healthy foods. Additionally, cultural differences and beliefs about weight can be barriers to change and treatment success. In some cultures, a healthy weight may be negatively construed as underweight, which can trigger concerns about malnutrition, particularly for impoverished families. Further, cultural values related to body shape and size may influence lifestyle and behaviors (Peña, Dixon, & Taveras, 2012). Finally, educational level has been found to be an important variable; obesity rates among children living with a head of household who completed college were nearly half the obesity rates among children living with a head of household who did not complete high school (May, Freedman,

Sherry, & Blanck, 2013). This, coupled with the challenge of understanding and interpreting conflicting messages and misleading information about food and physical activity, may put families from disadvantaged backgrounds at increased risk. Again, it is imperative that school professionals approach families dealing with obesity, especially those from underrepresented ethnic groups and those with low socioeconomic resources, in a nonjudgmental, nonstigmatizing, and nonblaming manner.

LEGAL AND POLICY ISSUES

Legal Protections for Students with Obesity

Youth with obesity may be eligible to receive accommodations and modifications in school if obesity affects their academic performance. The Individuals with Disabilities Education Act (IDEA) is a federal special education law for children with disabilities, while Section 504 of the Rehabilitation Act of 1973 is a federal civil rights law that prohibits discrimination against individuals with disabilities. Students can be eligible to receive special education services within the other health impairment (OHI) category if two criteria are met: (1) they have a condition that limits their strength, energy, or alertness; and (2) the condition adversely affects the student's educational performance. Having obesity does not automatically qualify a child as disabled under the OHI category; however, students with obesity along with related physical fitness or motor skill deficiencies may be eligible for special education services under the OHI category. Examples of accommodations and modifications include special seating modifications or furniture, dietary modifications based on physician recommendation, adapted physical education program per physician recommendation, ensuring that the student has privacy when changing clothes for physical education, allowing extra time to get to classes, and arranging opportunities for the student to participate in intramural and extracurricular events.

Policies Related to Weight-Based Discrimination, Bullying, and Victimization

No federal laws exist that explicitly prohibit discrimination against individuals with obesity. While schools often have general anti-bullying policies and may prohibit discrimination based on gender, race, ethnicity, or sexual orientation, discrimination based on size is not explicitly named. The Rudd Center for Food Policy and Obesity (http://www.uconnruddcenter.org) recommends that both students and educators be included in efforts to eliminate weight bias. Implementing legal protections that specifically apply to students with obesity can combat the adverse academic, social, physical, and psychological outcomes associated with weight-based discrimination and bias.

CONCLUSION

Given the amount of time children spend in school, and the opportunity for nutrition, physical activity, and social-emotional programming in the school setting, schools are an appropriate venue for obesity prevention and intervention. When school professionals promote healthy changes to nutrition and physical activity, they can positively impact the physical and mental health of students, particularly those students already challenged by their weight. Further, academic success may be enhanced, particularly when peer victimization is addressed. It is of vital importance for schools to take a nonjudgmental, nonblaming approach with children and families when addressing the issue of childhood obesity, given the weight stigma and bias that are both prevalent and counterproductive for health behavior change.

WEBSITES AND RESOURCES

Physical Activity

- *Fit* Kids: The Place for Kids to Play and Learn Healthy Habits: http://fit.webmd.com/default.htm
- Move: Fitness Activities: http://www.kidnetic.com/kore/
- BAM! Body and Mind: http://www.cdc.gov/bam/activity/cards.html
- Why Exercise is Cool: http://kidshealth.org/en/kids/work-it-out.html
- Marathon Kids: https://marathonkids.org/
- President's Council on Fitness and Nutrition: www.fitness.gov
- Let's Go: www.letsgo.org
- National Wildlife Federation Outdoor Activities: http://www.nwf.org/kids/family-fun.aspx

Nutrition

- Choose MyPlate: http://www.choosemyplate.gov
- Best Bones Forever!: http://www.bestbonesforever.org/
- ChopChop Cooking Club: http://www.chopchopmag.org/
- Kids Eat Right: http://www.kidseatright.org/
- Fresh for Kids: http://www.freshforkids.com.au/
- Calorie King: www.calorieking.com
- Spark People: www.sparkteen.com
- Ellyn Satter Institute: http://www.ellynsatterinstitute.org/
- Super Healthy Kids: http://www.superhealthykids.com/
- Sustainable Food Center: www.sustainablefoodcenter.org

Recipes

- www.allrecipes.com
- www.cookinglight.com
- www.sparkrecipes.com
- www.superhealthykids.com/healthy-kids-recipes/

Parent Resources

- Healthy Children (English): https://www.healthychildren.org/English/Pages/default.aspx
- Healthy Children (Spanish): https://www.healthychildren.org/spanish/paginas/default.aspx
- Kids Health: http://www.kidshealth.org/
- 5-2-1-0 Handout (English): http://www.ohsu.edu/xd/health/services/doernbecher/patients-families/healthy-lifestyles/upload/brochure-Kohls-diabetes-5-2-1-0_for-BB-FINAL2.pdf
- 5-2-1-0 Handout (Spanish): http://www.ohsu.edu/xd/health/services/doernbecher/patients-families/healthy-lifestyles/upload/brochure-Kohls-5-2-1-0spanish-1.pdf

Educator Resources

- Rudd Center for Food Policy and Obesity: http://www.uconnruddcenter.org/
- Rudd Center Resources on bullying: http://www.uconnruddcenter.org/files/Pdfs/Educators-WebResources_rev%207-11-16.pdf

REFERENCES

American Academy of Pediatrics (2013). *Strength based approach: Healthy active living for families implementation guide.* Retrieved from http://www.aap.org/en-us/advocacy-and-policy/aap-health-initiatives/HALF-Implementation-Guide/communicating-with-families/Pages/Strength-Based-Approach.aspx

Anderson, S. E., He, X., Schoppe-Sullivan, S., & Must, A. (2010). Externalizing behavior in early childhood and body mass index from age 2 to 12 years: Longitudinal analyses of a prospective cohort study. *BMC Pediatrics, 10*(49), 1–8.

Bammann, K., Peplies, J., De Henauw, S., Hunsberger, M., Molnar, D., Moreno, L. A., . . . Göteborgs universitet. (2014). Early life course risk factors for childhood obesity: The IDEFICS case-control study. *PloS One, 9*(2), e86914.

Barlow, S. E. (2007). Expert committee recommendations regarding the prevention, assessment, and treatment of child and adolescent overweight and obesity: Summary report. *Pediatrics,120*(Suppl.), S164–S192.

Basch, C. E. (2011). Healthier students are better learners: A missing link in school reforms to close the achievement gap. *Journal of School Health, 81*(10), 593–598.

Berry, D. C., Schwartz, T. A., McMurray, R. G., Skelly, A. H., Neal, M., Hall, E. G., . . . Melkus, G. (2014). The family partners for health study: a cluster randomized controlled trial for child and parent weight management. *Nutrition & Diabetes,* 4(1), e101.

Bradley, B. J., & Greene, A. C. (2013). Do health and education agencies in the United States share responsibility for academic achievement and health? A review of 25 years of evidence about the relationship of adolescents' academic achievement and health behaviors. *The Journal of Adolescent Health: Official Publication of the Society for Adolescent Medicine, 52*(5), 523–532.

Busch, V., Loyen, A., Lodder, M., Schrijvers, A. J. P., van Yperen, T. A., & de Leeuw, J. R. J. (2014). The effects of adolescent health-related behavior on academic performance: A systematic review of the longitudinal evidence. *Review of Educational Research, 84*(2), 245–274.

Centers for Disease Control and Prevention. (2013). Make a difference at your school. *Chronic Disease, 31.* Retrieved from http://digitalcommons.hsc.unt.edu/disease/31

Coppins, D. F., Margetts, B. M., Fa, J. L., Brown, M., Garrett, F., & Huelin, S. (2011). Effectiveness of a multi-disciplinary family-based programme for treating childhood obesity (the Family Project). *European Journal of Clinical Nutrition, 65*(8), 903–909.

Eaton, D. K., Lowry, R., Brener, N. D., Galuska, D. A., & Crosby, A. E. (2005). Associations of body mass index and perceived weight with suicide ideation and suicide attempts among US high school students. *Archives of Pediatrics & Adolescent Medicine, 159*(6), 513–519.

Eisenberg, M. E., Neumark-Sztainer, D., & Story, M. (2003). Associations of weight-based teasing and emotional well-being among adolescents. *Archives of Pediatrics & Adolescent Medicine, 157*(8), 733–738.

Flaherty, E., Stirling, J., & The Committee on Child Abuse and Neglect. (2010). The pediatrician's role in child maltreatment prevention. *Pediatrics, 126,* 833–841.

Geier, A., Foster, G., Womble, L., McLaughlin, J., Borradaile, K., Nachmani, J., . . . Shults, J. (2007). The relationship between relative weight and school attendance among elementary schoolchildren. *Obesity, 15*(8), 2157–2161.

Geoffroy, M. C., Boivin, M., Arseneault, L., Turecki, G., Vitaro, F., Brendgen, M., . . . Cote, S. (2016). Associations between peer victimization and suicidal ideation and suicide attempt during adolescence: Results from a prospective population-based birth cohort. *Journal of the American Academy of Child & Adolescent Psychiatry, 55*(2), 99–105.

Goldfield, G., Moore, C., Henderson, K., Buchholz, A., Obeid, N., & Flament, M. (2010). The relation between weight-based teasing and psychological adjustment in adolescents. *Paediatrics & Child Health, 15*(5), 283–288.

Haines, J., Neumark-Sztainer, D., Eisenberg, M. E., & Hannan, P. J. (2006). Weight teasing and disordered eating behaviors in adolescents: Longitudinal findings from project EAT (Eating Among Teens). *Pediatrics, 117*(2), e209–E215.

Hommel, K. A., Odell, S., Sander, E., Baldassano, R. N., & Barg, F. K. (2011). Treatment adherence in paediatric inflammatory bowel disease: Perceptions from adolescent patients and their families. *Health & Social Care in the Community, 19*(1), 80.

Hunte, H. E. R., & Williams, D. R. (2009). The association between perceived discrimination and obesity in a population-based multiracial and multiethnic adult sample. *American Journal of Public Health, 99*(7), 1285–1292.

Jackson, S. E., Beeken, R. J., & Wardle, J. (2014). Perceived weight discrimination and changes in weight, waist circumference, and weight status. *Obesity, 22*(12), 2485–2488.

Jensen, C. D., & Steele, R. G. (2009). Body dissatisfaction, weight criticism, and self-reported physical activity in preadolescent children. *Journal of Pediatric Psychology, 34*(8), 822–826.

Johnston, C. A., Moreno, J. P., Gallagher, M. R., Wang, J., Papaioannou, M. A., Tyler, C., & Foreyt, J. P. (2013). Achieving long-term weight maintenance in Mexican-American adolescents with a school-based intervention. *Journal of Adolescent Health, 53*(3), 335–341.

Kenney, E. L., Gortmaker, S. L., Davison, K. K., & Austin, S. B. (2015). The academic penalty for gaining weight: A longitudinal, change-in-change analysis of BMI and perceived academic ability in middle school students. *International Journal of Obesity, 39*(9), 1408–1413.

Lampard, A. M., Franckle, R. L., & Davison, K. K. (2014). Maternal depression and childhood obesity: A systematic review. *Preventive Medicine, 59*, 60–67.

Losekam, S., Goetzky, B., Kraeling, S., Rief, W., & Hilbert, A. (2010). Physical activity in normal-weight and overweight youth: Associations with weight teasing and self-efficacy. *Obesity Facts, 3*(4), 239–244.

Lumeng, J. C., Forrest, P., Appugliese, D. P., Kaciroti, N., Corwyn, R. F., & Bradley, R. H. (2010). Weight status as a predictor of being bullied in third through sixth grades. *Pediatrics, 125*(6), e1301–e1307.

Magee, L., & Hale, L. (2012). Longitudinal associations between sleep duration and subsequent weight gain: A systematic review. *Sleep Medicine Reviews, 16*(3), 231–241.

Mamun, A. A., O'Callaghan, M. J., Williams, G. M., & Najman, J. M. (2013). Adolescents bullying and young adults body mass index and obesity: A longitudinal study. *International Journal of Obesity (2005), 37*(8), 1140.

May, A. L., Freedman, D., Sherry, B., & Blanck, H. M. (2013). Obesity—United States, 1999–2010. *Morbidity and Mortality Weekly Report, 62*(3), 120–128.

Michael, S. L., Merlo, C. L., Basch, C. E., Wentzel, K. R., & Wechsler, H. (2015). Critical connections: Health and academics. *Journal of School Health, 85*(11), 740–758.

O'Connor, E. A., Evans, C. V., Burda, B. U., Walsh, E. S., Eder, M., & Lozano, P. (2017). Screening for obesity and intervention for weight management in children and adolescents: Evidence report and systematic review for the US preventive services task force. *Journal of the American Medical Association, 317*(23), 2427–2444.

Ogden, C. L., Carroll, M. D., Flegal, K. M., & Kit, B. K. (2014). Prevalence of childhood and adult obesity in the United States, 2011–2012. *Journal of the American Medical Association, 311*(8), 806–814.

Ogden, C. L., Carroll, M. D., Fryar, C. D., & Flegal, K. M. (2015). *Prevalence of obesity among adults and youth: United States, 2011–2014.* Hyattsville, MD: U.S. Department of Health and Human Services, Centers for Disease Control and Prevention, National Center for Health Statistics.

Payne, R. K. (2005). *A framework for understanding poverty* (4th revised ed.). Highlands, TX: aha! Process, Inc.

Peña, M.-M., Dixon, B., & Taveras, E. M. (2012). Are you talking to ME? The importance of ethnicity and culture in childhood obesity prevention and management. *Childhood Obesity, 8*(1), 23–27.

Peterson, J. L., Puhl, R. M., & Luedicke, J. (2012). An experimental assessment of physical educators' expectations and attitudes: The importance of student weight and gender. *Journal of School Health, 82*(9), 432–440.

Pulgarón, E. R. (2013). Childhood obesity: A review of increased risk for physical and psychological comorbidities. *Clinical Therapeutics, 35*(1), A18–32.

Puhl, R. M., Andreyeva, T., & Brownell, K. D. (2008). Perceptions of weight discrimination: Prevalence and comparison to race and gender discrimination in America. *International Journal of Obesity, 32*(6), 992–1000.

Puhl, R. M., & Latner, J. D. (2007). Stigma, obesity, and the health of the nation's children. *Psychological Bulletin, 133*(4), 557–580.

Puhl, R. M., & Luedicke, J. (2012). Weight-based victimization among adolescents in the school setting: Emotional reactions and coping behaviors. *Journal of Youth and Adolescence, 41*(1), 27–40.

Puhl, R. M., Luedicke, J., & Heuer, C. (2011). Weight-based victimization toward overweight adolescents: Observations and reactions of peers. *Journal of School Health, 81*(11), 696–703.

Puhl, R. M., Peterson, J. L., & Luedicke, J. (2011). Parental perceptions of weight terminology that providers use with youth. *Pediatrics, 128*(4), e786–e793.

Puhl, R., Peterson, J. L., & Luedicke, J. (2013). Motivating or stigmatizing? Public perceptions of weight-related language used by health providers. *International Journal of Obesity (2005), 37*(4), 612.

Puhl, R., & Suh, Y. (2015). Health consequences of weight stigma: Implications for obesity prevention and treatment. *Current Obesity Reports, 4*(2), 182.

Rasberry, C. N., Lee, S. M., Robin, L., Laris, B. A., Russell, L. A., Coyle, K. K., & Nihiser, A. J. (2011). The association between school-based physical activity, including physical education, and academic performance: A systematic review of the literature. *Preventive Medicine, 52*, S10–S20.

Rasberry, C. N., Tiu, G. F., Kann, L., McManus, T., Michael, S. L., Merlo, C. L., . . . Ethier, K. A. (2017). Health-related behaviors and academic achievement among high school students—United States, 2015. *Morbidity and Mortality Weekly Report, 66*(35), 921–927.

Schwartz, D., Gorman, A. H., Nakamoto, J., & Toblin, R. L. (2005). Victimization in the peer group and children's academic functioning. *Journal of Educational Psychology, 97*(3), 425–435.

Shi, L., Krupp, D., & Remer, T. (2014). Salt, fruit and vegetable consumption and blood pressure development: A longitudinal investigation in healthy children. *British Journal of Nutrition, 111*, 662–671.

Shore, S., Sachs, M., Lidicker, J., Brett, S., Wright, A., & Libonati, J. (2008). Decreased scholastic achievement in overweight middle school students. *Obesity, 16*(7), 1535–1538.

Skinner, A., Perrin, E., & Skelton, J. (2016). Prevalence of obesity and severe obesity in US children, 1999–2014. *Obesity, 24*(5), 1116–1123.

Small, L., & Aplasca, A. (2016). Child obesity and mental health: A complex interaction. *Child and Adolescent Psychiatric Clinics, 25*(2), 269–282.

Sobol-Goldberg, S., Rabinowitz, J., & Gross, R. (2013). School-based obesity prevention programs: A meta-analysis of randomized controlled trials. *Obesity, 21*(12), 2422–2428.

Spear, B. A., Barlow, S. E., Ervin, C., Ludwig, D. S., Saelens, B. E., Schetzina, K. E., & Taveras, E. M. (2007). Recommendations for treatment of child and adolescent overweight and obesity. *Pediatrics, 120*(Suppl.), S254–S288.

Spiel, E., Paxton, S., & Yager, Z. (2012). Weight attitudes in 3- to 5-year-old children: Age differences and cross-sectional predictors. *Body Image, 9*(4), 524–527.

Su, W., & Aurelia, D. S. (2012). Preschool children's perceptions of overweight peers. *Journal of Early Childhood Research, 10*(1), 19.

Tamayo, T., Christian, H., & Rathmann, W. (2010). Impact of early psychosocial factors (childhood socioeconomic factors and adversities) on future risk of type 2 diabetes, metabolic disturbances and obesity: A systematic review. *BMC Public Health, 10*(1), 525–525.

Toruner, E. K., & Savaser, S. (2010). A controlled evaluation of a school-based obesity prevention in Turkish school children. *The Journal of School Nursing, 26*(6), 473–482.

Wang, L., Collins, C., Ratliff, M., Xie, B., & Wang, Y. (2017). Breastfeeding reduces childhood obesity risks. *Childhood Obesity, 13*(3), 197–204.

Wang, Y., Wu, Y., Wilson, R. F., Bleich, S., Cheskin L, Weston, C. B., . . . Segal J. (2015). What childhood obesity prevention programmes work? A systematic review and meta-analysis. *Obesity Reviews, 16*(7), 547–565.

Zeller, M., Kirk, S., Claytor, R., Khoury, P., Grieme, J., Santangelo, M., & Daniels, S. (2004). Predictors of attrition from a pediatric weight management program. *The Journal of Pediatrics, 144*(4), 466–470.

HANDOUT 21.1.

SETTING SMART GOALS FOR YOUR HEALTH!

What is a general goal that you have for your health?

_____

(Example: Eat more vegetables)

Now let's make it a SMART goal! Take your general goal and answer the following questions:

Specific: What types of things can I try? Think about specific things you want to change. (Example: Which types of vegetables could I try?)

_____

Measurable: How much am I going to do? How many times per day or per week? Think about how you can measure if you have reached the goal. (Example: How many times a day do I want to try vegetables?)

_____

Achievable: Can I actually do this? Am I setting myself up for success? Think about what you are doing now and how you can challenge yourself to do a little bit more. (Example: If I don't eat any vegetables now, would trying one vegetable each week be a better starting place than every day?)

_____

Resources/Rewards: Who can help me? What can I give myself as a reward for completing my goal? Think about something that will motivate you to keep trying.

_____

Timely: How long will I give myself to try to accomplish this goal? When should I start?

_____

Examples of a SMART Goal:

By the end of the month, I will be eating colorful vegetables at least three times a week. I will start this week by trying carrots. I will ask Mom to buy some carrots (or go with her to the store). If I'm successful at the end of the month, I get to choose any colorful vegetable I want for dinner the next week.

What is your new SMART Goal?

Handout prepared by Gray and Pont on behalf of the Texas Center for the Prevention and Treatment of Childhood Obesity and shared with permission.

22

Sleep Disorders

**MICHELLE M. PERFECT, SARA S. FRYE,
AND ROBIN J. SAKAKINI** ■

Sleep is an essential human behavior that has physiological underpinnings. Sleep deficiency comprises sleep difficulties, including insufficient sleep, inconsistent sleep, daytime sleepiness, sleep-disordered breathing (SDB), and insomnia (El-Sheikh, Kelly, Buckhalt, & Hinnant, 2010; Perfect, Levine-Donnerstein, Archbold, Goodwin, & Quan, 2014). The purpose of this chapter is to provide an overview of the assessment and treatment of sleep and sleep-related disorders in children and adolescents.

OVERVIEW OF SLEEP CONDITIONS

Inadequate Sleep

Although not a disorder per se, inadequate sleep is perhaps the most pervasive sleep challenge in school-age youth. Obtaining sufficient sleep is critical throughout the lifespan, but the amount of sleep needed varies as a function of age. The current recommendations for sleep duration by the American Academy of Sleep Medicine (AASM) is 10 to 13 hours for preschool children, 9 to 12 hours for children ages 6 through 12, and 8 to 10 hours for adolescents 13 years old and older (AASM, 2014). Research has shown that over the years, the amount of sleep youth obtain has been steadily declining. This downward trend in total sleep time (TST) during adolescence across the last several decades has been equated with a "recession" (Keyes, Maslowsky, Hamilton, & Schulenberg, 2015).

Insomnia and Daytime Sleepiness

Insomnia symptoms include difficulties initiating and maintaining sleep. Approximately 1% to 6% of children and adolescents experience insomnia symptoms, with considerably higher rates among youth with mental health or developmental complications (Mindell et al., 2006; Roberts, Roberts, & Duong, 2008). Over one third of youth report daytime sleepiness, which manifests as difficulties staying awake or by falling asleep during daytime activities (Dewald, Meijer, Oort, Kerkof, & Bogels, 2010). Sleepiness can be a symptom of insufficient sleep as well as an indicator of an underlying sleep disorder.

Circadian Rhythm Disorders

Circadian rhythm disorders are conditions that result from a disruption of a person's natural biological cycle. Sleep need remains steady into adolescence; however, physiological and social changes result in a preference for later sleep onset and awakening times (Jenni & Carskadon, 2007). This can lead to delayed sleep–wake phase disorder (DSPD), which is one of the most common disorders in adolescents (AASM, 2014). Despite going to sleep later, youth usually are required to wake up prematurely because of early school start times, resulting in insufficient sleep. To compensate for insufficient sleep on school nights, adolescents may sleep longer on weekends (Moore et al., 2009).

Sleep-Disordered Breathing

Although the criteria for SDB used in previous studies has varied, SDB affects between 3% and 23% of youth (Goodwin, Vasquez, Silva, & Quan, 2010; O'Brien et al., 2004). SDB is diagnosed when breathing is partially or completely obstructed in the upper airway for brief periods during sleep.

Parasomnias

Parasomnias are experiences or events that occur during sleep, such as abnormal body movements, night terrors, or sleep walking. Although parasomnias are common in childhood, most cases resolve without treatment by adolescence (Laberge, Tremblay, Vitaro, & Montplaisir, 2000). A summary of the various sleep disorders is provided in Handout 22.1.

CASE EXAMPLE

Jordan is 15 years old. She is an average student, but recently her grades have begun to slip. She often asks to go to the nurse's office because she doesn't feel well. Jordan's teachers have noticed she is sluggish and seems withdrawn. Classroom observations indicate that Jordan appears uninterested and does not participate much in the classroom. She was observed putting her head down on the desk and not completing her work. Jordan's parents report that nothing has changed at home; however, her parents do report that Jordan snores loudly and complains of a dry throat and headache in the morning. They are very concerned about Jordan's well-being.

IMPLICATIONS FOR SCHOOL FUNCTIONING

Sleep and sleep-related disorders have broad implications for school functioning, including academic and psychosocial outcomes. As is illustrated in the case above, clinicians might initially think Jordan has depression or learning difficulties. However, information about her sleep suggests that she may have SDB, which can cause sleepiness and interfere with learning.

Academic Outcomes

Research has supported that less TST is associated with worse school-related outcomes and poorer academic performance (Fredriksen, Rhodes, Reddy, & Way, 2004; Roberts, Roberts, & Duong, 2009; Wolfson & Carskadon, 1998). In an epidemiological study, the Tucson Children's Assessment of Sleep Apnea (TuCASA) study, children who slept 9 or more hours during home polysomnography (PSG; an objective measure of sleep stages, duration, and respiration), had lower rates of parent-reported learning problems 5 years later than children who slept less than 7.5 hours (Silva et al., 2011). Youth from the TuCASA cohort (Perfect et al., 2014) and another study (Wolfson & Carskadon, 1998) showed that even 30 minutes less sleep can impact academic performance. Students with less sleep disproportionately displayed grades C or lower.

With regard to sleepiness, studies have revealed that students who reported feeling sleepier performed worse in school or showed less academic growth over time (Dewald et al., 2010; Pagel & Kwiatkowski, 2010; Perfect et al., 2012, 2014). Insomnia symptoms have also been found to associate with lower or failing grades (Pagel & Kwiatkowski, 2010; Perfect et al., 2014).

In a longitudinal study, self-reported sleep disturbances in elementary students predicted worse performance on state standardized tests 2 years later, with maternal education, socioeconomic status, and race moderating these relationships (Buckhalt, El-Sheikh, Keller, & Kelley, 2009; El-Sheikh, Buckhalt, Keller, Cummings, & Acebo, 2007). Inconsistent bed and wake times and daytime sleepiness also predicted performance on the SAT math and language subtests, and sleepiness also contributed significant variance to performance on SAT reading subtests (Buckhalt et al., 2009). Although most studies on sleep and academic outcomes have adopted observational study designs, an emerging area of research is use of experimental sleep manipulation to determine cause–effect relations of sleep duration. A recent systematic review (de Bruin, van Run, Staaks, & Meijer, 2016) identified 16 studies that examined the effects of sleep restriction on cognitive performance in youth. Few studies have focused on the potential benefits of sleep extension. In a cross-over study, scores on tests of attention, memory, and problem-solving were significantly higher when children obtained more sleep than their typical sleep duration compared to when they obtained less sleep (Sadeh, Gruber, & Raviv, 2003).

There have been mixed findings with regard to academic and cognitive outcomes among students with SDB. For instance, in TuCASA, concurrent SDB was related to parent-reported learning problems and parent-rated cognitive problems on the Conner's Parent Rating Scale–Revised (Goodwin et al., 2003; Mulvaney et al., 2006; Silva et al., 2011). However, performance did not appear to differ significantly on reading, writing, and math achievement standardized tests using the Woodcock-Johnson Tests of Achievement–Third Edition (Kaemingk et al., 2003). A follow-up study examining the TuCASA cohort at two time points found that, despite cognitive functioning in the average range, youth with persistent SDB (SDB at both time points) were more likely to show impairments in adaptive functioning (Perfect, Archbold, Goodwin, Levine-Donnerstein, & Quan, 2013). Beebe, Ris, Kramer, Long, and Amin (2010) found similar patterns, in that youth with SDB had lower grades and teacher-reported learning problems, although their performance was comparable to those without SDB on standardized tests. Thus, it may be critical for school-based practitioners to consider daily performance and reports of caregivers rather than rely solely on norm-based tests to determine the impact of untreated SDB on school functioning.

Social-Emotional Outcomes

In the TuCASA study, anxious and depressive symptoms were higher among children who slept less than 7.5 hours than those who slept the recommended number of hours (i.e., 9 hours; Silva et al., 2011). Other studies also reported that inadequate sleep related to internalizing symptoms and behavioral difficulties both cross-sectionally and longitudinally (El-Sheikh et al., 2010; Moore et al., 2009; Pasch, Nelson, Lytle, & Moe, 2010 Perfect et al., 2014; Wolfson & Carskadon, 1998). Longitudinal findings have suggested that insomnia symptoms predicted several social-emotional outcomes, including low self-esteem, depression, somatization, somatic complaints, peer-relationship problems, and overall mental health symptoms (Roberts, Roberts, & Chen, 2002; Roberts et al., 2008).

Several publications have highlighted social-emotional outcomes associated with SDB, including disruptive behaviors and social challenges (Mulvaney et al., 2006; Perfect et al., 2013). Perfect et al. (2013) further reported that, even when youth with SDB had cognitive functioning in the average or above-average range, they exhibited adaptive functioning difficulties in decision-making, effective communication, self-care, and social engagement. Beebe et al. (2010) found decreased teacher-reported attentiveness and higher levels of parent-reported hyperactivity, anxiety symptoms, depression symptoms, and inattention among youth with SDB.

BEHAVIORAL HEALTH COMORBIDITIES

Sleep problems are highly comorbid with psychiatric conditions; additionally, sleep disturbance is listed in the diagnostic criteria for multiple disorders (American Psychological Association, 2013). Thus, the relationship between sleep problems and mental health is considered to be bidirectional, because individuals with psychiatric diagnoses are at increased risk for sleep problems, and, conversely, sleep problems are associated with mood and behavioral dysregulation (Perfect et al., 2014). For example, youth with attention deficit hyperactivity disorder (ADHD) and autism spectrum disorder (ASD) experience high rates of sleep disruption, which may further exacerbate symptoms associated with these disorders (Cortese, Faraone, Konofal, & Lecendreux, 2009; Richdale & Schreck, 2009). This association is further complicated by the sleep-related side effects of medications like the stimulants that are commonly prescribed for children with ADHD, such as insomnia (Cohen-Zion & Ancoli-Israel, 2004). Given the overlap between sleep problems and other conditions that are being assessed or treated in a school setting, it is crucial that school-based practitioners be aware of the symptoms associated with sleep disorders and the potential impact on school functioning.

RISK FACTORS

Certain intrinsic risk factors may predispose a child to develop a more chronic sleep disturbance, such as difficult temperament, chronic illness, mental illness, and neurodevelopmental delay (Owens, 2004; Stein, Mendelsohn, Obermeyer, Amromin, & Benca, 2001). Some sleep disorders are associated with specific risk factors. For example, risk factors for SDB include upper airway abnormalities and obesity (Verhulst, Van Gaal, De Backer, & Desager, 2008).

Family and environmental variables also contribute to the development of healthy sleep hygiene. Sleep patterns have been found to vary among individuals from different racial, ethnic, and cultural backgrounds. Risk factors for sleep problems in youth include inconsistent bedtimes, family stressors, negative home environments, and low socioeconomic status (Allen, Howlett, Coulombe, & Corkum, 2016; Buckhalt, 2011). Alternatively, parent-set bedtimes, positive familial relationships, and good sleep hygiene serve as protective factors against sleep problems (Bartel, Gradisar, & Williamson, 2015).

Social and behavioral factors that negatively affect children's sleep include overscheduling, early school start times, heavy homework loads, and technology use (Bartel et al., 2015; Cain & Gradisar, 2010). The use of interactive technology (i.e., computer, phone, video games) in the hour before bed is associated with more difficulties falling asleep and reported unrefreshing sleep (Gradisar et al., 2013). Tobacco use, computer use, evening light, video games, cell phone use,

Internet time, caffeine, and pre-sleep worry have a negative impact on adolescents' sleep (Bartel et al., 2015).

ASSESSMENT OF SLEEP

Given the negative educational outcomes associated with sleep problems, assessment of sleep is a critical component of comprehensive evaluation procedures. Unfortunately, school-based practitioners are often not adequately trained in the assessment of sleep problems. At a minimum, school-based evaluations should inquire about sleep as part of the initial interview process. There are also numerous, well-established questionnaires that can be used by school-based practitioners to assess for sleep-related issues from both the parents' and youth's perspectives, such as the School Sleep Habits Survey (Owens, Spirito, & McGuinn, 2000) and Sleep Disorders Inventory for Students (SDIS; Luginbuehl, 2005). Other subjective measures of sleep include sleep diaries, which are used to gather information about the youth's sleep–wake schedule and collect intervention data. (An sample sleep diary is provided in Handout 22.2.) Technology can be utilized to obtain objective measures of sleep using devices like the actigraph, which is a wristwatch-type device that records movement to estimate sleep–wake behaviors (Meltzer, Walsh, Traylor, & Westin, 2012). Previously, the use of these devices outside a research or clinical setting was limited, due to cost. However, recent development of wearable technology has produced more affordable options.

SLEEP-BASED INTERVENTIONS

Although sleep is a biological process, it is also highly influenced by a multitude of external factors. Thus, treatment of sleep problems can target the underlying physiological causes, environmental influences, or behavioral factors. When pediatric sleep problems arise, one of the first steps is to ensure that the child is practicing good sleep hygiene. Sleep hygiene recommendations are provided in Handout 22.3.

Although sleep hygiene is important, it may not be sufficient to address sleep-related problems, particularly if the behavior has been reinforced over time (e.g., getting out of bed in the middle of the night has become positively associated with gaining parental attention). Thus, parent-led management strategies might be warranted. Research has demonstrated that parent-driven interventions are effective in treating pediatric behavioral sleep disorders (Sakakini, 2011). Bedtime fading (Meltzer, 2010) is appropriate for children who have difficulty with sleep initiation and maintenance. For 1 to 2 weeks prior to intervention, the family keeps a sleep diary. For those who have difficulty falling asleep, the average TST becomes the prescribed time in bed for the first week of intervention. For children who have difficulty falling asleep (but not staying asleep), their baseline sleep-onset time becomes their new bedtime. Positive bedtime routines are simultaneously implemented. After 1 to 2 weeks of implementing the new sleep schedule, children's sleep-onset latency and nighttime awakenings will be reduced. Additionally, their bedtime can be gradually "faded" earlier in 15- to 30-minute increments, until reaching the ideal bedtime for the child.

Graded exposure, which is also referred to as graduated extinction, is ideal for children who need a parent present to fall asleep. Similar to treatment for anxiety, graded exposure involves creating an exposure "hierarchy" in which the parent gradually withdraws from the bedroom (if the parent has been present in the child's room at bedtime) or the child is removed the parent's bedroom. Positive reinforcement (reward) is typically utilized when each step is accomplished. Graded exposure has been shown to be effective with both children and adolescents (Paine & Gradisar, 2011).

Graduated extinction also involves gradually withdrawing the parent's presence at bedtime. This technique is most often utilized for children under age 5, but it can also be useful with school-age children still struggling to sleep independently (Quach, Hiscock, Ukoumunne, & Wake, 2011). After saying goodnight, the parent ignores the child's protests (e.g., crying, calling out) in order to not reinforce the behavior. Instead, reinforcement is provided at predetermined intervals, in which the parent briefly visits the child in bed to give reassurance without actively engaging the child. The frequency of the brief visits is gradually decreased until the child is able to fall asleep without having a parent present.

Limit-setting is appropriate for children with bedtime resistance. It involves developing and consistently implementing clear rules for appropriate bedtime behaviors. The Bedtime Pass Program (Moore, Friman, Fruzzetti, & MacAleese, 2007) is a limit-setting intervention that provides the child with a set number of "passes" that can be exchanged for appropriate requests (e.g., drink, toilet, cuddle). After the child uses all the passes, the parent needs to ignore any further requests from the child. Unused passes may be exchanged for a tangible reward.

In older adolescents, treatment is more client-centered, as opposed to parent-led. Cognitive-behavioral therapy for insomnia (CBT-I) is an evidence-based treatment in adults (Okajima, Komada, & Inoue, 2011). There is emerging evidence that CBT-I is also effective for treating insomnia in adolescents (de Bruin, Bögels, Oort, & Meijer, 2015). CBT-I is generally provided in person over the course of 6 to 8 sessions and involves psychoeducation, sleep hygiene recommendations, modification of the sleep–wake schedule (e.g., sleep restriction), stimulus control (e.g., associating the bed with sleep only), cognitive therapy, and relaxation techniques. Internet-delivered CBT-I has also been shown to be effective, with only minimal differences in effect size as compared to in-person CBT-I (de Bruin et al., 2015). Furthermore, application-based delivery can be utilized at home with parental supervision.

The treatment of sleep disorders like SDB and circadian rhythm disorders often takes place under the supervision of a physician or certified sleep medicine specialist. SDB is generally treated by use of a continuous positive airway pressure (CPAP) device, surgical interventions (e.g., adenotonsillectomy), or weight loss (Verhulst et al., 2008). Bright light therapy is an evidence-based treatment for DSPD, in which the adolescent is exposed to natural light or a light box for 30 to 60 minutes upon awakening while following a strict sleep–wake schedule based on their natural rising time. Over the course of days or weeks, they advance their bedtime and waketime until the desired sleep–wake schedule is reached (Gradisar, Smits, & Bjorvatn, 2014).

Although school-based practitioners may not be directly delivering these interventions, they can support students while they are at school by ensuring they receive appropriate accommodations to address educational impacts. For example, schools should be flexible when students are undergoing treatment for DSPD, as it may require the student to comply with a strict sleep–wake schedule that could overlap with school start time or require the use of a light box at their desk in the morning.

CULTURAL CONSIDERATIONS

Sleep behaviors are determined by biological and cultural factors. It is the interaction between these two factors that contribute to behavioral and developmental norms and expectations regarding normal and problematic children's sleep (Jenni & O'Connor, 2005). Sleep patterns, parental behaviors, and sleep environments show significant variations across countries and cultures (Sadeh, Mindell, & Rivera, 2011). Culture impacts where children sleep, how they sleep, with whom, and for how long. For example, co-sleeping and bed sharing are common among many ethnic groups, including African American, Hispanic, and Asian families, but less common in Caucasian families (Liu, Liu, Owens, & Kaplan, 2005; Mindell & Owens, 2015). Sleep habits also vary, with Asian children and adolescents having a later bedtime compared to children and adolescents from North America and Europe, resulting in less TST on school nights (Gradisar, Gardner, & Dohnt, 2011; Sadeh et al., 2011). Furthermore, 75% of adolescents in the United States report sleeping less than 8 hours on weekdays, whereas South Korean adolescents report sleeping an average of 4.9 hours (Owens & Adolescent Sleep Working Group, 2014).

Parents' sleep expectations and perceptions of sleep problems are influenced by cultural norms. Parents from predominantly Asian countries or regions are more likely to endorse childhood sleep problems than are parents from predominantly Caucasian countries and regions (Sadeh et al., 2011). The TuCASA study found that, compared to youth of Caucasian ethnicity, youth who identified as Hispanic had significantly shorter sleep on weekends when they were younger, and significantly later bedtimes across the week during the adolescent period (Combs, Goodwin, Quan, Morgan, & Parthasarathy, 2016).

POLICY ISSUES RELATED TO SLEEP

As is the case with other health-related conditions, if a student has a sleep disorder, he or she may require accommodations or modifications. However, on a systemic level, school start times, especially at the middle- and high-school levels, contribute to the insufficient sleep trends. A policy statement from the American Academy of Pediatrics (2014) urged schools to consider the solid research evidence that shows not only the harmful effects of short sleep duration but also the benefit of later school start times. In particular, studies have shown better attendance, improved academic performance, and reduced vehicular accidents resulting from later school start times. Adolescents tend to get greater than 30 minutes more sleep when their first class begins later. Schools should also consider the impact of out-of-school workload requirements. For example, one study found that performance did not increase proportionally to time spent studying if the studying was in place of sleep (Gillen-O'Neel, Huynh, & Fuligni, 2013).

IMPLICATIONS FOR SCHOOL-BASED PRACTITIONERS

Schools serve as the optimal primary care facilities for identifying sleep problems. Addressing sleep issues in students may mitigate the negative academic, behavioral, emotional, and health outcomes associated with sleep problems. Universal screenings can be utilized to identify students at risk. School-based practitioners need to be able to recognize the signs and symptoms of sleep problems in order to facilitate early identification. Furthermore, school-based practitioners should ask about sleep habits early on in the assessment process. Evidence-based assessment tools to identify sleep problems are available to help make accurate diagnoses and proper referrals for treatment when necessary.

As part of developing an intervention to target sleep, school psychologists should adopt a multidisciplinary perspective, with particular collaboration with the school nurse, due the physiological factors that influence sleep. School-based practitioners need to be aware of potential resources and referrals for students whose sleep problems are more severe and require medical evaluation or treatment (e.g., SDB and movement disorders). Families should be encouraged to discuss the student's sleep issues with his or her pediatrician to coordinate referrals to appropriate specialists.

Through use of a problem-solving process, an intervention plan for students who are identified as having a behavioral sleep problem can be designed and implemented. School-based practitioners can consult and collaborate with parents to implement sleep interventions and can facilitate data collection to monitor progress to foster positive student outcomes.

CONCLUSIONS

In conclusion, sleep and sleep-related disorders are prevalent in school-age populations and can have broad impacts for students. It is imperative that school-based practitioners be aware of these issues and consider the impact of sleep when evaluating students.

RESOURCES FOR PRACTITIONERS, PARENTS, AND CHILDREN

Practitioners

- http://www.nationwidechildrens.org/sleep-disorders
- http://school.sleepeducation.com/
- https://schoolstarttime.org/
- http://www.childrenshospital.org/centers-and-services/programs/o-_-z/ pediatric-sleep-disorders-center-program/clinician-resources
- https://www.nasponline.org/Documents/Resources%20and%20 Publications/Handouts/Families%20and%20Educators/Sleep%20 Disorders%20WEB.pdf
- Book: Mindell, J., & Owens, J. A. (2015). *A Clinical Guide to Pediatric Sleep: Diagnosis and Management of Sleep Problems* (3rd ed.). Philadelphia, PA: Lippincott Williams & Wilkins.

Parents and Practitioners

- https://sleepfoundation.org/category/children-teens-sleep
- http://www.sleepeducation.org/news/-in-Category/Categories/ pediatrics/children
- http://sleepcenter.ucla.edu/patient-education
- http://www.apa.org/topics/sleep/why.aspx
- https://teensneedsleep.files.wordpress.com/2011/03/dawson-sleep-and-sleep-disorders-in-children-and-adolescents.pdf
- https://www.nhlbi.nih.gov/about/org/ncsdr/patpub/
- https://www.healthychildren.org/English/healthy-living/sleep/Pages/ default.aspx
- http://kidshealth.org/en/parents/sleep.html

Children

- http://www.sleepforkids.org/

REFERENCES

Allen, S. L, Howlett, M. D., Coulombe, J. A., & Corkum, P. V. (2016). ABCs of SLEEPING: A review of the evidence behind pediatric sleep practice recommendations. *Sleep Medicine Reviews, 29,* 1–14

American Academy of Pediatrics. (2014). School start times for adolescents. *Pediatrics, 134,* 642–649. doi:10.1542/peds.2014-1697

American Academy of Sleep Medicine. (2014). *International classification of sleep disorders.* Darien, IL: Author.

American Psychiatric Association. (2013). *Diagnostic and statistical manual of mental disorders* (DSM-5®). Arlington, VA: Author.

Bartel, K. A., Gradisar, M., & Williamson, P. (2015). Protective and risk factors for adolescent sleep: A meta-analytic review. *Sleep Medicine Reviews, 21,* 72–85. doi:10.1016/j.smrv.2014.08.002

Beebe, D. W., Ris, M. D., Kramer, M. E., Long, E., & Amin, R. (2010). The association between sleep disordered breathing, academic grades, and cognitive and behavioral functioning among overweight subjects during middle to late childhood. *Sleep, 33,* 1447–1456.

Buckhalt, J. A. (2011). Insufficient sleep and the socioeconomic status achievement gap. *Child Development Perspectives, 5,* 59–65. doi:10.1111/j.1750-8606.2010.00151.x

Buckhalt, J. A., El-Sheikh, M., Keller, P., & Kelley, R. (2009). Concurrent and longitudinal relations between children's sleep and cognitive functioning. *Child Development, 80,* 875–892. doi:10.1111/j.1467-8624.2009.01303.x

Cain, N., & Gradisar, M. (2010). Electronic media use and sleep in school-aged children and adolescents: A review. *Sleep Medicine, 11*(8), 735–742.

Cohen-Zion, M., & Ancoli-Israel, S. (2004). Sleep in children with attention-deficit hyperactivity disorder (ADHD): A review of naturalistic and stimulant intervention studies. *Sleep Medicine Reviews, 8,* 379–402. doi:10.1016/j.smrv.2004.06.002

Combs, D., Goodwin, J. L., Quan, S. F., Morgan, W. J., & Parthasarathy, S. (2016). Longitudinal differences in sleep duration in Hispanic and Caucasian children. *Sleep Medicine, 18,* 61–66. doi:10.1016/j.sleep.2015.06.008

Cortese, S., Faraone, S. V., Konofal, E., & Lecendreux, M. (2009). Sleep in children with attention-deficit/hyperactivity disorder: Meta-analysis of subjective and objective studies. *Journal of the American Academy of Child & Adolescent Psychiatry, 48,* 894–908. doi:10.1097/CHI.0b013e3181ac09c9

de Bruin, E. J., Bögels, S. M., Oort, F. J., & Meijer, A. M. (2015). Efficacy of cognitive behavioral therapy for insomnia in adolescents: A randomized controlled trial with internet therapy, group therapy and a waiting list condition. *Sleep, 38,* 1913–1926. doi:10.5665/sleep.5240

de Bruin, E. J., van Run, C., Staaks, J., & Meijer, A. M. (2016). Effects of sleep manipulation on cognitive functioning of adolescents: A systematic review. *Sleep Medicine Reviews, 32,* 45–57. doi:10.1016/j.smrv.2016.02.006

Dewald, J. F., Meijer, A. M., Oort, F. J., Kerkof, G. A., & Bogels, S. M. (2010). The influence of sleep quality, sleep duration and sleepiness on school performance in children and adolescents: A meta-analytic review. *Sleep Medicine Reviews, 14,* 179–189. doi:10.1016/j.smrv.2009.10.004

El-Sheikh, M., Buckhalt, J. A., Keller, P. S., Cummings, E. M., & Acebo, C. (2007). Child emotional security and academic achievement: The role of sleep disruptions. *Journal of Family Psychology, 21,* 29–38. doi:10.1037/0893-3200.21.1.29

El-Sheikh, M., Kelly, R. J., Buckhalt, J. A., & Hinnant, J. B. (2010). Children's sleep and adjustment over time: The role of socioeconomic context. *Child Development, 81,* 870–883. doi:10.1111/j.1467-8624.2010.01439.x

Fredriksen, K., Rhodes, J., Reddy, R., & Way, N. (2004). Sleepless in Chicago: tracking the effects of adolescent sleep loss during the middle school years. *Child Development, 75(1),* 84–95.

Gillen-O'Neel, C., Huynh, V. W., & Fuligni, A. J. (2013). To study or to sleep? The academic costs of extra studying at the expense of sleep. *Child Development, 84,* 133–142. doi:10.1111/j.1467-8624.2012.01834.x

Goodwin, J., Kaemingk, K., Fregosi, R. F., Rosen, G., Morgan, W., . . . Quan, S. F. (2003). Clinical outcomes associated with sleep disordered breathing in Caucasian and Hispanic children—The Tucson Children's Assessment of Sleep Apnea Study (TuCASA). *Sleep, 26,* 587–591.

Goodwin, J. L., Vasquez, M. M., Silva, G. E., & Quan, S. F. (2010). Incidence and remission of sleep-disordered breathing and related symptoms in 6- to 17- year old children—The Tucson Children's Assessment of Sleep Apnea Study. *The Journal of Pediatrics, 157,* 57–61. doi:10.1016/j.jpeds.2010.01.033

Gradisar, M., Gardner, G., & Dohnt, H. (2011). Recent worldwide sleep patterns and problems during adolescence: A review and meta-analysis of age, region, and sleep. *Sleep Medicine, 12,* 110–118.doi:10.1016/j.sleep.2010.11.008

Gradisar, M., Smits, M. G., & Bjorvatn, B. (2014). Assessment and treatment of delayed sleep phase disorder in adolescents: Recent innovations and cautions. *Sleep Medicine Clinics, 9,* 199–210. doi:10.1016/j.jsmc.2014.02.005

Gradisar, M., Wolfson, A. R., Harvey, A. G., Hale, L., Rosenberg, R., & Czeisler, C. A. (2013). The sleep and technology use of Americans: Findings from the National Sleep Foundation's 2011 Sleep in America poll. *Journal of Clinical Sleep Medicine, 9(12),* 1291–1299. doi:10.5664/jcsm.3272

Jenni, O. G., & Carskadon, M. A. (2007). Sleep behavior and sleep regulation from infancy through adolescence: Normative aspects. *Sleep Medicine Clinics, 2,* 321–329. doi:10.1016/j.jsmc.2012.06.002

Jenni, O. G., & O'Connor, B. B. (2005). Children's sleep: An interplay between culture and biology. *Pediatrics, 115,* 204–216. doi:10.1542/peds.2004-0815B

Kaemingk, K. L., Pasvogel, A. E., Goodwin, J. L., Mulvaney, S. A., Martinez, F., Enright, P. L., . . . Quan, S. F. (2003). Learning in children and sleep disordered breathing: Findings of the Tucson Children's Assessment of Sleep Apnea (TuCASA) prospective cohort study. *Journal of the International Neuropsychological Society, 9,* 1016–1026. doi:10.1017/S1355617703970056

Keyes, K. M., Maslowsky, J., Hamilton, A., & Schulenberg, J. (2015). The great sleep recession: Changes in sleep duration among US adolescents, 1991–2012. *Pediatrics, 135,* 460–468. doi:10.1542/peds.2014-2707

Laberge, L., Tremblay, R. E., Vitaro, F., & Montplaisir, J. (2000). Development of parasomnias from childhood to early adolescence. *Pediatrics, 106,* 67–74. doi:10.1542/peds.2004-0815F

Liu, X., Liu, L., Owens, J. A., & Kaplan, D. L. (2005). Sleep patterns and sleep problems among schoolchildren in the United States and China. *Pediatrics, 115,* 241–249. doi:10.1542/peds.2004-0815F

Luginbuehl, M. (2005). *Sleep Disorders Inventory for Students—Children's Form.* Clearwater, FL: Child Uplift, Inc.

Meltzer, L. J. (2010). Clinical management of behavioral insomnia of childhood: Treatment of bedtime problems and night wakings in young children. *Behavioral Sleep Medicine,* 8, 172–189. doi:10.1080/15402002.2010.487464

Meltzer, L. J., Walsh, C. M., Traylor, J., & Westin, A. M. (2012). Direct comparison of two new actigraphs and polysomnography in children and adolescents. *Sleep, 35,* 159–166. doi:10.5665/sleep.1608

Mindell, J. A., Emslie, G., Blumer, J., Genel, M., Glaze, D., Ivanenko, A., ... Banas, B. (2006). Pharmacological management of insomnia in children and adolescents: Consensus statement. *Pediatrics, 117,* e1223–e1232. doi:10.1542/peds.2005-1693

Mindell, J., & Owens, J. (2015). *A clinical guide to pediatric sleep: Diagnosis and management of sleep problems* (3rd ed.). Philadelphia, PA: Lippincott Williams & Wilkins.

Moore, B. A., Friman, P. C., Fruzzetti, A. E., & MacAleese, K. (2007). Brief report: Evaluating the Bedtime Pass Program for child resistance to bedtime—A randomized, controlled trial. *Journal of Pediatric Psychology, 32,* 283–287. doi:10.1093/jpepsy/jsl025

Moore, H., Kirchner, H. L., Drotar, D., Johnson, N., Rosen, C., Ancoli-Israel, S., & Redline, S. (2009). Relationships among sleepiness, sleep time, and psychological functioning in adolescents. *Journal of Pediatric Psychology, 34,* 1175–1183. doi:10.1093/jpepsy/jsp039

Mulvaney, S. A., Goodwin, J. L., Morgan, W. J., Rosen, G. R., Quan, S. F., & Kaemingk, K. L. (2006). Behavior problems associated with sleep disordered breathing in school-aged children—The Tucson Children's Assessment of Sleep Apnea Study. *Journal of Pediatric Psychology, 31,* 322–330. doi:10.1093/jpepsy/jsj035

O'Brien, L. M., Mervis, C. B., Holbrook, C. R., Bruner, J. L., Smith, N. H., McNally, N., ... Gozal, D. (2004). Neurobehavioral correlates of sleep-disordered breathing in children. *Journal of Sleep Research, 13,* 165–172. doi:10.1111/j.1365-2869.2004.00395.x

Okajima, I., Komada, Y., & Inoue, Y. (2011). A meta-analysis on the treatment effectiveness of cognitive behavioral therapy for primary insomnia. *Sleep and Biological Rhythms, 9,* 24–34. doi:10.1111/j.1479-8425.2010.00481.x

Owens, J. (2004). Services and programs proven to be effective in managing infant/child sleeping disorders and their impact on the social and emotional development of young children (0–5). In R. E. Tremblay, R. G. Barr, & R. Peters (Eds.), *Encyclopedia of early childhood development.* Retrieved from http://www.child-encyclopedia.com/documents/OwensJANGxp.pdf

Owens, J., & Adolescent Sleep Working Group. (2014). Insufficient sleep in adolescents and young adults: an update on causes and consequences. *Pediatrics, 134*(3), e921–e932.

Owens, J. A., Spirito, A., & McGuinn, M. (2000). The Children's Sleep Habits Questionnaire (CSHQ): Psychometric properties of a survey instrument for school-aged children. *Sleep, 23,* 1–9.

Pagel, J. F., & Kwiatkowski, C. F. (2010). Sleep complaints affecting school performance at different educational levels. *Frontiers in Neurology, 1,* 1–6.

Paine, S., & Gradisar, M. (2011). A randomized controlled trial of cognitive-behavior therapy for behavioral insomnia of childhood in school-aged children. *Behavior Research & Therapy, 49,* 379–388. doi:10.1016/j.brat.2011.03.008

Pasch, K. E., Nelson, M. C., Lytle, L. A., & Moe, S. G. (2010). Adolescent sleep, risk behaviors, and depressive symptoms: Are they linked? *American Journal of Health Behavior, 34,* 237–248. doi:10.5993/AJHB.34.2.11

Perfect, M. M., Archbold, K., Goodwin, J., Levine-Donnerstein, D., & Quan, S. F. (2013). Risk of difficulties in behavioral and adaptive functioning in youth with persistent and current sleep-disordered breathing. *Sleep, 26,* 517–525.

Perfect, M. M., Levine-Donnerstein, D., Archbold, K., Goodwin, J. E., & Quan, S. F. (2014). The contribution of multiple sleep disturbances on school and psychosocial functioning. *Psychology in the Schools, 51,* 273–295. doi:10.1002/pits.21746

Perfect, M. M., Patel, P. G., Scott, R. E., Wheeler, M. D., Patel, C., . . . Quan, S. F. (2012). Sleep, glucose, and daytime functioning in youth with type 1 diabetes. *Sleep, 35,* 81–88. doi:10.5665/sleep.1590

Quach, J., Hiscock, H., Ukoumunne, O. C., & Wake, M. (2011). A brief sleep intervention improves outcomes in the school entry year: A randomized controlled trial. *Pediatrics, 128,* 692–701. doi:10.1542/peds.2011-0409

Richdale, A. L., & Schreck, K. A. (2009). Sleep problems in autism spectrum disorders: Prevalence, nature, & possible biopsychosocial aetiologies. *Sleep Medicine Reviews, 13,* 403–411. doi:10.1016/j.smrv.2009.02.003

Roberts, R. E., Roberts, C .R., & Chen, I. G. (2002). Impact of insomnia on future functioning of adolescents. *Journal of Psychosomatic Research, 53,* 561–569.

Roberts, R. E., Roberts, C. R., & Duong, H. T. (2008). Chronic insomnia and its negative consequences for health and functioning of adolescents: A 12-month prospective study. *Journal of Adolescent Health, 42,* 294–302. doi:10.1016/j.jadohealth.2007.09.016

Roberts, R. E., Roberts, C. R., & Duong, H. T. (2009). Sleepless in adolescence: Prospective data on sleep deprivation, health and functioning. *Journal of Adolescence, 32,* 1045–1057. PMID: 1936185

Sadeh, A., Gruber, R., & Raviv, A. (2003). The effects of sleep restriction and extension on school-age children: What a difference an hour makes. *Child Development, 74,* 444–455.

Sadeh, A., Mindell, J., & Rivera, L. (2011). "My child has a sleep problem": A cross-cultural comparison of parental definitions. *Sleep Medicine, 12,* 478–482. doi:10.1016/j.sleep.2010.10.008

Sakakini, R. (2011). *Behavioral treatments for sleep problems in youth: A meta-analytic review* (Doctoral dissertation). Retrieved from ProQuest (3452590).

Shin, C., Kim, J., Lee, S., Ahn, Y., & Joo, S. (2003). Sleep habits, excessive daytime sleepiness and school performance in high school students. *Psychiatry and Clinical Neurosciences, 57,* 451–453. doi:10.1046/j.1440-1819.2003.01146.x

Silva, G. E., Goodwin, J. L., Parthasarathy, S., Sherrill, D. L., Vana, K. D., Drescher, A. A., & Quan, S. F. (2011). Longitudinal association between short sleep, body weight, and emotional and learning problems in Hispanic and Caucasian children. *Sleep, 34,* 1197–1205. doi:10.5665/SLEEP.1238

Stein, M. A., Mendelsohn, J., Obermeyer, W. H., Amromin, J., & Benca, R. (2001). Sleep and behavior problems in school-aged children. *Pediatrics, 107,* 60–69. doi:10.1542/peds.107.4.e60

Verhulst, S. L., Van Gaal, L., De Backer, W., & Desager, K. (2008). The prevalence, anatomical correlates and treatment of sleep-disordered breathing in obese children and adolescents. *Sleep Medicine Reviews, 12*, 339–346. doi:10.1016/j.smrv.2007.11.002

Wolfson, A. R., & Carskadon, M. A. (1998). Sleep schedules and daytime functioning in adolescents. *Child Development, 69*, 875–887.

HANDOUT 22.1.

SYMPTOMS AND CHALLENGES FOR SCHOOL-BASED PROFESSIONALS AND PARENTS

Possible symptoms in youth with sleep problems:

Cognitive: Difficulty remembering things, problems with concentration, inattention, poor judgment, poor decision-making, rigid thinking, disorganization, poor planning, lack of inhibition, memory problems, and low motivation.

Behavioral: Hyperactivity, impulsivity, tantrums, disruptive behavior, and aggression.

Social/Emotional: Poor emotional regulation, difficult temperament, increased negative mood, irritability, and increased anxiety

Specific sleep-related complaints:

Daytime Sleepiness: Reported fatigue and/or falling asleep in class.

SBD: Morning headaches, fatigue, dry mouth upon awakening, loud snoring, gasping for air/breathing pauses, choking or snorting in sleep, sleeping in odd positions, and open-mouthed breathing during the day.

Periodic Limb Movement Disorder (PLMD): Restless sleep, waking up in different positions, tangled in covers, daytime fatigue, and inattention.

DSPD: Difficulty falling asleep and waking up at typical/expected times.

Next steps for school-based practitioners:

- Facilitate universal screenings.
- Routinely assess for sleep problems in youth (informal questions, standardized questionnaires, sleep diary, actigraph, etc.).
- Become familiar with referrals for more serious sleep problems as well as medical assessment and treatment.
- Consult and collaborate with parents to assist with design, implementation, and monitoring of behavioral sleep interventions.

WEEKLY SLEEP DIARY

TODAY'S DATE:	8/23						
1. How many naps did you take today?	1						
2. How long did you nap for (**total**)?	1.5 hours						
3. What time did you try to fall asleep?	11:00 PM						
4. How long did it take you to fall asleep?	20 min						
5. How many times did you wake up during the night?	2						
6. How long were you awake during the night (**total**)?	10 min						
7. What time was your final awakening?	7:00 AM						
9. How did you sleep last night?	☐ Very bad ☐ Bad ☐ Fair ☐ Good ☐ Very good	☐ Very bad ☐ Bad ☐ Fair ☐ Good ☐ Very good	☐ Very bad ☐ Bad ☐ Fair ☐ Good ☐ Very good	☐ Very bad ☐ Bad ☐ Fair ☐ Good ☐ Very good	☐ Very bad ☐ Bad ☐ Fair ☐ Good ☐ Very good	☐ Very bad ☐ Bad ☐ Fair ☐ Good ☐ Very good	☐ Very bad ☐ Bad ☐ Fair ☐ Good ☐ Very good
10. NOTES	Stayed up late for home-work						

HANDOUT 22.3.

SLEEP HYGIENE RECOMMENDATIONS FOR PARENTS OF CHILDREN AND ADOLESCENTS

1. **Keep a consistent sleep–wake schedule:** Developing a stable sleep pattern across weekdays and weekends helps regulate a person's internal clock and makes going to bed and waking up easier.
2. **Control lighting conditions:** Sleep is regulated by exposure to light and darkness. Bedrooms should have low light at bedtime and be dark for sleep. If a nightlight is needed, choose a small one and place it away from the bed. In the morning, children should be exposed to daylight upon awakening.
3. **Beds should be for sleeping only:** Engaging in activities in bed not only interferes with sleep, but also trains children to stay awake in bed by associating their bed with those activities. The bed should be a place that is easy to go to sleep in and to stay asleep in.
4. **Create a sleep** Bedrooms should quiet and kept at a comfortable temperature. Sound machines or soft music can help reduce outside noises.
5. **Do not watch the clock:** Children may be tempted to watch the clock when they cannot sleep. Remove clocks from the bedroom or turn the clock in another direction to prevent children from worrying what time it is.
6. **No-phone zone:** Technology creates distractions, and the light from screens can actually interfere with the way the brain regulates sleep and induce wakefulness, making it difficult to fall asleep. Limit exposure to phones, television, and other screens at least an hour before bedtime.
7. **Limit caffeine use:** Consuming caffeine can keep children awake and interfere with the quality of their sleep. Coffee, soda, tea, and chocolate should be avoided after dinner.
8. **Get regular exercise:** Regularly engaging in physical activity can also improve sleep. It is important for overall health, which also affects sleep. Children should avoid vigorous exercise close to bedtime because it may make it more difficult to fall asleep.
9. **Create a bedtime routine:** Developing a routine helps make the process of going to bed easier and more familiar. Encourage children to do quiet, relaxing activities before bedtime followed by preparing to go to sleep.
10. **Don't reinforce nighttime awakenings:** Getting attention from a parent after getting out of bed can be unintentionally rewarding to children. Direct them back to bed using a calm, unemotional voice.
11. **Praise good sleep habits:** It is important to acknowledge good sleep habits and to praise children for making an effort to get better sleep.

23

Chronic Pain Disorders

GRACE S. KAO, EVELYN C. MONICO, RASHMI P. BHANDARI,
AND SAMANTHA E. HUESTIS ■

For many children pain is a short-term, typical part of daily life. It can come in the form of a bruise incurred while playing on the playground, an impulsive grab for a still-too-hot mug, or a stomachache after eating too much dessert. Pain is an important, useful component of the childhood experience; however, for some youth (i.e., children and adolescents) who experience discomfort chronically, pain can become a debilitating symptom that limits multiple aspects of daily living, including in the school environment. Chronic pain is defined as recurrent or persistent pain that lasts beyond the time expected for healing, generally defined as 3 months. What can be the most disconcerting aspect of chronic pain is that often the etiology of the pain is unknown, causing confusion, frustration, and prolonged pursuit of anatomical causes. In the past few decades, pediatric chronic pain has been increasingly acknowledged as a clinical problem, and it is estimated to affect 20% to 30% of youth worldwide (King et al., 2011). An estimated 5% to 15% of youth are likely to experience more severe pain-related disability and require supports for improved functioning, such as school accommodations (Huguet & Miró, 2008; von Baeyer, 2011).

Pain research over the last 30 years has generated mounting evidence that pain is a biopsychosocial experience, affected by behavioral (e.g., avoidance, activation), cognitive (e.g., catastrophizing), affective (e.g., anxiety, depression), sociocultural, and neurosensory (i.e., nerve sensitivity) factors (Liossi & Howard, 2016). Environmentally, pain is also affected by family, peer, and school factors. Youth with chronic pain should therefore be evaluated by an interdisciplinary team of physicians, nurse practitioners, physical and occupational therapists, and behavioral health psychologists who specialize in pediatric pain. This integrated team approach allows both identification of applicable diagnoses and comprehensive recommendations. Physicians and nurse practitioners may recommend further testing, medications, procedures (e.g., nerve blocks), or other interventions (e.g., medical acupuncture); physical and occupational therapists may highlight the importance of daily physical activity and nerve desensitization training; and psychologists may emphasize constructive use of behavioral health support through cognitive-behavioral therapy, caregiver/parent management training, and family systems work. After an integrated team evaluation is completed, in most cases multidisciplinary follow-up is needed to encourage adherence to recommendations and determine helpfulness of such treatments over time. Overall, the primary goal of treatment is improvement of functioning and quality of life (Bruce et al., 2017).

The implications of chronic pain are far-reaching, and in the pediatric population school engagement is perhaps the most universal measure of daily functioning. Multiple school challenges may unfold, including frequent school absences, decreased school satisfaction and academic performance, and increased peer victimization (Vervoort, Logan, Goubert, De Clercq, & Hublet, 2014). Teachers and school staff are often at the front lines of supporting students with chronic medical conditions. Thus, it is crucial for families and medical providers to form a healthy partnership with school providers to optimize management of pain and ensure sound rehabilitative efforts. The school-based behavioral health professional is well positioned to serve as the liaison between these two systems.

COMMON PEDIATRIC CHRONIC PAIN CONDITIONS

Common pediatric chronic pain conditions are defined and described below. A multimodal approach to treatment is optimal for almost all chronic pain conditions. Modalities include both pharmacological and nonpharmacological therapies and are described in detail in the Pediatric Chronic Pain Intervention and Management section of this chapter.

Chronic Abdominal Pain (CAP)

Chronic abdominal pain (CAP) is a common problem among children and adolescents. In the United States 13% to 17% of youth report abdominal pain that occurs at least once a week, and of this group 21% report that pain interferes with daily activities (Sprenger, Gerhards, & Goldbeck, 2011). Abdominal pain can occur in different areas (i.e., upper, central, or lower regions), differ in sensation (e.g., cramplike, sharp, dull, throbbing), and be generalized or localized. When abdominal pain is persistent, pediatricians may refer patients to a gastroenterologist or pain specialist.

Sometimes, it may be difficult to determine an exact cause for CAP, especially in youth. Biological factors may include atypical motility or bowel activity, food sensitivities, infections, ulcers, menstrual cramps, medication side effects, or any disturbances that might exist in the enteric nervous system (ENT), the part of the autonomic nervous system that governs the gastrointestinal tract. Psychosocial contributors may include stress, anxiety, and reinforcement from external factors, such as school avoidance or escape from family conflict. Intervention for abdominal pain management may incorporate dietary changes (e.g., consideration of an anti-inflammatory diet) along with pharmacological and other nonpharmacological interventions (Sprenger et al., 2011).

Chronic Headaches

Chronic daily headache is a diagnostic category that clinicians utilize in addition to categorizing headaches as either migraine or tension types. More recent and comprehensive models of classification have emphasized a headache continuum that spans the spectrum between autonomic nervous system and muscular tension symptoms. Pediatric migraines may occur more acutely and differ in presentation according to developmental age (Bigal, Rapoport, Sheftell, Tepper, & Lipton, 2007). The prevalence of frequent or severe headaches, including migraines, ranges from 12% to 22% during the elementary-school years, although by the high-school years, it gradually rises to 22% (Lateef et al., 2009).

Headaches can be caused by illness, infections, colds, fevers, and inflammation. Chronic or severe headaches or migraines may also result from unknown etiologies related to changes in the brain or genetic influences. Headache and migraine triggers can include bright lights, loud sounds, weather changes, stress, anxiety, depression, changes in routine, impaired or variable sleep patterns, specific foods, or, in females, changes in the menstrual cycle. Tension headaches have been linked to pressure and stress, as well as to eyestrain and neck and back pain. Neurocognitively, school-age youth with headache may be particularly apt to report difficulties with concentration and attention, which can affect their learning in the classroom or completion of work outside of the classroom. Headaches can be functionally impairing and limit participation in academic, physical, social, extracurricular, and family activities, leading to chronic disability. Chronic or recurrent headaches have also been associated with occurrence of mental health disorders and poor quality of life (Blume, Brockman, & Breuner, 2012).

Complex Regional Pain Syndrome (Neuropathic Pain)

Complex regional pain syndrome (CRPS) is a chronic pain condition in a limb (e.g., arm, leg, hand, or foot) and is thought to be caused by malfunctioning of the central nervous system (brain and spinal cord) and peripheral nervous system (nerves signaling from brain and spinal cord to the rest of the body). CRPS type I—formerly known as reflex sympathetic dystrophy (RSD)—is diagnosed when no evidence of nerve injury has been identified; CRPS II is diagnosed when patients have confirmed nerve injury or injuries. Currently, there is limited information regarding the prevalence and incidence of pediatric CRPS. CRPS I is known to occur more commonly in girls, and a lower extremity is more commonly affected than an upper extremity (Weissmann & Uziel, 2016).

Multiple factors may contribute to CRPS development. In some cases, CRPS is triggered by a clear event of trauma or injury (e.g., during sports). For some individuals, their bodily response to trauma is a maintained and amplified perception of pain. Nerve fibers that carry pain signals throughout the body may become injured (as in CRPS II) or dysfunctional, leading to symptoms of CRPS. In an individual with CRPS pain can radiate to include an entire arm or leg, even if a triggering trauma or injury affected only a smaller portion of the limb. The main symptoms of CRPS include prolonged and substantial pain, changes in skin color, changes in skin temperature, swelling in the affected limb, and sensitivity to touch or cold. Other symptoms may include changes in skin texture, changes in hair and nail growth, muscle spasms, or weakness and decreased ability to move the affected body part. Symptoms may sometimes also spread from one limb to another (e.g., from one arm or leg to the opposite one).

Fortunately, many youth recover fully from CRPS, especially with a multimodal, rehabilitative approach to treatment. Functional rehabilitation, which involves progression from gentle to more progressive movements in order to reset altered central nervous system processing, is thought to be the most effective form of treatment (Wilder, 2006). To complement the rehabilitation process patients may receive nerve blocks, medications, and additional skills training with a pediatric pain psychologist (Logan et al., 2012).

Chronic Low Back Pain (Musculoskeletal Pain)

Low back pain (LBP) is one of the most common chronic musculoskeletal pain complaints among adolescents, with prevalence increasing with age: 1% at age 7 years, 6% at age 10 years, and 18% at ages 14 to 16 years. It is estimated that just 7% of youth seek medical attention, as most cases of LBP are self-limited (less than 6 weeks) and benign (MacDonald, Stuart, & Rodenberg, 2017). Youth with LBP may report tightness, pressure, stiffness, or pain that moves toward the buttocks or down one or both legs. The pain can develop acutely (over 1–2 days), subacutely (over a week), or chronically (over 3 months).

There are many etiologies of LBP in the pediatric population. Underlying musculoskeletal or biomechanical causes may be present, and other contributors, such as infectious, oncologic, or rheumatologic etiologies, should also be considered (Taxter, Chauvin, & Weiss, 2014). As with other musculoskeletal pains, lifestyle, psychological factors, and behavioral factors are also often a part of chronic LBP presentation, and evaluations include assessment of pain interference with sleep, physical activities, academics, social and family life, and mood. A child with nonspecific and self-limiting back pain will be treated first with conservative measures, such as nonsteroidal anti-inflammatory drugs (NSAIDs), physical therapy, and rest from activities that acutely heighten current pain (MacDonald et al., 2017).

Fibromyalgia (Central Sensitization)

Fibromyalgia causes widespread body pain, fatigue, sleep difficulties, mood disturbances (anxiety and depression most commonly), and multiple somatic complaints, like headaches, abdominal pain, and dizziness. Fibromyalgia typically occurs more commonly in adults, but it can also affect youth. Between 1% and 7% of youth are thought to be affected by fibromyalgia, and the condition is more likely to be found in girls than in boys. Overall, adolescent females are the demographic group with the highest prevalence of juvenile fibromyalgia (Kimura, 2000).

Researchers believe that individuals with fibromyalgia experience increased sensitivities to pain signals in the central nervous system, a process termed *central sensitization* (Kashikar-Zuck & Ting, 2014). Biologically, there may be an increase in the chemical process that signifies pain in the brain. Pain receptors may then begin to remember, and become hypersensitive to, these pain signals. Psychosocially, stress and effects of trauma are also important in this process, as they affect how pain signals are created and transmitted.

A subset of youth with fibromyalgia may also evidence issues with hypermobility (i.e., joint laxity) and dysautonomia, which typically presents as orthostatic dizziness, sweating, passing out, constipation, nausea, and diarrhea. These symptoms add a complex layer to the physical impairment of juvenile fibromyalgia and may contribute to frequent school absenteeism. It can be particularly hard for students with fibromyalgia to ensure attendance if their school environments have reduced or no disability service access (e.g., elevators) or school personnel do not feel equipped for medical management of dizziness or fainting spells. These youth not only may miss school, but also may give up on sports or other extracurricular activities (e.g., missing theater productions due to fainting spells). This causes them to experience even more social isolation, leading to more negative quality of life than age-matched peers with migraines, juvenile arthritis, and systemic lupus erythematosus (SLE; Kashikar-Zuck & Ting, 2014).

Disease-Related Pain Disorders (Sickle Cell Disease)

Chronic pain may also occur as a symptom of a chronic disease (e.g., juvenile arthritis, cancer, and pancreatitis), and sickle cell disease (SCD) is discussed here as the example. SCD affects between 70,000 and 100,000 individuals in the United States, most of whom are of African descent or self-identify as black. Individuals with SCD experience vaso-occlusive or acute pain crises which can occur in the extremities, chest, and back. SCD pain is reported to be present in youth with SCD approximately 10% of the time.

SCD results from a genetic substitution mutation in hemoglobin. This small substitution makes red blood cells prone to sickling (changing to sickle shape) when hemoglobin is deoxygenated. When in this crescent shape red blood cells are inflexible and blood is more viscous, which makes red cells interact abnormally with the blood vessel lining. Over time, youth can experience both acute pain crises and chronic pain. Functionally, the crises can lead to more frequent or lengthy hospital stays for pain management, consequently resulting in frequent school absences. Pain can occur both in and outside of the context of SCD. A multidisciplinary team may educate the patient's family about the biology of SCD and chronic pain. Understanding the relationship between chronic illness and chronic pain can curtail unnecessary disease-related clinical testing or diagnostic investigations, decrease pain episodes, increase pain thresholds, and enhance functioning (Yawn et al., 2014).

PEDIATRIC CHRONIC PAIN INTERVENTION AND MANAGEMENT

Nonpharmacological Strategies

BEHAVIORAL HEALTH INTERVENTIONS

Youth who experience chronic pain benefit from weekly treatment with a mental health provider to learn how to manage chronic discomfort, resume and maintain function, and receive support around the impact of pain on mood. The mental health provider may also work closely with a student's school to ensure gradual reintegration, incorporate accommodations for academic success, assist with establishing reward plans to promote academic function, and inform school personnel about ways that the student can be supported. Behavioral health treatment may incorporate the following interventions.

Cognitive-behavioral therapy (CBT) has been shown to enhance long-term rehabilitation for individuals with chronic pain by shifting behavior and thoughts related to the experience of pain and its impact on function (Palermo, 2012). In fact, some research shows that these skills are even more effective for youth than medication in terms of restoring functioning and reducing pain. The main goals of CBT are to: help youth change their view of the pain experience from overwhelming to manageable; motivate them to engage in their lives and treatment, despite discomfort, with appropriate pacing, utilization of self-regulations skills, and pursuit of adaptive management techniques; and shift maladaptive thoughts that exacerbate the pain experiences (e.g., catastrophizing) through gradual exposure to activities that improve quality of life.

Stress management and self-regulation skills training are useful for youth with chronic pain because the experience of chronic pain can be stressful, affecting all aspects of life, and stress in turn is known to exacerbate the experience of pain. Stress and pain can influence sleep quality, worsen fatigue, trigger gastrointestinal disturbances and headaches, increase concentration problems, heighten irritability, cause anger and agitation, lower immunity, and reduce academic productivity. Learning how to manage stress is therefore a critically important part of managing pain. Skills that are taught—and can be practiced at school by giving the child some time at the nurses' office or in a quiet space—include breathing exercises, progressive muscle relaxation, imagery, self-hypnosis (i.e., mobilizing imagination to shift the sensory experience of discomfort), mindfulness (i.e., the act of paying careful attention to the present experience) and biofeedback. (Handouts 23.3 and 23.4 have information helpful for teaching relaxed breathing for pain management.)

Nervous system responses become activated with pain, triggering increased muscle tension, elevating heart rate, and decreasing body temperature. Learning to better regulate these aspects of the nervous system can help reduce pain. Biofeedback involves using one or more sensors to examine the body's physiology. The sensors convert the body's information into a sound or an image on a computer or portable electronic device that allows for increased awareness and more active control of physiological factors that contribute to pain.

The experience of chronic pain can result in decreased ability to enjoy and to engage in rewarding social interactions, thereby inadvertently increasing, in some youth, a need for even more attention from healthcare providers, teachers, family members, and peers. This dynamic can sometimes convert health-related care and attention to a secondary reinforcement for continued functional impairment. Secondary reinforcements may also come in the form of a child's being able to avoid unwanted responsibilities (e.g., chores), academic stressors, unpleasant social interactions and bullying, and conflict-laden family dynamics. Mental health providers work closely with schools and parents to modify the behavioral contingencies related to the experience of pain. Useful strategies include requesting that school personnel and family members provide attention and positive reinforcement for non-pain-related behaviors while diminishing attention to and reinforcement of pain-related interactions. That is, celebrating a child's engagement in school activities (even when enduring pain) can be more helpful than criticizing the child on the days he or she misses school. Other recommended approaches include reducing unnecessary inquiries about the experience of pain, encouraging pacing, and advocating use of self-regulation skills and distraction when pain complaints arise.

OPTIMIZING LIFESTYLE FACTORS (E.G., Sleep, Exercise, Diet, Hydration)
Pain and insomnia negatively affect each other. As an individual gets less sleep, pain worsens; as pain worsens, sleep disturbances become more likely. Adequate sleep, exercise, diet, and hydration are critically important to health, because they allow the body time to heal, replenish the immune system, and improve mood and pain. Temporarily modified school schedules may be considered for students who are challenged by nightly insomnia related to pain and consequent daytime fatigue. Regular exercise is also highly recommended, because it helps with stress management and increases endorphins that decrease the experience of pain. Physical education class activities may require modifications to support consistent and achievable exercise.

PHYSICAL AND OCCUPATIONAL THERAPY

Youth with chronic pain can become caught in a cycle of pain avoidance, inactivity, and sensitivity to pain, which leads to reduced strength, endurance, and confidence; therefore, these youth benefit from physical rehabilitation. The appointments usually occur on a weekly basis and then reduce in frequency. During and upon finishing treatments it is critical for youth to participate in their prescribed daily home exercise program (HEP). Consistent physical therapy sessions can often be counted for physical education credit. Alternatively, allowing students to engage in their HEP during PE class may be helpful.

Some students may also benefit from sitting at the back of the classroom in order to engage in stretches without disturbing the rest of the classroom. Others may use a prescribed transcutaneous electrical nerve stimulation (TENS) unit in class to help promote comfort. TENS is a low-intensity electrical stimulation of the skin and muscles on specific areas of the body in order to decrease the perception and intensity of pain. TENS is safe, does not pose a hazard for students in the classroom, and can be used without overt disturbance.

MEDICAL ACUPUNCTURE

Acupuncture uses stimulation via placement of thin needles in designated body areas to release the body's *chi* and to induce chemical changes that improve certain pain conditions, enhance sleep, and promote relaxation (National Institute of Health, 2011). The stimulation provided in classical acupuncture has been modernized recently by the application of low-frequency (<5 Hz) stimulation of the needles, which also produces tension-relieving muscle contractions. Acupuncture is generally administered weekly for 4 to 8 weeks, after which the frequency is reduced depending on efficacy.

Pharmacological Strategies

To date, there is limited empirical evidence to support specific pharmacological therapies in youth with chronic pain. When available, most recommendations are based on adult studies, pediatric case reports, expert opinion, and the skill of the treating pediatric pain physician (Finnerup et al., 2015). This is particularly appreciable in the management of pediatric headaches, where the placebo effect is substantial and only ibuprofen and triptans have sufficient evidence to support their use in pediatrics (Friedrichsdorf et al., 2016). Nonetheless, medications for pediatric chronic pain are sometimes prescribed, although they often do not singularly provide pain-free states. They are, however, utilized to provide pain relief to facilitate the initiation and maintenance of physiotherapy and physical function and in conjunction with nonpharmacological strategies. Common pain medications prescribed by a specialist may include nerve pain medications, such as gabapentin (Neurontin) or amitriptyline (Elavil). Nonprescription medications (e.g., Advil, Tylenol) may also be employed. Opioids are rarely indicated in nonmalignant pain and long-term treatment of pediatric chronic pain. It is important to clarify that medication regimens must be tailored to the individual patient, and there is no one-size-fits-all regimen. Factors such as maladaptive behavior, altered mood, or poor sleep must be addressed in tandem with prescribing medications.

Medications may be administered in the school setting if they enable a child to improve function and better manage pain. Measurable functional gains can be seen if a child is able to achieve consistent school attendance, remain in class, remain attentive while in the classroom, or participate in extracurricular activities (e.g., sports, drama, band, etc.). Schools should be prepared to safely administer pain medications to allow students to achieve these goals, in accordance with state guidelines on medication administration in schools. In general and at a minimum, appropriate parental consent for medication administration should first be obtained through a written request from the parent or legal guardian and should include the student's name, drug and dose to be administered, and time of administration. Many schools also require medication to be kept in its original container with a clear label.

Procedural Strategies

Pain blocks or nerve blocks are procedures that interrupt the flow of pain signals in the central nervous system, thereby alleviating pain. Most of these procedures involve injecting local anesthetics near nerves or into joints that cause pain. Chronic pain pathophysiology exists in the peripheral and central nervous systems, so nerve blocks that target only the periphery or the spinal cord may not yield complete pain relief. Where sympathetically mediated or maintained pain is evident, it may be appropriate to perform a sympathetic block. Nerve block procedures are not used as a "magic wand" to minimize or eliminate pain (but can), and more often serve as a means or "bridge" to facilitate paced physical therapies and improve function. Ideally, procedures should be performed only by pain specialists after a multidisciplinary evaluation of the child and family. Procedures can typically be performed on an outpatient basis and may require few if any days for recovery (Shah, Cappiello, & Suresh, 2016).

COMMON SCHOOL-RELATED CONCERNS

Educational Considerations

Chronic pain can lead to various school-related concerns and complications in academic, physical, and social realms. Academically and socially, the most challenging complication may be the high number of absences students with chronic pain incur (Gorodzinsky, Hainsworth, & Weisman, 2011). Frequent absences can lead to difficulties with missed schoolwork, lack of social interactions, truancy concerns, and risk for grade retention. Late arrivals at, and early departures from, school are also common. Moreover, because students with chronic pain may also experience co-occurring anxiety symptoms (often related to academics), extended periods of absences and resulting missed instruction can further add to academic anxiety.

Students with chronic pain also often experience peer difficulties (e.g., having fewer friends, increased peer victimization) that affect both pain and school functioning (Forgeron et al., 2010). Some students may also have a pre-existing history of peer difficulties that contribute to school avoidance being a reinforcing element of chronic pain disability. A common social stressor is the perception that others, including teachers and classmates, do not believe the pain is "real."

To target these educational concerns a variety of collaborative and educational steps may be taken. First, family and teacher conferences should be scheduled to provide reassurance that a student's chronic pain condition is acknowledged, to identify necessary accommodations, and to define expectations for the school environment to ensure school staff, family, and student are on the same page. Students may also prepare educational presentations for teachers and classmates, often in collaboration with a healthcare provider, regarding their chronic pain condition (e.g., CRPS) to promote understanding.

For teachers and other school personnel, variability in student functioning can be perplexing. They may observe differences in functioning between students with the same or similar chronic pain diagnoses or inconsistencies in pain-related functioning within the same individual (Logan & Curran, 2005). Although many students with chronic pain receive formal school accommodations, schools and teachers must acquaint themselves with students' individual needs, with pain triggers, and with indicated academic, functional, and behavioral recommendations to best optimize student participation. Given the variable course and impact of chronic pain and symptom occurrence, it is difficult to apply a one-size-fits-all school functioning plan; however, a basic guiding principle is to provide supports and expectations beneficial for progress in functioning. Often, restoration of functioning, rather than absolute pain relief, is the primary goal for successful management of chronic pain. With understanding, supportive teachers may curb the negative outcomes of school absenteeism and bullying associated with chronic pain (Vervoort et al., 2014) and help to promote resilience among youth striving to manage the daily effects of chronic pain on school functioning.

Legal, Policy, and Accommodation Considerations

Pediatric chronic pain can occur as a medical condition in and of itself and warrants provision of school accommodations under the Individuals with Disabilities Education Act or Section 504 of the Rehabilitation Act of 1973 (described in Chapter 5). Under these policies, students with chronic pain may receive a variety of accommodations operationalized through development of a 504 Plan or an individualized education plan (IEP) under the special education category of other health impaired (OHI). (Handouts 23.1 covers possible educational challenges and accommodations for pediatric chronic pain.)

Medical providers encourage students with chronic pain to attend school as consistently as possible. This helps to re-establish or reinforce adaptive pursuit of a structured lifestyle, to provide distraction from pain, and to promote opportunities for social interactions. For students who have become entrenched in a pattern of absenteeism, a temporary modified schedule and graduated attendance plan may be implemented to aid in reintegration to school and to build consistency. In most cases, full homebound schooling without a reintegration plan is not recommended for students with chronic pain, because spending more time at home can compound difficulties with school, socialization, and deconditioning, and can even lead to more pain. In the school environment, students often benefit from teacher flexibility, whether in use of adjusted timelines for turning in work; permission to stretch, change positions, or engage in relaxation exercises in the classroom; or provision of extra time between classes to accommodate potentially more difficult travel, particularly when the pain condition limits the child's mobility.

Effective communication and understanding among and between students, school personnel, healthcare providers, and parents and caregivers is an integral part of optimal pain management in schools. Teachers are important stakeholders in students' pain management plans, as they may aid healthcare teams in assessing student functioning and limitations due to pain in the classroom. Healthcare teams, in turn, may provide schools and parents with guidance about suitable accommodations, challenges to expect, and constructive expectations schools should set. Parents serve as expert observers of their child's functioning, interests, and goals. They consequently remain critical to ensuring that environmental and behavioral techniques (e.g., use of pain management strategies) implemented at school are also utilized at home. (The section "Helpful Websites and Resources" at the end of this chapter lists resources for understanding pediatric chronic pain.)

Risk and Protective Factors and Socioemotional Health Considerations

Many factors place youth at higher risk for chronic pain occurrence, exacerbation, and maintenance (McKillop & Banez, 2016). In the school setting, stress-related risks are particularly relevant, given the impact of school on stress, and of stress on the pain response. Maladaptive coping responses to stress, such as internalizing or catastrophizing, further add to pain risk. Notably, parental catastrophizing and protectiveness also negatively affect school attendance and global functioning. Additionally, fear of pain and resulting activity avoidance appear to perpetuate the pain–disability cycle, and sleep difficulties often contribute to pain exacerbation.

Protective factors are similarly multifaceted. In the school environment, social relationships may offset some of the negative impact of chronic pain. Specifically, supportive teacher and peer relationships have been found to be protective. Adaptive coping factors such as optimism, problem-solving, behavioral distraction, pursuit of valued activities, and maintenance of a healthy lifestyle (such as regular and sufficient sleep and consistent activity), have also been linked to positive outcomes in the face of chronic pain.

Mental and emotional difficulties frequently accompany chronic pain in youth, especially in the form of internalizing disorders, such as depression and anxiety. Mental and emotional stress can both prime an individual for pain exacerbation and maintenance and be reciprocally amplified by pain symptoms. For many youth with chronic pain limitations on desired activities, peer difficulties related to pain, and a sense of injustice contribute to the decline in mental and emotional health. Along with pain behaviors (e.g., grimacing, guarding affected areas), students with chronic pain may also evidence symptoms of depression and anxiety, such as heightened irritability, withdrawing from others, crying episodes, concentration difficulties, activity avoidance, and acting-out behaviors in the school environment (Noel, Groenewald, Beals-Erickson, Gebert, & Palermo, 2016).

Cultural Considerations

Culture and context play an important role in how youth and families understand and respond to pain. Cultural considerations may include racial and ethnic background, as well as religious, spiritual, philosophical, social, lifestyle, political, economic, and educational factors. For example, parental ethnicity has been linked to preference for, and use of, nonpharmacological versus pharmacological pain management, and religion has been linked to use of spiritual support or prayer as means of coping with pain. Lifestyle and family values toward health and illness may influence whether youth express their pain or hide it from others. Economic factors may also determine whether youth and families have access to specialized pain management, and which interventions may (or may not) be included in their treatment (Kankkunen, Vehviläinen-Julkunen, Pietilä, & Nikkonen, 2009). In achieving optimal pain management, cultural considerations should be factored into understanding, accommodating, and awareness of a student's chronic pain symptoms in the school environment.

CASE EXAMPLE

Beatrice was a 16-year-old female high-school junior when she presented for an interdisciplinary pain clinic evaluation. Her medical history was remarkable for asthma, acute allergies, bone tumor, nausea, and pain in her abdomen, low back, neck, knees, ankles, and heels. Concurrent anxiety and depression, worsened in part by family stressors, compounded her discomfort. While Beatrice had a 504 Plan for asthma and allergies, there were no accommodations for her chronic pain. Due to pain, she had missed over 2 months of school, was failing courses despite being a previously high-achieving student, and had been placed on a basic independent studies program. Her depression was quickly worsening, however, due to the isolation inherent to her 504 Plan, and Beatrice missed her in-class learning opportunities and time spent with friends on campus. She shared that she wanted to work with the pain clinic on a plan to "tolerate pain more, get to school more, and so it doesn't affect daily functioning."

Consequently, a medical letter of support from the pain clinic was provided that outlined the impact that Beatrice's chronic pain had on school functioning and that recommended Beatrice promptly return to school via revised programming. Recommended accommodations included provision of a modified/partial day, extended time for homework and exams, and access to an empathic independent studies teacher to guide Beatrice's progress and to complement time spent on campus. Beatrice had previously understood that her school had an all-or-none approach to independent studies, but the communication from the pain team helped her to acquire a more tailored program. In fact, Beatrice reported that implementation of flexible accommodations "was the light at the end of the tunnel" in her pain rehabilitation process, because it enabled her to return to academic achievement proportionate to her abilities.

Beatrice has since graduated from high school and is now in college, hoping to pursue graduate or medical school. She reflected that her academic success was, in part, facilitated by treatments like behavioral health therapy, acupuncture, physical therapy, and use of medications for pain and mood. Moreover, Beatrice found that, once school faculty took into account her medical team's recommendations, she felt empowered to communicate health information to her school.

In looking back, Beatrice suggested that all schools regularly provide a proactive academic liaison versed in health matters to students with accommodations. The liaison's role would be to facilitate program transitions (e.g., standard school to off-campus; modified schedule with dynamic home and campus components depending on need) and to enhance communication with healthcare provider(s), given the variable impact of pain (e.g., flares limiting physical education, hospitalizations preventing attendance) over time. Beatrice also reflected that schools that are overly proactive—such as those that provide college tours to ninth graders to increase excitement about applications—might unintentionally intensify pressure among those struggling with standard requirements. After Beatrice grappled with a bone tumor in middle school, this perceived pressure at the start of high school increased Beatrice's anxiety—a known pain amplifier—and discomfort. Given her overall success, however, Beatrice recently met with the school board to share how their flexible, personalized support was instrumental to her achieving her goals despite chronic pain.

HELPFUL WEBSITES AND RESOURCES

- American Pain Society List of Pediatric Pain Clinics (USA): http://americanpainsociety.org/uploads/get-involved/ped%20pain%20clinic%20list%2012292016.pdf

- Children's National Health System: What Is Pain?: http://www.interfacemedia.com/Portfolio/CNHS#pain
- How Does Your Brain Respond to Pain?: https://www.youtube.com/watch?v=I7wfDenj6CQ
- Pain and Your Child or Teen: http://www.med.umich.edu/yourchild/topics/pain.htm
- Pain Retreat: http://www.painretreat.net/mainbottom.htm
- Seattle Children's Hospital Pain Medicine Resources: http://www.seattlechildrens.org/clinics-programs/pain-medicine/resources/
- The Centre for Pediatric Pain Research: Science Helping Children: http://pediatric-pain.ca/resources/ and http://pediatric-pain.ca/for-health-professionals/
- The Coping Club: Pain: http://copingclub.com/category/condition/pain/
- Understanding Pain: What To Do About It In Less Than 5 Minutes: https://www.youtube.com/watch?v=vdM4dHefA4w

Books

Managing Your Child's Chronic Pain (2015), by Tonya Palermo and Emily F. Law
When Your Child Hurts: Effective Strategies to Increase Comfort, Reduce Stress, and Break the Cycle of Chronic Pain (2016), by Rachael Coakley

REFERENCES

Bigal, M. E., Rapoport, A. M., Sheftell, F. D., Tepper, S. J., & Lipton, R. B. (2007). The International Classification of Headache Disorders revised criteria for chronic migraine—Field testing in a headache specialty clinic. *Cephalalgia: An International Journal of Headache, 27*(3), 230–234. doi:10.1111/j.1468-2982.2006.01274.x

Blume, H., Brockman, L., & Breuner, C. (2012). Biofeedback therapy for pediatric headache: Factors associated with response. *Headache: The Journal of Head and Face Pain, 52*(9), 1377–1386. doi:10.1111/j.1526-4610.2012.02215.x

Bruce, B. K., Ale, C. M., Harrison, T. E., Bee, S., Luedtke, C., Geske, J., & Weiss, K. E. (2017). Getting back to living: Further evidence for the efficacy of an interdisciplinary pediatric pain treatment program. *The Clinical Journal of Pain, 33*(6), 535–542. doi:10.1097/AJP.0000000000000433

Finnerup, N. B., Attal, N., Haroutounian, S., McNicol, E., Baron, R., Dworkin, R. H., . . . Wallace, M. (2015). Pharmacotherapy for neuropathic pain in adults: A systematic review and meta-analysis. *The Lancet. Neurology, 14*(2), 162–173. doi:10.1016/S1474-4422(14)70251-0

Forgeron, P. A., King, S., Stinson, J. N., McGrath, P. J., MacDonald, A. J., & Chambers, C. T. (2010). Social functioning and peer relationships in children and adolescents with chronic pain: A systematic review. *Pain Research & Management, 15*(1), 27–41.

Friedrichsdorf, S., Sidman, J., & Krane, E. (2016). Prevention and treatment of pain in children: Toward a paradigm shift. *Otolaryngology–Head and Neck Surgery, 154*(5), 804–805. doi:10.1177/0194599816636100

Gorodzinsky, A. Y., Hainsworth, K. R., & Weisman, S. J. (2011). School functioning and chronic pain: A review of methods and measures. *Journal of Pediatric Psychology, 36*(9), 991–1002. doi:10.1093/jpepsy/jsr038

Huguet, A., & Miró, J. (2008). The severity of chronic pediatric pain: An epidemiological study. *Journal of Pain, 9*(3), 226–236. doi:10.1016/j.jpain.2007.10.015

Kankkunen, P., Vehviläinen-Julkunen, K., Pietilä, A.-M., & Nikkonen, M. (2009). Cultural factors influencing children's pain. *International Journal of Caring Sciences, 2*(3), 126–134.

Kashikar-Zuck, S., & Ting, T. V. (2014). Juvenile fibromyalgia: Current status of research and future developments. *Nature Reviews: Rheumatology, 10*(2), 89–96. doi:10.1038/nrrheum.2013.177

Kimura, Y. (2000). Fibromyalgia syndrome in children and adolescents. *The Journal of Musculoskeletal Medicine, 17*(3), 142–142.

King, S., Chambers, C. T., Huguet, A., MacNevin, R. C., McGrath, P. J., Parker, L., & MacDonald, A. J. (2011). The epidemiology of chronic pain in children and adolescents revisited: A systematic review. *Pain, 152*(12), 2729–2738. doi:10.1016/j.pain.2011.07.016

Lateef, T. M., Merikangas, K. R., He, J., Kalaydjian, A., Khoromi, S., Knight, E., & Nelson, K. B. (2009). Headache in a national sample of American children: Prevalence and co-morbidity. *Journal of Child Neurology, 24*(5), 536–543. doi:10.1177/0883073808327831

Liossi, C., & Howard, R. F. (2016). Pediatric chronic pain: Biopsychosocial assessment and formulation. *Pediatrics, 138*(5), e20160331. doi:10.1542/peds.2016-0331

Logan, D. E., Carpino, E. A., Chiang, G., Condon, M., Firn, E., Gaughan, V. J., . . . Berde, C. B. (2012). A day-hospital approach to treatment of pediatric complex regional pain syndrome: Initial functional outcomes. *The Clinical Journal of Pain, 28*(9), 766–774. doi:10.1097/AJP.0b013e3182457619

Logan, D. E., & Curran, J. A. (2005). Adolescent chronic pain problems in the school setting: Exploring the experiences and beliefs of selected school personnel through focus group methodology. *The Journal of Adolescent Health: Official Publication of the Society for Adolescent Medicine, 37*(4), 281–288. doi:10.1016/j.jadohealth.2004.11.134

MacDonald, J., Stuart, E., & Rodenberg, R. (2017). Musculoskeletal low back pain in school-aged children: A review. *JAMA Pediatrics, 171*(3), 280–287. doi:10.1001/jamapediatrics.2016.3334

McKillop, H. N., & Banez, G. A. (2016). A broad consideration of risk factors in pediatric chronic pain: Where to go from here? *Children, 3*(4), 38. doi:10.3390/children3040038

National Institutes of Health. (2011). Understanding acupuncture. *NIH News in Health.* Retrieved from https://newsinhealth.nih.gov/2011/02/understanding-acupuncture

Noel, M., Groenewald, C. B., Beals-Erickson, S. E., Gebert, J. T., & Palermo, T. M. (2016). Chronic pain in adolescence and internalizing mental health disorders: A nationally representative study. *Pain, 157*(6), 1333–1338. doi:10.1097/j.pain.0000000000000522

Palermo, T. M. (2012). *Cognitive-behavioral therapy for chronic pain in children and adolescents.* New York, NY: Oxford University Press.

Shah, R. D., Cappiello, D., & Suresh, S. (2016). Interventional procedures for chronic pain in children and adolescents: A review of the current evidence. *Pain Practice: The Official Journal of World Institute of Pain, 16*(3), 359–369. doi:10.1111/papr.12285

Sprenger, L., Gerhards, F., & Goldbeck, L. (2011). Effects of psychological treatment on recurrent abdominal pain in children—A meta-analysis. *Clinical Psychology Review, 31*(7), 1192–1197. doi:10.1016/j.cpr.2011.07.010

Taxter, A. J., Chauvin, N. A., & Weiss, P. F. (2014). Diagnosis and treatment of low back pain in the pediatric population. *The Physician and Sportsmedicine, 42*(1), 94–104. doi:10.3810/psm.2014.02.2052

Vervoort, T., Logan, D. E., Goubert, L., De Clercq, B., & Hublet, A. (2014). Severity of pediatric pain in relation to school-related functioning and teacher support: An epidemiological study among school-aged children and adolescents. *Pain, 155*(6), 1118–1127. doi:10.1016/j.pain.2014.02.021

von Baeyer, C. L. (2011). Interpreting the high prevalence of pediatric chronic pain revealed in community surveys. *Pain, 152*(12), 2683–2684. doi:10.1016/j.pain.2011.08.023

Weissmann, R., & Uziel, Y. (2016). Pediatric complex regional pain syndrome: A review. *Pediatric Rheumatology Online Journal, 14.* doi:10.1186/s12969-016-0090-8

Wilder, R. T. (2006). Management of pediatric patients with complex regional pain syndrome. *The Clinical Journal of Pain, 22*(5), 443–448. doi:10.1097/01.ajp.0000194283.59132.fb

Yawn, B. P., Buchanan, G. R., Afenyi-Annan, A. N., Ballas, S. K., Hassell, K. L., James, A. H., . . . John-Sowah, J. (2014). Management of sickle cell disease: Summary of the 2014 evidence-based report by expert panel members. *JAMA, 312*(10), 1033–1048. doi:10.1001/jama.2014.10517

Handout 23.1.

Symptoms, Educational Challenges, and School Accommodations: Pediatric Chronic Pain

Major Characteristics and Symptoms
- Recurrent or persistent pain that lasts beyond the time expected for healing, generally a 3-month period, and that may present as abdominal, musculoskeletal, neuropathic, and disease-related pain, as well as headache.
- Responds best to interdisciplinary treatment, which may include pain medicine, physical therapy, occupational therapy, and pain psychology.
- Often accompanied by mental health symptoms, such as depression and/or anxiety.
- Restoration of functioning, rather than absolute pain relief, serves as the primary goal for successful management.

Possible Educational Challenges	Possible School Accommodations
Frequent absences, delayed arrivals, and early dismissals due to pain flares	Modified school schedule, which will ensure regular school attendance (e.g., modified or reduced course load, including lunch on campus and supplementation of remaining courses as homebound or independent studies). Importantly, as functioning improves, so, too, should school attendance (i.e., reintegration into full-day attendance).
Impaired academic performance Difficulty concentrating on work (including pain-related challenges with writing, reading, sitting long period of time, etc.)	• Increased or extended time or deadlines for assignment completion. • Modified assignments to promote understanding while limiting repetitive work (e.g., completion of even or odd numbers only). • Ability to take exams in a quiet, isolated setting. • Possible provision of in-home educational support (e.g., tutors) and repetition of concepts or materials missed, along with additional academic support if indicated. • Audio books for class reading. • Access to laptop or outline for note taking and writing assignments. • Assistance with note taking. • Ability to move around the classroom or take a structured time out in a quiet setting when pain is elevated during the school day.

POSSIBLE EDUCATIONAL CHALLENGES	POSSIBLE SCHOOL ACCOMMODATIONS
Ambulation difficulties (e.g., walking from class to class, using stairs) Fear of pain motivates general activity avoidance	• Permission to leave class early to have sufficient time to travel between classes, thus preventing tardiness. • Provision of two sets of textbooks: one set for school and a second set for home to prevent carrying the extra weight, which may increase the student's pain.
Difficulties with performing all activities in physical education classes or with participating fully in athletic team practices and games	• Ability to limit participation in physical education when pain is elevated and symptomatic (e.g., walking instead of running and exclusion from contact sports, high-impact activities, and jumping). • Modifications to physical education requirements. Allowing physical therapy sessions and home program to count toward physical education credits or graduation requirements, or home program to be performed during physical education class.
Peer difficulties and vulnerability to teasing, especially when others do not believe the pain symptoms are real* Mood and/or behavioral changes in the classroom	• Promotion of involvement in other behavioral activities offered through the school in order to support social growth and connection to peers at school. • Ensuring that all teachers understand the need for flexibility, given the student's vulnerabilities due to chronic pain.

*It is important for school personnel to know that all pain, independent of cause, is real to the student, and should be supported accordingly.

HANDOUT 23.2.

BIOPSYCHOSOCIAL MODEL OF PAIN

Pain has many parts:

<u>Physical</u>—*Physical changes that lead to pain*
- growth of scar tissue
- nerve malfunction
- degenerative changes or loss of function in the affected area

<u>Cognitive</u>—*How you think about pain*
- pain becomes the focus of
  - attention
  - memory for pain
  - perceptions
  - expectations

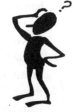

<u>Emotional</u>—*How pain makes you feel*
- sad
- anxious
- angry
- irritable

- afraid
- worried
- guilty
- stressed

<u>Actions</u>—*How you respond to pain*
- rubbing
- guarding
- limping
- reduced physical activity
- more rest

<u>Social</u>—*How others respond to your pain*
- giving you support, medicine, ice/heat
- changes in relationships with friends, family, teachers, and others due to pain

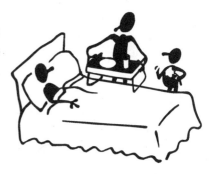

Handout 23.3.

Relaxed Breathing Procedure

1. Find a comfortable place, where you can be alone, with no distractions or interruptions, for about 10 minutes.
2. Complete the first part of your Relaxation Log (Handout 23.4).
3. Close your eyes and take a moment to get your breathing slowed down.
4. Place one hand on your chest and the other on your stomach. As you breathe in through your nose and out through your mouth, notice which hand is moving.
5. As you breathe in deeply, push your stomach out. Imagine warm air flowing into your lungs and to all parts of your body as you inhale.
6. Pause for one second, then breathe out to the count of four. As you are breathing out, your stomach should be going down.
7. Pause for one second, then breathe in deeply again.
8. Pause for one second, then breathe out to the count of four.
9. Continue breathing in and out, slowly. As you are breathing in, think the words *I am,* and as you are breathing out, think the word *Relaxed.*
10. Do the breathing exercise for about 5 to 10 minutes.
11. Complete your Relaxation Log.
12. Remember to practice at least two to four times per day.

HANDOUT 23.4.

RELAXATION LOG

DATE	TIME	LENGTH OF PRACTICE	COMFORT RATING* BEFORE RELAXATION	COMFORT RATING* AFTER RELAXATION	NOTES

*Comfort rating on a scale of 0 to 10, 0 = not comfortable at all; 10 = completely comfortable.

24

Eating and Feeding Disorders

CAROLYN HA, RACHEL WOLFE, AND REBECCA WAGNER ■

Eating disorders typically emerge in adolescence or young adulthood, with prevalence rates ranging from 0.3% to 2.7% in the general population (Merikangas et al., 2010; Swanson, Crow, Le Grange, Swendsen, & Merikangas, 2011). These disorders encompass a broad spectrum of diagnoses and have been classified under the heading Feeding and Eating Disorders in the *Diagnostic and Statistical Manual of Mental Disorders*, Fifth Edition (DSM-5; American Psychiatric Association [APA], 2013). An eating disorder is defined as "a persistent disturbance of eating or eating-related behavior that results in the altered consumption or absorption of food and that significantly impairs physical health or psychosocial functioning" (APA, 2013). There is evidence that eating disorders occur across all ethnic and cultural groups (Chisuwa & O'Dea, 2010; Jackson & Chen, 2010; Marques et al., 2011). Specific feeding and eating disorders listed in DSM-5 include pica, rumination disorder, anorexia nervosa (AN), bulimia nervosa (BN), binge eating disorder (BED), and avoidant restrictive food intake disorder (ARFID).

The present chapter focuses on eating or food-related disorders (AN, BN, BED, ARFID, orthorexia) and malnutrition in children and adolescents. This group of disorders is generally referred to as eating disorders throughout the chapter. The overall goals of the chapter are to provide a general description of eating disorders in children and adolescents, assessment and treatment considerations, and resources for school-based clinicians who work with children and adolescents diagnosed with an eating disorder.

OVERVIEW OF SPECIFIC EATING DISORDERS

Ongoing maturation and development across physical, social, emotional, and cognitive domains of functioning are expected during childhood and adolescence. Behaviors and symptoms representative of an eating disorder diagnosis in adults may present differently in children and adolescents due to developmental immaturity, therefore, it is important to consider developmental appropriateness for symptom presentations or when considering diagnostic criteria (Bravender et al., 2007; Knoll, Bulik, & Hebebrand, 2011). Behavioral observations provided by multiple sources is important, as children and adolescents may have limited insight into their own symptoms, a limited awareness of feelings and thoughts regarding weight or body image, limited verbal ability to express symptoms, and poorer abstract reasoning abilities (Bravender et al., 2007; Marini & Case, 1994).

Anorexia Nervosa

Characteristics of AN include a persistent restriction of energy intake, an intense fear of weight gain, engaging in behaviors that interfere with weight gain (i.e. excessive exercise, purging, laxatives), and a disturbance in the individual's self-evaluation of body weight or shape (APA, 2013). In children and adolescents, the DSM-5 criteria for restriction of energy intake may present as a failure to make expected weight gain or a failure to maintain a normal developmental trajectory for their age and sex (APA, 2013). Youth may display behaviors like food refusal or somatic complaints (e.g., stomach pains when eating) and may deny the significance of malnutrition (Lock & La Via, 2015). Depending on the child or adolescent's developmental and cognitive maturity, there may be a lack of insight into the fear of weight gain, and youth are less likely than adults to engage in binge eating or purging behaviors (APA, 2013; Lock & La Via, 2015; Peebles, Wilson, & Lock, 2006). Instead, children and adolescents may display behaviors like repeated weighing, engaging in excessive exercise or sports, or pinching skin (Lock & La Via, 2015).

There are two subtypes of AN: the restricting type and the binge-eating/ purging type. In the restricting subtype, individuals achieve weight loss through dieting, fasting, or excessive exercise (APA, 2013). Individuals with the binge-eating/purging subtype engage in recurrent episodes of binge eating and purging behavior, such as self-induced vomiting, laxative misuse, diuretic use, or enemas (APA, 2013). This subtype can be differentiated from BN because individuals with BN maintain their body weight at or above a minimally normal level (APA, 2013). However, the subtypes may not be useful in diagnosis of AN in children and adolescents because the majority of youth present with the restricting subtype (Knoll et al., 2011; Peat, Mitchell, Hoek, & Wonderlich, 2009) and there is evidence that subtype diagnoses are not stable over time (Hebebrand, Casper, Treasure, & Schweiger, 2004; Herpertz-Dahlmann et al., 2001).

Bulimia Nervosa

The DSM-5 criteria for BN include recurrent episodes of binge eating, characterized by eating an excessive amount of food in a discrete period of time (i.e., within a

2-hour time period) that is distinctly more than what most individuals would eat in a similar period of time under similar circumstances, as well as having a lack of control over eating during the episode (APA, 2013). Individuals with BN frequently engage in inappropriate compensatory behaviors to prevent weight gain (i.e., vomiting, excessive exercise, misuse of laxatives, etc.), and their self-evaluation is excessively influenced by body shape and weight (APA, 2013). Binge eating and compensatory behaviors must occur on average at least once a week for 3 months (APA, 2013).

In children and adolescents, binge eating may be better characterized as a loss of control over eating, rather than in terms of consuming an excessive amount of food in a 2-hour period, because youth may have limited access to, and control over, food in comparison to adults (Bravender et al. 2007; Peebles et al., 2006). Shame and guilt often lead children and adolescents to engage in binge eating and compensatory behaviors in secrecy, and these behaviors may interfere with typical social development in this age group (APA, 2013; Lock & La Via, 2015). For individuals with dual diagnoses of type 1 diabetes mellitus and BN, it is important to recognize that youth may engage in "diabulimia" (National Eating Disorders Association [NEDA], 2008), which involves manipulation of insulin doses in order to lose weight (APA, 2013; NEDA, 2008).

Binge Eating Disorder

Symptoms of BED include recurring episodes of binge eating at least once a week for 3 months without inappropriate compensatory behaviors like those seen in BN. Furthermore, BED does not occur during a course of either BN or AN (APA, 2013). Binge eating episodes occur with at least three of the following behaviors: eating much more rapidly than usual; eating until feeling uncomfortably full, eating large amounts of food when not feeling physically hungry, eating alone because of embarrassment about how much one is eating, and feeling disgusted with oneself, depressed, or very guilty afterward (APA, 2013). In children and adolescents, symptoms may present as a loss of control over eating rather than consuming an excessive amount of food (Lock & La Via, 2015; Marcus & Kalarchian, 2003). A lower threshold has been recommended for the frequency and duration of binge-eating episodes in children and adolescents, at a rate of once a month over a 3-month period instead of once per week (Bravender et al., 2007).

Avoidant Restrictive Food Intake Disorder

The DSM-5 category of ARFID is a revision of the DSM-IV category feeding disorder of infancy or early childhood (APA, 2013). ARFID is characterized by an avoidance or restriction of food intake to the extent of failing to meet nutritional requirements or insufficient energy intake through oral intake of food. Symptoms may include significant weight loss (failing to achieve expected weight or growth in children and adolescents), significant nutritional deficiency, dependence on enteral feeding or oral nutritional supplements, or marked interference with psychosocial functioning (APA, 2013). Unlike patients with AN or BN, children and adolescents with ARFID have no concerns about weight or body image (Kreipe & Palomaki, 2012; Nicely, Lane-Loney, Masciulli, Hollenbeak, & Ornstein, 2014). Physical symptoms may appear very similar to those of AN due to malnutrition/starvation (Nicely et al., 2014). ARFID may develop in early infancy and childhood and continue into adolescence and adulthood (APA, 2013). Individuals may present with highly selective or restrictive intake of food and fear of trying new foods (neophobia), or they may be hypersensitive to textures, tastes, smells, appearance, or color of certain food types (APA, 2013). ARFID may also be a result of food dysphagia, which is the fear of swallowing or an inability to eat or swallow food, typically due to a fear of gagging, choking, or vomiting as a result of experiencing or witnessing these events (Nicely et al., 2014).

Orthorexia Nervosa

Orthorexia nervosa (ON) is not an official DSM-5 clinical diagnosis but involves problematic eating behaviors in which individuals focus excessively on eating healthy foods or focus on consuming only biologically pure foods. These behaviors often lead to a restriction of food intake and severe malnutrition and weight loss (Bratman & Knight, 2000; Dell'Osso et al., 2016; Dunn & Bratman, 2016; Zamora, Bonaechea, Sanchez & Rial, 2005). Weight and body shape may not be a motivation for this problematic eating behavior, but there is an excessive focus on promoting good health (Dunn & Bratman, 2016). Individuals with ON may exclude foods due to a belief about the impurity of certain foods or excessive worry about the techniques and materials used to produce foods (Zamora et al., 2005). There is a great deal of energy invested in worrying about food quality and its effects on health (Dell'Osso et al., 2016; Zamora et al., 2005). While ON would be classified under ARFID in DSM-5, diagnostic criteria for ON have been proposed as: a preoccupation with "healthy foods" that focuses on quality of food and composition of meals; impairment in physical health or severe distress in social, academic, or work functioning due to obsessions about "healthy" eating; the disturbance is not an exacerbation of symptoms of another disorder; and the behavior is not better accounted for by a religious food observance, or by obsessions about adherence to a specific food type that are related to medically diagnosed food allergies or medical conditions (Moroze, Dunn, Holland, Yager, & Weintraub, 2015).

Malnutrition

Malnutrition is of particular concern in individuals with eating disorders and can lead to serious medical complications affecting almost every organ of the body (for a review, see Mehler, Birmingham, Crow, & Jahraus, 2010). The cardiovascular system can be affected in multiple ways, including unstable orthostatic vital signs, such as low heart rate and low blood pressure (Mehler et al. 2010). These complications place individuals with malnutrition at risk for heart failure. Bone density is reduced (i.e., patients have osteoporosis) and there is associated amenorrhea (Baker, Roberts & Towell, 2000). Reduced bone density places individuals at risk for injury, such as stress fractures. This is particularly of concern with student athletes. Growth retardation in children and adolescents with significant malnutrition is also noted in some cases (Golden et al., 2003; Lantzouni, Frank, Golden, & Shenker, 2002), as is pubertal delay. The brain can also be affected by malnutrition, with several studies indicating that malnutrition causes structural changes in the brain (Golden et al., 2003). One such study revealed through MRI that individuals with malnutrition secondary to AN had significant deficits in both gray and white matter volume of the brain, some of which was irreversible after recovery (Katzman, Zipursky, Lambe, & Mikulis, 1997). In some serious cases, the renal system may also be affected, resulting in chronic renal disease (Herzog, Deter, Fiehn, & Petzold, 1997). Lastly, individuals with malnutrition may experience dermatologic issues, such as dry skin, dry hair, hair loss, and lanugo (Mehler et al., 2010).

It is important to note that a child may experience malnutrition and still appear to be a normal or healthy weight. Therefore, thinness is not always the most accurate indicator of an eating disorder or the severity of medical complications related to an eating disorder. If a child is identified as potentially having an eating disorder or disordered eating, appropriate referral is recommended regardless of apparent weight status. Similarly, many individuals with eating disorders may experience malnutrition and still appear well. They may seem to have energy, be happy, and be doing well in school. These are not helpful indicators in identifying malnutrition and referral is still recommended if an eating disorder is suspected.

CASE EXAMPLE

Sarah is a 16-year-old female with strong genetic history of AN, including her mother, who is likely still active in her eating disorder. Sarah's parents are divorced, and Sarah spends alternate weeks with each parent. Sarah restricts heavily, at times consuming only Jell-O throughout the day. She has severe constipation and was recently hospitalized for bradycardia (slowed heart rate) with a heart rate of 45 beats per minute. Sarah fears maturing, beginning her menstrual cycle, and becoming bigger than her mother. The degree of Sarah's restricting is so severe that she has trouble concentrating, is physically weak, and feels faint often. Sarah's parents noticed that she is withdrawn from friends and family and that her grades are slipping at school. Sarah has been a straight-A student her whole life and is now receiving B's and C's in her classes. However, Sarah's parents have been reluctant to address her grades due to fears of upsetting her even more.

Since her weight loss was difficult to see due to the baggy clothes Sarah has been wearing, her parents were unaware of the severity of her condition. In addition, Sarah's parents have had a hard time keeping a close eye on her, given that she is in school all day, where she is able to restrict by throwing her packed lunch in the trash or not buying lunch with the money her parents give her. In the evenings, Sarah is able to restrict by claiming she is too busy studying or that she had a late lunch at school. Given her alternating weeks at each parent's house, Sarah's extreme restricting has gone unnoticed for some time. Although Sarah has not yet received treatment for an eating disorder, it was agreed that she forgo outpatient treatment and start at a higher level of care. This decision was based on the APA's criteria for treatment of an eating disorder, and included her degree of medical complications, BMI, difficulty at school, and need for family support to effect change.

At admission to partial hospital treatment, Sarah was 5'4" and weighed 100 pounds. Early treatment efforts were aimed at medical stabilization, such as normalizing heart rate, blood pressure, and blood work, as well as weight restoration through balanced regular meals. Once stable, Sarah worked with her treatment team to understand her fears and to begin creating a meaningful life. Intense family work concurrently addressed dynamics that perpetuated her eating disorder and ways her parents could support Sarah's recovery. During treatment, Sarah's clinical team was in close contact with her school regarding class assignments, for which she was provided time to complete during programming hours with the aid of a tutor. Despite the fact that Sarah was able to keep up with some of her classes via the tutor, Sarah's family, with the help of the treatment team, was able to receive 504 accommodations to help support her educational needs moving forward. Following partial hospital treatment, Sarah's longer-term plan is to step down to intensive outpatient treatment (3 days a week for 3 hours each day), where she will continue to meet with her therapist and dietitian, as well as engage in psychoeducational and meal support groups to further support her recovery, and to eventually to receive ongoing support from a psychiatrist, therapist, and dietitian on an outpatient basis. The family also plans for Sarah to attend summer school to make up the classes she was unable to complete while in partial hospital treatment so that she will not fall behind her classmates.

MENTAL HEALTH/BEHAVIORAL HEALTH COMORBIDITIES

According to the DSM-5, AN is associated with a number of psychiatric comorbidities, including anxiety disorders (e.g., obsessive-compulsive disorder), depression, and substance abuse disorders. Obsessive-compulsive disorder (OCD) is particularly prevalent among individuals diagnosed with AN, restricting subtype. Substance abuse disorders are more commonly associated with the binge-eating/purging subtype. Additionally, adolescents with AN have been shown to fall into three different personality subtypes, including perfectionistic, emotionally dysregulated, and overcontrolled/constricted (Gazillo et al., 2013). These findings suggest that children in schools who have AN may present in a variety of ways, ranging from being perfectionistic (restricting type) to quite impulsive (binge-eating/purging subtype).

Individuals with BN often experience comorbid psychiatric conditions. According to DSM-5, most will have at least one other mental disorder diagnosed. Mood disorders are most commonly associated with BN. Anxiety and substance use disorders are also often co-diagnosed. A study examining adolescents with BN also noted that a high percentage (25%) of adolescents in the sample had previous suicide attempts and/or self-injurious behavior (Fischer & le Grange, 2007). In schools, these students may present as withdrawn, anxious, or depressed and may engage in substance abuse.

Children and adolescents diagnosed with ARFID also experience a higher risk of psychiatric comorbidities. Specifically, they are more likely to have diagnoses of anxiety disorders, OCD, and neurodevelopmental disorders (e.g., autism spectrum disorder, attention deficit hyperactivity disorder). Children with ARFID may present in school as anxious, have school refusal, and have frequent stomach complaints (vomiting, abdominal cramps, etc., with no known medical conditions), or they may refuse or avoid foods based on sensory characteristics (i.e., texture).

There is some research suggesting that ON is correlated with higher levels of obsessive-compulsive behaviors (Asil & Surucuoglu, 2015; Dell'Osso et al., 2016; Koven & Senbonmatsu, 2013), and it has been suggested that individuals with ON also may experience heightened levels of depressive symptoms (Gleaves, Graham, & Ambwani, 2013). There is also some research correlating ON with the personality subtypes of perfectionism and narcissism (Oberle, Samaghabadi, & Hughes, 2017). Further, there is evidence of overlapping traits between ON and other disorders (AN, OCD, and ASD), perfectionism, rigid thinking, and preoccupation with rules and details (Dell'Osso et al., 2016). In the school setting, students with ON may appear withdrawn or distant from peers, may refuse to eat food prepared by the school cafeteria or others, may show rigid thinking in only selecting healthy foods (e.g., adhering to veganism or raw or "pure" food diets), or be fixated on the nutritional properties of foods (i.e., genetically modified ingredients, sugar, fat, etc.).

COMMON SCHOOL-RELATED CONCERNS

Cognition

It is widely accepted that eating disorders are likely to contribute to difficulties in academic performance, albeit the level of impairment can vary greatly (APA, 2013). Difficulties in a school setting may arise for a variety of reasons. Impaired cognitive functioning is one potential explanation for academic difficulties in adolescents with eating disorders. A body of literature suggests at least some cognitive performance discrepancies between individuals with eating disorders and their nonclinical peers in domains like cognitive flexibility, executive function, problem-solving, and attention. For example, in a study of adolescents with AN, it was demonstrated that cognitive impairment (e.g., impaired processing speed and memory) improved significantly with refeeding (Lozano-Serra, Andres-Perpina, Lazaro-Garcia, & Castro-Fornieles, 2013). A study examining individuals with diagnoses of BN or AN suggested that impairment in attention was similar between the two groups (Bosanac et al., 2007). Other correlates of eating disorders may also explain academic difficulties. One study revealed that eating disturbance (the impact of eating problems on school attendance, attention in class, and ability to complete homework) and body dissatisfaction (overall dissatisfaction with one's weight and body) were associated with higher levels of academic impairment (Yanover & Thompson, 2008).

School Absences

Another common concern that may arise in students with eating disorders is the issue of frequent school absences. Absences may occur due to the student's social anxiety with regard to body image or eating in front of peers, illness secondary to the eating disorder (stomach pains, fatigue), and frequent medical appointments for students who have already been diagnosed with an eating disorder. Some students may even experience extended absences due to the need to attend residential or partial-hospitalization treatment programs. This in turn can impact academic performance and will require significant communication and cooperation among the school and the patient and his or her family and treatment team to help the student stay caught up.

Physical Education and Sports

Students involved in specific sports are considered to be at higher risk for the development of an eating disorder. The sports generally emphasize the importance of thin or lean body types and may include gymnastics, cheerleading, distance running, and swimming, among others (Carney & Scott, 2012). For students struggling with eating disorders and already participating in sports, the most significant concern is the student's physical safety, given the various medical conditions that can arise secondary to eating disorder behaviors. For students who have been identified as having an eating disorder, it is imperative that school personnel comply with medical restrictions on physical activity related to athletic participation.

Nutritional Intake

Although it is uncommon, at times, students with eating disorders may require supervision during meals. This can create a conundrum for schools about who the appropriate staff person is to provide this service. Schools may provide a nurse or school counselor to supervise the meal. In other instances, parents are allowed to attend the school at the designated meal time to sit with their child and provide appropriate supervision. Similarly, some students with identified eating disorders will need to eat snacks during the school day. It is important for school personnel to discuss these needs directly with the students' parents and treatment team in order to come up with a plan that works best for both parties.

In each of the instances discussed above, the key is communication among the school and the student's parents and treatment team, which can facilitate accommodating a child with an eating disorder in the school setting. There are a number of resources for schools, including the *Educator Toolkit*, a free online handbook that provides eating disorder information and strategies for schools and educators (NEDA, 2008). General guidelines for developing an individualized education plan (IEP) and 504 accommodations are provided in Table 24.1.

RISK AND PROTECTIVE FACTORS

The risk for development of an eating disorder is multifactorial, with complex interplay among various biological, sociocultural, familial, and psychological variables (Steiner & Lock, 1998). Biological factors that may influence the development of an eating disorder include puberty and genetic predispositions (Mazzeo & Bulik, 2009). Personality traits, such as neuroticism and perfectionism (Cassin & von Ranson, 2005; McVey, Pepler, Davis, Flett, & Abdolell, 2002; Steiger, Leung, Puentes-Neuman, & Gottheil, 1992), have also been linked to risk for eating disorders. Environmental factors may include social pressures, family attitudes toward body image, or maladaptive parental behaviors (Johnson, Cohen, Kasen, & Brook, 2002; Rodgers & Chabrol, 2009). Various personal, socio-environmental, and behavioral protective factors have been identified in adolescent eating disorders (Neumark-Sztainer et al., 2007). High self-esteem has also been found to be a protective factor for AN (Nicholls & Viner, 2009).

CONSIDERATIONS FOR ASSESSMENT AND INTERVENTION

Diagnosis of an eating disorder ideally requires a full DSM-5 psychological interview with the individual and his or her family, accompanied by psychometrically sound rating measures. In addition, individuals suspected of having an eating disorder should be evaluated medically and undergo a nutritional assessment (Grilo & Mitchell, 2011). For the purpose of the school setting, it is recommended that brief screening tools be used to identify a potential eating disorder, followed by referral to an appropriate treatment facility where a more in-depth evaluation can take place.

Table 24.1. GUIDELINES FOR DEVELOPING AN INDIVIDUALIZED EDUCATION PROGRAM (IEP) AND 504 ACCOMMODATIONS

In-School Advocate	Supportive Counseling
• Coordinates care among teachers, school counselor, nursing, and family members • Helps to resolve conflicts between school attendance and medical/therapy appointments • Provides education to teachers about possible effects of medications on student's behaviors	• Provides safe place to eat meals and snacks • Teaches relaxation techniques • Suggests coping strategies • Suggest short-term solutions focused on problem-solving techniques for in-school issues • Consults with faculty, administrators, and staff • Educates school administrators, teachers, and staff about eating disorders
Medical/Nursing Support	**Academic Support**

• Provides release from physical education classes
• Assists with meal monitoring
• Provides alternatives to, or eliminates requirements for, in-school weight assessment and BMI measurements
  ○ Weight and measurements should be assessed individually in a private location with students (if necessary)
	• Provides adequate time to eat lunch
	• Releases child from physical education classes
	• Provides alternative to class activities that may trigger eating-disorder behaviors (i.e., calorie counting, classroom discussions of food, weight, exercise, and dieting)
	• Provides flexible scheduling and deadlines on projects and assignments, including:
	  • Reduced homework load
	  • Extended times for tests and assignments
	  • Breaking down assignments into smaller chunks
	• Excuses absences caused by medical or therapy appointments
	• Supports child in returning to typical extracurricular and social activities

Social Support	
• Works with administrators to provide a supportive environment (i.e., zero tolerance for bullying) • Educates peers about eating disorders	

Note. Guidelines adapted from the *National Eating Disorders Association Educator Toolkit* (available from https://www.nationaleatingdisorders.org/sites/default/files/Toolkits/EducatorToolkit.pdf).

Several brief self-report measures have been described in the research literature that would be appropriate for eating disorder screening in the school setting. The Eating Disorder Inventory (EDI; Garner, Olmsted, & Polivy, 1983; Garner, 1991) is appropriate for individuals 12 years old and older and assesses for a number of characteristics often associated with eating disorders, including a drive for thinness, bulimia, body dissatisfaction, and more. The Eating Disorder Examination Questionnaire (EDE-Q; Carter, Stewart, & Fairburn, 2001; Fairburn & Beglin, 2008) can be used for individuals 12 years old and older as well and explores a range of eating disorder characteristics, including restraint, shape concern, and weight concern. The SCOFF Questionnaire is a five-item screening measure of eating disorder symptoms that has been validated primarily in adults (Hill, Reid, Morgan, & Lacey, 2010), but it is also being utilized to screen for eating disorders in adolescents in primary care settings (Campbell & Peebles, 2014). It has been translated into Finnish and has been widely studied in Finnish-speaking adolescents (Hautala, Helenius, Karukivi, et al., 2011; Hautala, Junnila, Alin, et al., 2009). Of note, the above measures are focused on behaviors more commonly associated with AN and BN. The two commonly used scales to assess ARFID in children are the Behavioral Pediatrics Feeding Assessment Scale (BPFAS; Crist et al., 1994), and the Child Food Neophobia Scale (CFNS; Dovey, Martin, Aldridge, Haycraft, & Meyer, 2011). The BPFAS can differentiate individuals with ARFID from individuals in a nonclinical sample (Dovey, Aldridge, Martin, Wilken, & Meyer, 2016). This scale is a 35-item questionnaire that requires response by the parent or caregiver and examines feeding behavior and parent or caregiver experience of mealtimes. The CFNS is a six-item parent-report questionnaire assessing children's response to new foods. It has similar psychometric properties to those of the BPFAS and can also differentiate between children with ARFID from children in a community sample (Dovey et al., 2016).

Schools should implement specific guidelines and protocols to follow when a student is suspected of having an eating disorder (NEDA, 2008). School professionals may refer students and families to appropriate specialists, including medical professionals or licensed clinical psychologists who are familiar with eating disorders, for further evaluation. Treatment of an eating disorder requires a multidisciplinary team of specialists; school professionals may coordinate with the team in assisting the student with transition back to school.

EVIDENCE-BASED INTERVENTIONS

Given the complex nature of eating disorders, interventions targeting the symptoms of eating disorders should be carried out by a specialized multidisciplinary team, including medical, behavioral health, and nutrition professionals, among others. The interventions described here focus specifically on the psychological treatments that are supported by the research literature.

Behavioral family therapy (Eisler, 2005; Lock & Le Grange, 2005; Lock & le Grange, 2013) has the strongest research support for the treatment of AN and has some support in treatment of BN in adolescents (Lock, 2015). The Maudsley approach is an example of this type of therapy. While individual therapy may not be as effective as family-based therapy, there is some evidence of its usefulness for treatment of eating disorders in adolescents. Cognitive-behavioral therapy (CBT) has been shown to be a cost-effective treatment for adolescents with an eating disorder (Dalle Grave, Calugi, Doll, & Fairburn, 2013). Acceptance and commitment therapy is a third-wave CBT intervention that has also been used in treatment of adults with AN or BN, although research on its effectiveness is currently limited.

Eating disorder recovery is a long-term process and students will require ongoing monitoring and accommodations as they transition back to school. During the recovery process, students may miss significant amounts of time from school due to treatment and ongoing appointments (NEDA, 2008). It is important for school professionals to coordinate care with the student's multidisciplinary team and family in order to support the student's recovery process. Table 24.1 provides guidelines for developing an individualized education program (IEP) or 504 accommodations in support of students with an eating disorder.

Other considerations may include a designated staff member or "safety person" (i.e. teacher, school counselor, or nurse) who should take responsibility for supporting and monitoring the student upon his or her return to school and communicate changes appropriately (NEDA, 2008). It is recommended that school professionals review their protocols for antiharassment and antidiscrimination polices to ensure they cover harassment based on physical appearance and body shape, and the policies should be communicated clearly to students and staff (NEDA, 2008). Peers should be encouraged to seek support or discuss concerns about eating disorders with trusted school staff, and educational opportunities to learn about supporting individuals with an eating disorder and prevention of eating disorders should be provided (NEDA, 2008). Additional recommendations for school professionals may be found in the *National Eating Disorders Association Educator Toolkit* (NEDA, 2008).

LEGAL AND POLICY ISSUES

Legal and ethical issues often arise around patients with AN who refuse treatment and are at a critical stage of impairment with a high risk for death, requiring involuntary treatment (Kendall, 2014). In adults, issues like competence to provide consent, autonomy, and resistance to treatment are considered (Kendall, 2014). However, in children and adolescents, parents and legal guardians provide legal consent for treatment and collaborate with the child's treatment team to provide care and intervention. Even so, treatment refusal may occur in children and adolescents.

Several school-based policies have been proposed for prevention of eating disorders, including screening for eating disorders, implementation of antibullying policies that specifically address weight-based bullying, training coaches on early identification of eating disorders and prevention, and health courses to include material aimed at prevention of eating disorders (Puhl, Neumark-Sztainer, Austin, Luedicke, & King, 2014). Guidelines for schools in prevention and treatment of eating disorders have been published by the National Association of Anorexia Nervosa and Associated Disorders (ANAD) and NEDA.

Students with an eating disorder often require additional accommodations or modifications of their educational services during treatment and recovery. Many school districts have policies in place to provide students with necessary accommodations and services under special education, or Section 504 of the Rehabilitation Act, which protects students from discrimination due to a disability. Schools typically have a specific team or coordinator (i.e., 504 coordinator, special education coordinator, etc.) who may refer students for evaluations and determine eligibility for services or accommodations under Section 504 (Bryant & Strabavy, 2015). In some cases, students may require services through special education, and an IEP may be developed after eligibility is determined. Once a referral is made for evaluation, parental consent must be obtained.

WEBSITES AND RESOURCES

- National Eating Disorders Association: www.nationaleatingdisorders.org
  https://www.nationaleatingdisorders.org/sites/default/files/Toolkits/ParentToolkit.pdf
- F.E.A.S.T.: http://www.feast-ed.org/
  http://www.feast-ed.org/news/253577/Addressing-Eating-Disorders-in-Middle-and-High-Schools.htm
- Project Heal: http://theprojectheal.org/
- Eating Recovery Center: https://www.eatingrecoverycenter.com/
- The Emily Program Foundation: http://emilyprogramfoundation.org/about-us/history/
- Child Mind Institute: https://childmind.org/article/when-to-worry-about-an-eating-disorder/ (Helpful articles for parents and teachers)
- Family-based intervention for eating disorder—Maudsley Parents: http://www.maudsleyparents.org/
- Bodywise—Eating Disorders Information for Middle School Personnel: https://www1.maine.gov/education/sh/eatingdisorders/bodywise.pdf

REFERENCES

American Psychiatric Association. (2013). *Diagnostic and statistical manual of mental disorders* (DSM-5). Arlington, VA: Author.

Asil, E., & Surucuoglu, M.S. (2015). Orthorexia nervosa in Turkish dietitians. *Ecology of Food and Nutrition, 4*, 303–313.

Baker, D., Roberts, R., & Towell, T. (2000). Factors predictive of bone mineral density in eating-disordered women: A longitudinal study. *International Journal of Eating Disorders, 27*, 29–35.

Bosanac, P., Kurlender, S., Stojanovska, L., Hallam, K., Norman, T., McGrath, C., . . . Olver, J. (2007). Neuropsychological study of underweight and "weight-recovered" anorexia nervosa compared with bulimia nervosa and normal controls. *International Journal of Eating Disorders, 40*(7), 613–621.

Bratman, S., & Knight, D. (2000). Health food junkies: Overcoming the obsession with healthful eating. New York, NY: Broadway Books.

Bravender, T., Bryant-Waugh, R., Herzog, D., Katzman, D., Kreipe, R. D., Lask, B., . . . Nicholls, D. (2007). Classification of child and adolescent eating disturbances: Workgroup for Classification of Eating Disorders in Children and Adolescents (WCEDCA). *International Journal of Eating Disorders, 40*, S117–S122.

Bryant, J. K., & Strabavy, D. J. (2015). Section 504 considerations for students with internalizing disorders experiencing academic difficulties. *VISTAS Online, American Counseling Association, 23*, 1–14.

Campbell, K., & Peebles, R. (2014). Eating disorders in children and adolescents: State of the art review. *Pediatrics, 134*(3), 582–592.

Carney, J. M., & Scott, H. L. (2012). Eating issues in schools: Detection, management, and consultation with allied professionals. *Journal of Counseling and Development, 90*, 290–297.

Carter, J. C., Stewart, D. A., & Fairburn, C. G. (2001). Eating disorder examination questionnaire: Norms for young adolescent girls. *Behaviour Research and Therapy, 39*(5), 625–632.

Cassin, S. E., & von Ranson, K. M. (2005). Personality and eating disorders: A decade in review. *Clinical Psychology Review, 25*(7), 895–916.

Chisuwa, N., & O'Dea, J. A. (2010). Body image and eating disorders amongst Japanese adolescents: A review of the literature. *Appetite, 54*(1), 5–15.

Crist, W., McDonnell, P., Beck, M., Gillespie, C., Barrett, P., & Mathews, J. (1994). Behaviour at mealtimes and the young child with cystic fibrosis. *Journal of Developmental and Behavioral Pediatrics, 15*, 157–161.

Dalle Grave, R., Calugi, S., Doll, H. A., & Fairburn, C. G. (2013). Enhanced cognitive behaviour therapy for adolescents with anorexia nervosa: an alternative to family therapy?. *Behaviour Research and Therapy, 51*(1), R9–R12.

Dell'Osso, L., Abelli, M., Carpita, B., Pini, S., Castellini, G., Carmassi, C., & Ricca, V. (2016). Historical evolution of the concept of anorexia nervosa and relationships with orthorexia nervosa, autism, and obsessive–compulsive spectrum. *Neuropsychiatric Disease and Treatment, 12*, 1651.

Dovey, T. M., Aldridge, V. K., Martin, C. I., Wilken, M., & Meyer, C. (2016). Screening avoidant/restrictive food intake disorder (ARFID) in children: Outcomes from utilitarian versus specialist psychometrics. *Eating Behaviors, 23*, 162–167.

Dovey, T. M., Martin, C. I., Aldridge, V. K., Haycraft, E., & Meyer, C. (2011). Measures, measures everywhere, but which ones should I use? *The Feeding News, 6*(1), 1–13.

Dunn, T. M., & Bratman, S. (2016). On orthorexia nervosa: A review of the literature and proposed diagnostic criteria. *Eating Behaviors, 21*, 11–17.

Eisler, I. (2005). The empirical and theoretical base of family therapy and multiple family therapy for adolescent anorexia nervosa. *Journal of Family Therapy, 27*, 104–131.

Fairburn, C. G. (1997). Interpersonal psychotherapy for bulimia nervosa. In D. M. Garner & P. E. Garfinkle (Eds.), *Handbook of Treatment for Eating Disorders* (pp. 278–294). New York, NY: The Guilford Press.

Fairburn, C. G. (2008). *Cognitive behavior therapy and eating disorders*. New York, NY: The Guilford Press.

Fischer, S., & le Grange, D. (2007). Comorbidity and high-risk behaviors in treatment-seeking adolescents with bulimia nervosa. *International Journal of Eating Disorders, 40*, 751–753.

Garner, D. M. (1991). *Eating Disorder Inventory-2. Professional manual*. Odessa, FL: Psychological Research, Inc.

Garner, D. M., Olmstead, M. P., & Polivy, J. (1983). Development and validation of a multidimensional eating disorder inventory for anorexia nervosa and bulimia. *International Journal of Eating Disorders, 2*(2), 15–34.

Gazillo, F., Lingiardi, V., Peloso, A., Giordani, S., Vesco, S., Zanna, V., . . . Vicari, S. (2013). Personality subtypes in adolescents with anorexia nervosa. *Comprehensive Psychiatry, 54*, 702–712.

Gleaves, G. H., Graham, E. C., & Ambwani, S. (2013). Development of the Eating Habits Questionnaire. *International Journal of Educational and Psychological Assessment, 12*, 1–18.

Golden, N. H., Katzman, D. K., Kreipe, R. E., Stevens, S. L., Sawyer, S. M., Rees, J., . . . Rome, E. S. (2003). Eating disorders in adolescents: Position paper of the Society for Adolescent Medicine. *Journal of Adolescent Health, 33*, 496–503.

Grilo, C. M., & Mitchell, J. E. (Eds.). (2011). *The treatment of eating disorders: A clinical handbook*. New York, NY: Guilford Press.

Hautala, L., Helenius, H., Karukivi, M., Maunula, A. M., Nieminen, J., Aromaa, M., . . . Saarijärvi, S. (2011). The role of gender, affectivity and parenting in the course of disordered eating: A 4-year prospective case-control study among adolescents. *International Journal of Nursing Studies, 48*(8), 959–972.

Hautala, L., Junnila, J., Alin, J., Grönroos, M., Maunula, A. M., Karukivi, M., . . . Saarijärvi, S. (2009). Uncovering hidden eating disorders using the SCOFF questionnaire: Cross-sectional survey of adolescents and comparison with nurse assessments. *International Journal of Nursing Studies, 46*(11), 1439–1447.

Hebebrand, J., Casper, R., Treasure, J., & Schweiger, U. (2004). The need to revise the diagnostic criteria for anorexia nervosa. *Journal of Neural Transmission, 111*(7), 827–840.

Herpertz-Dahlmann, B., Hebebrand, J., Müller, B., Herpertz, S., Heussen, N., & Remschmidt, H. (2001). Prospective 10-year follow-up in adolescent anorexia nervosa—Course, outcome, psychiatric comorbidity, and psychosocial adaptation. *Journal of Child Psychology and Psychiatry and Allied Disciplines, 42*(5), 603–612.

Herzog, W., Deter, H. C., Fiehn, W., & Petzold, E. (1997). Medical findings and predictors of long term physical outcome in anorexia nervosa: A prospective, 12-year follow-up study. *International Journal of Eating Disorders, 27*, 269–279.

Hill, L. S., Reid, F., Morgan, J. F., & Lacey, J. H. (2010). SCOFF, the development of an eating disorder screening questionnaire. *International Journal of Eating Disorders, 43*(4), 344–351.

Jackson, T., & Chen, H. (2010). Sociocultural experiences of bulimic and non-bulimic adolescents in a school-based Chinese sample. *Journal of Abnormal Child Psychology, 38*(1), 69–76.

Johnson, J. G., Cohen, P., Kasen, S., & Brook, J. S. (2002). Childhood adversities associated with risk for eating disorders or weight problems during adolescence or early adulthood. *American Journal of Psychiatry, 159*(3), 394–400.

Katzman, D. K., Zipursky, R. B., Lambe, E. K., & Mikulis, D. J. (1997). A longitudinal magnetic resonance imaging study of brain changes in adolescents with anorexia nervosa. *Archives of Pediatric Adolescent Medicine, 151*, 793–797.

Kendall, S. (2014). Anorexia nervosa: The diagnosis. *Journal of Bioethical Inquiry, 11*(1), 31–40.

Knoll, S., Bulik, C. M., & Hebebrand, J. (2011). Do the currently proposed DSM-5 criteria for anorexia nervosa adequately consider developmental aspects in children and adolescents?. *European Child & Adolescent Psychiatry, 20*(2), 95–101.

Koven, N. S., & Senbonmatsu, R. (2013). A neuropsychological evaluation of orthorexia nervosa. *Open Journal of Psychiatry, 3*, 214–222.

Kreipe, R. E., & Palomaki, A. (2012). Beyond picky eating: Avoidant/restrictive food intake disorder. *Current Psychiatry Reports, 14*(4), 421–431.

Lantzouni, E., Frank, G. R., Golden, N. H., & Shenker, R. I. (2002). Reversibility of growth stunting in early onset anorexia nervosa: A prospective study. *Journal of Adolescent Health, 31*, 162–165.

Lock, J., & Le Grange, D. (2005). Family-based treatment of eating disorders. *International Journal of Eating Disorders, 37*, S64–S67.

Lock, J. (2015). An update on evidence-based psychosocial treatments for eating disorders in children and adolescents. *Journal of Clinical Child and Adolescent Psychology, 44*, 707–721.

Lock, J., & La Via, M. C. (2015). American Academy of Child and Adolescent Psychiatry (AACAP) Committee on Quality Issues (CQI): Practice parameter for the assessment and treatment of children and adolescents with eating disorders. *Journal of the American Academy of Child & Adolescent Psychiatry, 54*(5), 412–425.

Lock, J., & le Grange, D. (2013). *Treatment manual for anorexia nervosa: A family-based approach.* New York, NY: Guilford Press.

Lozano-Serra, E., Andres-Perpina, S., Lazaro-Garcia, L., & Castro-Fornieles, J. (2013). Adolescent anorexia nervosa: Cognitive performance after weight recovery. *Journal of Psychosomatic Research, 76*, 6–11.

Marcus, M. D., & Kalarchian, M. A. (2003). Binge eating in children and adolescents. *International Journal of Eating Disorders, 34*(S1).

Marini, Z., & Case, R. (1994). The development of abstract reasoning about the physical and social world. *Child Development, 65*(1), 147–159.

Marques, L., Alegria, M., Becker, A. E., Chen, C. N., Fang, A., Chosak, A., & Diniz, J. B. (2011). Comparative prevalence, correlates of impairment, and service utilization for eating disorders across US ethnic groups: Implications for reducing ethnic disparities in health care access for eating disorders. *International Journal of Eating Disorders, 44*(5), 412–420.

Mazzeo, S. E., & Bulik, C. M. (2009). Environmental and genetic risk factors for eating disorders: What the clinician needs to know. *Child and Adolescent Psychiatric Clinics of North America, 18*(1), 67–82.

McVey, G. L., Pepler, D., Davis, R., Flett, G. L., & Abdolell, M. (2002). Risk and protective factors associated with disordered eating during early adolescence. *The Journal of Early Adolescence, 22*(1), 75–95.

Mehler, P. S., Birmingham, L. C., Crow, S. J., & Jahraus, J. P. (2010). Medical complications of eating disorders. In C.M. Grilo & J.E. Mitchell (Eds.), *The treatment of eating disorders: A clinical handbook* (pp. 66–80). New York, NY: The Guildford Press.

Merikangas, K. R., He, J. P., Burstein, M., Swanson, S. A., Avenevoli, S., Cui, L., . . . Swendsen, J. (2010). Lifetime prevalence of mental disorders in US adolescents: results from the National Comorbidity Survey Replication–Adolescent Supplement (NCS-A). *Journal of the American Academy of Child & Adolescent Psychiatry, 49*(10), 980–989.

Moroze, R. M., Dunn, T. M., Holland, J. C., Yager, J., & Weintraub, P. (2015). Microthinking about micronutrients: A case of transition from obsessions about healthy eating to near-fatal "orthorexia nervosa" and proposed diagnostic criteria. *Psychosomatics, 56*(4), 397–403.

National Eating Disorders Association (NEDA). (2008). *The National Eating Disorders Association Educator Toolkit*. Retrieved from http://www.nationaleatingdisorders.org

Neumark-Sztainer, D. R., Wall, M. M., Haines, J. I., Story, M. T., Sherwood, N. E., & van den Berg, P. A. (2007). Shared risk and protective factors for overweight and disordered eating in adolescents. *American Journal of Preventive Medicine, 33*(5), 359–369.

Nicely, T. A., Lane-Loney, S., Masciulli, E., Hollenbeak, C. S., & Ornstein, R. M. (2014). Prevalence and characteristics of avoidant/restrictive food intake disorder in a cohort of young patients in day treatment for eating disorders. *Journal of Eating Disorders, 2*(1), 21.

Nicholls, D. E., & Viner, R. M. (2009). Childhood risk factors for lifetime anorexia nervosa by age 30 years in a national birth cohort. *Journal of the American Academy of Child & Adolescent Psychiatry, 48*(8), 791–799.

Oberle, C. D., Samaghabadi, R. O., & Hughes, E. M. (2017). Orthorexia nervosa: Assessment and correlates with gender, BMI, and personality. *Appetite, 108*, 303–310.

Peat, C., Mitchell, J. E., Hoek, H. W., & Wonderlich, S. A. (2009). Validity and utility of subtyping anorexia nervosa. *International Journal of Eating Disorders, 42*(7), 590–594.

Peebles, R., Wilson, J. L., & Lock, J. D. (2006). How do children with eating disorders differ from adolescents with eating disorders at initial evaluation? *Journal of Adolescent Health, 39*(6), 800–805.

Puhl, R. M., Neumark-Sztainer, D., Austin, S. B., Luedicke, J., & King, K. M. (2014). Setting policy priorities to address eating disorders and weight stigma: Views from the field of eating disorders and the US general public. *BMC Public Health, 14*(1), 524.

Rodgers, R., & Chabrol, H. (2009). Parental attitudes, body image disturbance and disordered eating amongst adolescents and young adults: A review. *European Eating Disorders Review, 17*(2), 137–151.

Steiger, H., Leung, F. Y., Puentes-Neuman, G., & Gottheil, N. (1992). Psychosocial profiles of adolescent girls with varying degrees of eating and mood disturbances. *International Journal of Eating Disorders, 11*(2), 121–131.

Steiner, H., & Lock, J. (1998). Anorexia nervosa and bulimia nervosa in children and adolescents: a review of the past 10 years. *Journal of the American Academy of Child and Adolescent Psychiatry, 37*, 352–359.

Swanson, S. A., Crow, S. J., Le Grange, D., Swendsen, J., & Merikangas, K. R. (2011). Prevalence and correlates of eating disorders in adolescents: Results from the national comorbidity survey replication adolescent supplement. *Archives of General Psychiatry*, *68*(7), 714–723.

Yanover, T., & Thompson, J. K. (2008). Eating problems, body image disturbances, and academic achievement: Preliminary evaluation of the Eating and Body Image Disturbances Academic Interference Scale. *International Journal of Eating Disorders*, *41*, 184–187.

Zamora, M. L., Bonaechea, B. B., Sánchez, F. G., & Rial, B. R. (2005). Orthorexia nervosa: A new eating behavior disorder? *Actas Esp Psiquiatr*, *33*(1), 66–68.

Page references to tables and figures and boxes are indicated by *t's*, *f's*, and *b's* respectively. *For the benefit of digital users, indexed terms that span two pages (e.g., 52–53) may, on occasion, appear on only one of those pages.*